Concepts and Pharmaceutical Applications of Antioxidants

Concepts and Pharmaceutical Applications of Antioxidants

Edited by **Nick Gilmour**

SYRAWOOD
PUBLISHING HOUSE
New York

Published by Syrawood Publishing House,
750 Third Avenue, 9th Floor,
New York, NY 10017, USA
www.syrawoodpublishinghouse.com

Concepts and Pharmaceutical Applications of Antioxidants
Edited by Nick Gilmour

International Standard Book Number: 978-1-68286-295-7 (Hardback)

Printed in China.

Contents

Preface

Antioxidants play a major role in preventing oxidative stress which is responsible for cell damage and other fatal diseases. This book is a collective contribution of specialists and experts associated with the field of antioxidants and their applications. The chapters included herein aim to provide significant information on some of the major concepts and pharmaceutical applications of antioxidants such as, activity of antioxidant compounds and substances, extraction and production of antioxidants from different sources, etc. This book would prove to be an invaluable source of reference for students and professionals alike.

This book has been the outcome of endless efforts put in by authors and researchers on various issues and topics within the field. The book is a comprehensive collection of significant researches that are addressed in a variety of chapters. It will surely enhance the knowledge of the field among readers across the globe.

It gives us an immense pleasure to thank our researchers and authors for their efforts to submit their piece of writing before the deadlines. Finally in the end, I would like to thank my family and colleagues who have been a great source of inspiration and support.

Editor

Oxidative Stress Is Associated with Neuroinflammation in Animal Models of HIV-1 Tat Neurotoxicity

Jean-Pierre Louboutin [1,*], Lokesh Agrawal [1], Beverly A. S. Reyes [2,†], Elisabeth J. Van Bockstaele [2,†] and David S. Strayer [1]

[1] Department of Pathology, Anatomy and Cell Biology, Thomas Jefferson University, Philadelphia, PA 19107, USA; E-Mails: lokagrawal@gmail.com (L.A.); David.Strayer@jefferson.edu (D.S.S.)

[2] Department of Neurosurgery, Farber Institute for Neurosciences, Thomas Jefferson University, Philadelphia, PA 19107, USA; E-Mails: beverly.reyes@drexelmed.edu (B.A.S.R.); elisabeth.vanbockstaele@drexelmed.edu (E.J.B.)

[†] Current address: Department of Pharmacology and Physiology, Drexel University College of Medicine, Philadelphia, PA 19102, USA.

[*] Author to whom correspondence should be addressed; E-Mail: jplouboutin@hotmail.com

---

Abstract: HIV-1 *trans*-acting protein Tat, an essential protein for viral replication, is a key mediator of neurotoxicity. If Tat oxidant injury and neurotoxicity have been described, consequent neuroinflammation is less understood. Rat caudate-putamens (CPs) were challenged with Tat, with or without prior rSV40-delivered superoxide dismutase or glutathione peroxidase. Tat injection caused oxidative stress. Administration of Tat in the CP induced an increase in numbers of Iba-1- and CD68-positive cells, as well as an infiltration of astrocytes. We also tested the effect of more protracted Tat exposure on neuroinflammation using an experimental model of chronic Tat exposure. SV(Tat): a recombinant SV40-derived gene transfer vector was inoculated into the rat CP, leading to chronic expression of Tat, oxidative stress, and ongoing apoptosis, mainly located in neurons. Intra-CP SV(Tat) injection induced an increase in microglia and astrocytes, suggesting that protracted Tat production increased neuroinflammation. SV(SOD1) or SV(GPx1) significantly reduced neuroinflammation following Tat administration into the CP. Thus, Tat-induced oxidative stress, CNS injury, neuron loss and inflammation may be mitigated by antioxidant gene delivery.

Keywords: HIV-1; Tat; oxidative stress ; brain; antioxidant enzymes; gene therapy; SV40; neuroinflammation; microglia; astrocytes

1. Introduction

Under normal physiologic conditions, reactive oxygen species (ROS), which include superoxide (O_2^-), hydrogen peroxide (H_2O_2) and hydroxyl radical (OH^-), are generated at low levels and play important roles in signaling and metabolic pathways [1]. ROS levels are controlled by antioxidants such as superoxide dismutases (SOD), glutathione peroxidase (GPx1), glutathione and catalase. The tripeptide glutathione (γ-L-glutamyl-L-cysteinylglycine, GSH) is the key low molecular thiol antioxidant involved in the defense of brain cells against oxidative stress. Oxidative stress arises due to the disturbances of the balance in pro-oxidant/antioxidant homeostasis that further causes the generation of ROS which are potentially toxic for neurons.

Abnormalities in oxidative metabolism have been reported in many nervous system diseases. These include neurodegenerative diseases (Parkinson's disease, Alzheimer's disease, Huntington's disease, amyotrophic lateral sclerosis and cerebellar degeneration) [2–6], vascular diseases (ischemia-reperfusion) [7] or toxic reactions (chronic alcoholism) [8], as well as aging [9].

Similarly, neuroinflammation plays an important role in the pathophysiology of numerous chronic neurodegenerative diseases like Parkinson's disease (PD), and Alzheimer's disease (AD) [10,11]. Neuroinflammation is also observed in acute brain insults like stroke and status epilepticus (SE) [12–14]. Activation of microglial cells, the brain's resident phagocytes, which both produce and respond to proinflammatory factors during the inflammation process, might result in subsequent neurodegeneration. Anti-inflammatory treatment can protect from onset or progression of AD in patients [15].

Oxidative stress and neuroinflammation are involved as well in Human Immunodeficiency Virus-1-(HIV-1)-associated neurocognitive disorder (HAND) [16]. HAND covers a range of HIV-related CNS dysfunction. HIV-1 enters the Central Nervous System (CNS) soon after it enters the body. There, it is largely impervious to highly active anti-retroviral therapeutic drugs (HAART). The brain may be an important reservoir for the virus, and neurodegenerative and neuroinflammatory changes may continue despite use of HAART [17–19]. As survival with chronic HIV-1 infection improves, the number of people harboring the virus in their CNS increases. The prevalence of HAND therefore continues to rise. HAND remains a significant independent risk factor for AIDS mortality [17–20].

In the brain, HIV-1 mainly infects microglia and perivascular macrophages, and rare astrocytes, leading to increased production of cytokines, such as interleukin-6 (IL-6), IL-1β and tumor necrosis factor-α (TNF-α), and chemokines such as monocyte chemotactic protein-1 (MCP-1) [21]. Macrophages and microglia release HIV-1 proteins, several of which are neurotoxins, including the envelope (Env) protein gp120 and Tat [22–25]. Neurons themselves are rarely infected by HIV-1, and neuronal damage is mainly indirect. HAND involves ROS-mediated damage to cellular protein and lipids, and neuronal apoptosis.

The pathogenesis of HAND largely reflects the neurotoxicity of HIV-1 proteins. The HIV-1 *trans*-acting protein Tat, an essential protein for viral replication, is a key mediator of neurotoxicity.

Brain areas that are particularly susceptible to Tat toxicity include the CA3 region and the dentate gyrus of the hippocampus and the striatum. Tat is internalized by neurons primarily through lipoprotein related protein receptor (LRP) and by activation of NMDA receptor [26]. It also interacts with several cell membrane receptors, including integrins, VEGF receptor in endothelial cells and possibly (C-X-C motif) receptor 4 (CXCR4) [27].

Tat can promote excitotoxic neuronal apoptosis [28,29] by activating endoplasmic reticulum pathways to release intracellular calcium ($[Ca^{2+}]i$) [30]. Consequent dysregulation of calcium homeostasis [28,31,32] leads to mitochondrial calcium uptake, caspase activation and, finally, neuronal death. Tat can directly depolarize neuron membranes, independently of Na^+ flux [33] and may potentiate glutamate- and NMDA-triggered calcium fluxes and neurotoxicity [32]. Tat also triggers lipid peroxidation [29] by generating the ROS superoxide (O_2^-) and hydrogen peroxide (H_2O_2). It activates inducible nitric oxide synthase (iNOS) to produce nitric oxide (NO), which binds superoxide anion to form the highly reactive peroxynitrite ($ONOO^-$) [34]. The latter may attack lipids, proteins and DNA, enhancing oxidant-related injury.

Tat neurotoxicity has been reported in cultured cells, but few studies have demonstrated its neurotoxic properties *in vivo* [24,35–37]. Tat-induced protein oxidation is well documented [36,37] but little is known about its effects on lipid peroxidation. We demonstrated that Tat activates multiple signaling pathways. In one of these, Tat-induced superoxide acts as an intermediate, while the other utilizes peroxide as a signal transducer [38]. We asked here if direct injection of Tat into the caudate-putamen (CP) can induce neuroinflammation and oxidative stress. We also tested the consequences of protracted exposure to Tat, by expressing Tat over time in neurons. Finally, we assessed the effects of prior gene delivery of antioxidant enzymes Cu/Zn superoxide dismutase (SOD1) or glutathione peroxidase (GPx1) into the CP before injecting Tat.

2. Material and Methods

2.1. Animals

Female Sprague-Dawley rats (300–350 g) were purchased from Charles River Laboratories (Wilmington, MA, USA). Protocols for injecting and euthanizing animals were approved by the Thomas Jefferson University Institutional Animal Care and Use Committee (IACUC), and are consistent with Association for Assessment and Accreditation of Laboratory Animal Care (AAALAC) standards. Because estrogens can influence inflammation in the brain and attenuate Tat-induced oxidative stress, experiments were done in female rats at similar points of their estrous cycle determined by vaginal smears. Animals were preferably injected during the diestrus stage of the estrous cycle. Oestrogens are typically low during this stage. In any case, animals were not injected during the estrus stage of the cycle when oestrogens levels are elevated. The diet that the animals received was a standard commercial, regular powdered rodent diet without any component that might cause oxidative stress (e.g., high fat diet, or high manganese) and was not folate/methyl or iron deficient. Animals had free access to water and diet. Numbers of animals used in experiments are indicated in the "Experimental Design" section.

2.2. Reagents

Recombinant Tat was obtained through the NIH AIDS Research and Reference Reagent Program, Division of AIDS, NIAID, NIH, Germantown, MD. Tat was reconstituted in PBS containing 1 mg/mL BSA and 0.1 mM DTT, then aliquoted and stored in dark bottles to avoid oxidation. Endotoxin levels of Tat was also determined using E-Toxate kit (ET0200) (Sigma Chemical Co., St Louis, MO, USA). Tat protein was found to be endotoxin free with concentration below 0.015 Endotoxin units (EU)/mL, which was below the lowest concentration of endotoxin standard.

2.3. Antibodies

Diverse primary antibodies were used: rabbit anti-Iba1 (IgG; 1:100), a marker of quiescent and active microglia (Waco Chemicals, Osaka, Japan), mouse anti-glial fibrillary acidic protein (GFAP) (IgG2b; 1:100) (BD Pharmingen Franklin Lakes, NJ, USA), mouse anti-neuN (IgG1; 1:100), mouse anti-rat CD68/ED1 (IgG1; 1:100), a marker of activated microglial cells in a phagocytic state (Serotec, Oxford, UK). Secondary antibodies were used at 1:100 dilution: FITC and Tetramethyl Rhodamine IsoThioCyanate (TRITC)-conjugated goat anti-mouse IgG (γ-chain specific and against whole molecule respectively), TRITC-conjugated goat anti-rabbit IgG (whole molecule), FITC-conjugated sheep anti-rabbit IgG (whole molecule) (Sigma, Saint-Louis, MO, USA), FITC and TRITC-conjugated donkey anti-mouse IgG (whole molecule), FITC and TRITC-conjugated donkey anti-sheep IgG (whole molecule), Cy3-conjugated donkey anti-rabbit IgG (whole molecule) and anti-goat IgG (whole molecule) (Jackson ImmunoResearch Laboratories, Inc., WestGrove, PA, USA).

2.4. Vector Production

The general principles for making recombinant, *Tag*-deleted, replication-defective SV40 viral vectors have been previously reported [39,40]. Cu/Zn superoxide dismutase (SOD1) or glutathione peroxidase (GPx1) transgenes were subcloned into pT7[RSVLTR], in which transgene expression is driven by the Rous Sarcoma Virus long terminal repeat (RSV-LTR). Tat expression in SV(Tat) is driven by RSV-LTR. The cloned rSV40 genome was excised from its carrier plasmid, gel-purified and recircularized, then transfected into COS-7 cells. These cells supply large T-antigen (Tag) and SV40 capsid proteins *in trans*, which are needed to produce recombinant replication-defective SV40 viral vectors [41]. Crude virus stocks were prepared as cell lysates, then band-purified by discontinuous sucrose density gradient ultracentrifugation and titered by quantitative (Q)-PCR [42]. SV(human bilirubin-uridine 5′-diphosphate-glucuronosyl-transferase) (BUGT), which was used here as negative control vector, with a non-toxic byproduct, has been reported [43].

2.5. Experimental Design

2.5.1. Tat Injection

It is difficult to know what concentration of Tat in the brain is sufficient to produce pathogenesis [24]. The amount of Tat injected was decided after previous experiments showing that 10 ng Tat was the optimal amount of Tat necessary for inducing neuronal apoptosis *in vitro* [38]. In this previous study, cells were incubated with 0, 1, 10 and 100 ng/mL of recombinant soluble Tat for 48 h. Apoptotic bodies were analyzed using terminal deoxynucleotidyl transferase-mediated nick end labeling (TUNEL). Neurons were identified by their expression of MAP-2. The intensity and frequency of TUNEL+ cells were significantly higher ($p < 0.001$) as compared to untreated cultures. Increasing Tat concentration above 10 ng/mL did not increase apoptosis significantly. Thus, 10 ng/mL of Tat was used in all subsequent *in vitro* studies [33].

For *in vivo* studies, Tat was suspended in saline at a concentration of 10 ng/µL. The volume of solution containing Tat that was injected into the striatum was 1 µL. By comparison, the concentration of Tat injected in the striatum ranged from 1–50 µg/µL [24], to 20 µg/µL [44], and 50 µg/µL [37].

In order to study Tat-induced abnormalities, 1 µL saline containing 10 ng Tat was injected stereotaxically into the CP of rats whose brains were harvested at different time points after the injection (6, 24, 48 h and 1, 2, 4 week, with 4 rats at each time point total: $n = 24$ rats).

Controls ($n = 2$ for each time point) received saline instead of Tat in the CP (total: $n = 12$ rats). In order to test the specificity of the effects of Tat, 1 µL saline containing 10 ng rat IgG (Sigma) was injected into the CP as a control unrelated protein ($n = 2$ for each time point, total = 12). Saline and saline containing rat IgG were used as negative controls, as was the contralateral side of the unilaterally injected brains.

2.5.2. Injection of SV(Tat)

To assess the effects of more protracted exposure to Tat, we used a system in which Tat is expressed over time in CNS cells. Rats were injected intra-CP with SV(Tat), which allows for continued Tat production by transduced cells. The brains from the animals were then studied 1, 2 and 4 weeks after injection of SV(Tat) for Tat expression and apoptosis. SV(Tat) was injected into the CP of Sprague-Dawley rats ($n = 5$ at each time, total = 15). Controls received an unrelated vector, SV(BUGT), instead of SV(Tat) in the CP ($n = 5$ at each time point, $n = 15$).

2.5.3. Challenge with Tat after Administration of SV(GPx1) or/and SV(SOD1)

To study possible protection by rSV40-mediated overexpression of SOD1 and/or GPx1 from Tat-related injury, we first injected the CP of rats with SV(SOD1) ($n = 10$), SV(GPx1) ($n = 10$) and a mixture 50:50 SV(SOD1)/SV(GPx1) ($n = 10$). One month later, the CP in which SV(SOD1) or/and SV(GPx1) has been administered was injected with 10 ng Tat. Half of the brains were harvested 2 days after injection of Tat into the CP and studied for apoptosis and malondialdehyde (MDA) level at d2 ($n = 5$ for each vector, total = 15 rat). Other brains ($n = 15$) were harvested two weeks after injection of Tat in the CP and studied for neuroinflammation (e.g., immunostaining for microglial cells and astrocytes), In all cases, controls received SV(BUGT) in the CP instead of SV(SOD1), SV(GPx1) or SV(SOD1)/SV(GPx1) ($n = 10$).

2.6. *In Vivo Injection of Tat and Vectors*

Rats were anesthetized with isofluorane UPS (BaxterHealthcare Corp., Deerfield, IL, USA) (1.0 unit isofluorane/1.5 L O_2 per min) and placed in a stereotaxic apparatus (Stoelting Corp.,

Wood Dale, IL, USA) for cranial surgery. Body temperature was maintained at 37 °C by using a feedback-controlled heater (Harvard Apparatus, Boston, MA, USA). Glass micropipettes (1.2 mm outer diameter; World Precisions Instruments, Inc., Sarasota, FL, USA) with tip diameters of 15 μm were backfilled with either 5 μL of SV(BUGT), SV(SOD1), SV(GPx1), or a mixture 50:50 SV(SOD1)/SV(GPx1) viral vector, which contains approximately 10^7 particles. The vector-filled micropipettes were placed in the CP using coordinates obtained from the rat brain atlas of Paxinos and Watson [45]. For injection into the CP, a burr hole was placed +0.48 mm anterior to bregma and −3.0 mm lateral to the sagittal suture. Once centered, the micropipette was placed 6.0 mm ventral from the top of the brain. The same coordinates were used for injecting 10 ng Tat in 1 μL saline, as well as for injecting saline and 1 μL saline containing 10 ng rat IgG. Tat or the vector were given by a Picospritzer II (General Valve Corp., Fairfield, NJ, USA) pulse of compressed N2 duration 10 ms at 20 psi until the fluid was completely ejected from the pipette. Following surgery, animals were housed individually with free access to water and food.

2.7. Procedure for Harvesting the Tissue

After a variable survival period, the rats were anesthetized by intraperitoneal injection of sodium pentobarbital (Abbott Laboratories, North Chicago, IL, USA) at 60 mg/kg and perfused transcardially though the ascending aorta with 10 mL heparinized saline followed by ice cold 4% paraformaldehyde (Electron Microscopy Sciences, Fort Washington, PA, USA) in 0.1M phosphate buffer (pH 7.4). Immediately following perfusion-fixation, the rat brains were removed, placed in 4% paraformaldehyde for 24 h, then in a 30% sucrose solution for 24 h, then frozen in methyl butane cooled in liquid nitrogen. Samples were cut on a cryostat (10 μm sections).

2.8. Immunocytochemistry

For immunofluorescence, coronal cryostat sections (10 μm thick) were processed for indirect immunofluorescence. Blocking was performed by incubating 60 min with 10% goat, or 10% donkey, serum in phosphate buffer saline (PBS; pH 7.4). Then, sections were incubated with antibodies diluted according to the manufacturer's recommendations: 1h with primary antibody, then 1 h with secondary antibody diluted 1:100, all at room temperature. Double immunofluorescence was performed as previously described [46]. All incubations were followed by extensive washing with PBS. To stain nuclei, we used mounting medium containing 4′,6-diamidino-2-phenylindole (DAPI) (Vector Laboratories, Burlingame, CA, USA). Specimens were finally examined under a Leica DMRBE microscope (Leica Microsystems, Wetzlar, Germany). Negative controls were performed each time and immunostaining was done, which consisted of preincubation with PBS, a substitution of non-immune isotype-matched control antibodies for the primary antibody, and/or omission of the primary antibody.

2.9. Staining of Neurons Using NeuroTrace

Neurotrace (NT) staining has been used as a neuronal marker in studies focusing on the characterization of neurons [47] and NT staining has been performed as previously reported [48–50]. After rehydration in 0.1 M PBS, pH 7.4, sections were treated with PBS plus 0.1% Triton X-100 10 min, washed twice for 5 min in PBS then stained by NT (Molecular Probes, Inc., Eugene, OR) (1:100), for 20 min at room temperature. Sections were washed in PBS plus 0.1% Triton X-100 then × 2 with PBS, then let stand for 2 h at room temperature in PBS before being counterstained with DAPI. Combination NT + antibody staining was performed using primary and secondary antibodies staining first (see above), followed by staining with the NT fluorescent Nissl stain. All experiments were repeated 3 times and test and control slides were stained the same day.

2.10. TUNEL Assay

Terminal deoxynucleotidyl transferase-mediated biotinylated UTP nick end labeling (TUNEL) assay was performed according to the manufacturer's recommendations (Roche, Indianapolis, IN, USA) and following a previously described protocol [25]. We used two assays: end-labeling of DNA with fluorescein-dUTP and tetramethylrhodamine-dUTP (TMR-dUTP). To quantitate the TUNEL assay, TUNEL-positive cells were expressed as a total number per CP measured in at least 5 consecutive sections, using the same computerized system as described in the Morphometry section. The final number was an average of results measured in the different sections.

2.11. Morphometry

NeuN-, NT-, CD68/ED1-, GFAP-, and Iba-1-positive cells were enumerated manually on the injected and uninjected sides in the whole CP of animals injected with Tat, or saline, in at least 5 consecutive sections using a computerized imaging system (Image-Pro Plus, MediaCybernetics, Bethesda, MD, USA) as previously described [49,51]. In all cases, the final number was an average of results measured in the different sections. This procedure already described for assessment of numbers of transgene-positive cells in the brain [49,52] allows quantitative and relative comparisons among different time points, although it does not reflect the total number of transduced cells *in vivo*. The results were expressed as percentages of NT-positive cells.

Tat- and TUNEL-positive cells were enumerated as previously described in SV(Tat) recipients. Neuronal loss was estimated by calculating the ratio of the number of NT-positive cells on the injected side compared with the number of NT-positive cells on the uninjected side.

2.12. Measurement of Malondialdehyde

The measurement of malondialdehyde (MDA) was used as an indicator of lipid peroxidation. The MDA assay was performed using lipid peroxidation kit (Oxford Biochemical Research, Oxford, MI, USA). The assay is based on reaction of chromogenic reagent *N*-methyl-2-phenylindole, with MDA and 4-hydroxyalkenals at 45 °C to form a stable chromophore at 586 nm. MDA standards were prepared with target concentration in reaction mixture ranging from 0 to 4 μM, and the assay was performed following manufacturer's instructions and as previously reported [53]. Cryostat sections (50 μm thick) of the striatum areas injected with Tat or saline were harvested then homogenized in buffer, and lysates were prepared as previously reported [25,53]. Briefly, for 200 μL of sample, 650 μL of reagent R1 and 150 μL of 12 N HCL were added and incubated at 45 °C for 60 min. The absorbance was measured at 586 nm, and the MDA levels of unknown samples were deduced from the standard curve. MDA levels of samples from CPs injected with Tat after prior administration of SV(BUGT), SV(SOD1), SV(GPx1) or SV(SOD1) and SV(GPx1) were measured the same way.

2.13. Statistical Analysis

Comparison of medians between 2 groups was achieved by using the Mann-Whitney test (with a two-tail p value). Comparison of medians between more than 2 groups was done by using the Kruskall-Wallis test. The difference between the groups was considered significant when $p < 0.05$. On graphs, values are represented as means ± SEM.

3. Results

3.1. Injection of Tat Induces Oxidative Damage

Because oxidative injury is seen in the brains of patients with HAND, we tested for oxidative damage occurring after Tat injection. Lipid peroxidation was measured by calorimetric MDA assay. Injection of Tat elicited more MDA than did the control saline at the different times considered ($p < 0.001$) (Figure 1).

Figure 1. Graph showing the evolution of malondialdehyde (MDA) levels with time after injection of Tat in the caudate-putamen. Levels of MDA increased 6 h after injection of Tat in the CP and remained significantly elevated at the different times considered, even 2 weeks later (** $p < 0.01$).

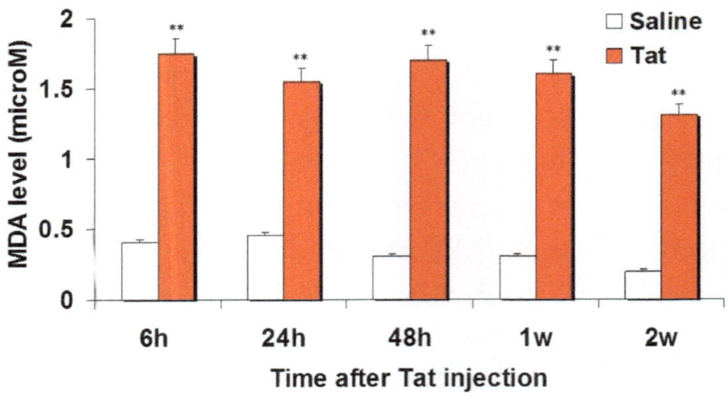

3.2. Injection of Tat into the CP Elicits Apoptosis

After injection of 10 ng Tat into the CP, TUNEL assays were performed to detect apoptosis between 6 h and 4 weeks. TUNEL-positive cells were enumerated in the whole CP, at least in five different sections for each animal. Extremely rare TUNEL-positive cells were seen when the CP was injected with saline or rat IgG (negative controls). Numbers of TUNEL-positive cells peaked 2 days after injection of Tat (Figure 2A,B).

3.3. Tat-Induced Apoptotic Cells Are Mainly Neurons

Sections from the CP obtained 2 days after Tat injection were double-stained for TUNEL and neuN, a marker of neurons, or Iba-1, a marker of microglial cells. Most of TUNEL-positive cells were immunopositive for neuN, identifying them as neurons (Figure 2C). Rare TUNEL-positive cells also co-immunostained for Iba-1, a microglial marker (Figure 2D). About 96% of TUNEL-positive cells were neuN-positive, 4% were microglial cells.

3.4. HIV-1 Tat Triggers Increases in Microglial Cells and Astrocytes

We first characterized different populations of microglial cells by immunocytochemistry to assess if Tat induced an increase of microglial cells. Immunostaining for Iba-1, a marker of quiescent and activated microglial cells, and for CD68/ED1, a marker of activated microglial cells (mainly in the phagocytic state), showed an increase in the numbers of Iba-1- and CD68/ED1-positive cells 7 and 14 days after injection of Tat into the CP. No increase in the number of microglial cells was seen in the contralateral uninjected side or after injection of saline into the CP (Figure 3A,B) ($p < 0.01$: Tat *vs.* saline, both for Iba-1 and CD68/ED1, at d7 and d14). We then enumerated the number of astrocytes by immunostaining for GFAP. An increase in the number of GFAP-positive cells was observed in the CPs injected with Tat. There were more astrocytes 14 days after injection of Tat into the CP than at 7 days ($p < 0.05$). There were significantly fewer astrocytes in the contralateral CP or after injection of saline into the CP ($p < 0.01$: Tat *vs.* saline, at d7 and d14) (Figure 3A,B).

3.5. Transgene Expression of Tat by Intra-CP Injection of SV(Tat) Induces Oxidative Stress, Apoptosis and Neuroinflammation

HIV-1 infection of the brain is a long-term disease that is characterized by production of HIV-1 proteins for extended periods of time. We previously reported the use of an SV40-derived expression vector, SV(gp120), to provide ongoing expression of HIV-1 envelope glycoprotein gp120 as a model to study more chronic CNS consequences of protracted production of neurotoxic HIV-1 gene products [53]. We tested whether a similar system could be used to study the effects of Tat production in the CNS for a protracted period of time. We injected SV(Tat) into the CNS. Expression of Tat protein, which is produced as a result of transduction, was demonstrated by immunocytochemistry at different time points after injection of SV(Tat). One month after SV(Tat)injection, Tat-positive cells were still present in the CP. Tat was localized mainly within neurons. The expression of Tat protein was sustained after injection of SV(Tat). However, there was a decrease in the number of Tat-positive cells with time, probably because of the neuronal death following Tat expression. No Tat was detected in the contralateral uninjected side (not shown) or after injection of SV(BUGT), a control vector, into the CP (Table 1).

Figure 2. Tat injection in the caudate-putamen induces neuronal apoptosis. (**A**) TUNEL-positive cells were observed in the caudate-putamen (CP) after injection of Tat in the same structure. Number of TUNEL-positive cells peaked 2 days after Tat injection. No TUNEL-positive cells could be seen in CP injected with saline or in the uninjected side; (**B**) Graph showing that TUNEL-positive cells peaked 2 days after injection of Tat in CP; (**C**) TUNEL-positive cells were positive for neuN, a neuronal marker, suggesting that most of apoptotic cells were neurons; (**D**) Rare Iba-1-positive cells were TUNEL-positive (arrow).

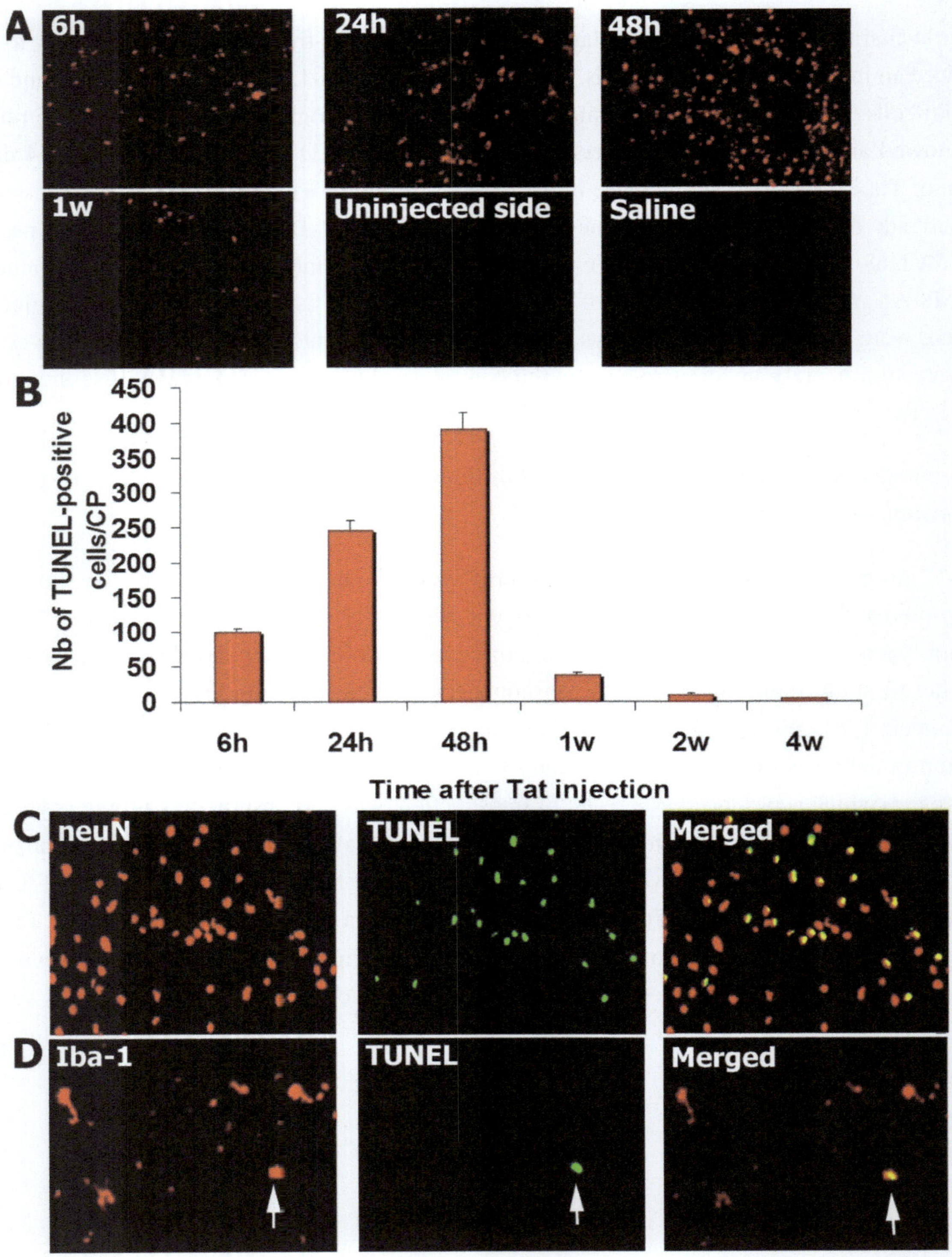

Figure 3. Injection of Tat in the caudate-putamen (CP) triggers neuroinflammation. (**A**) Activated (CD68-positive) microglial cells and proliferating astrocytes were observed in the CP of rats injected with Tat; (**B**) Graph showing an increase in the number of microglial cells (Iba-1 and activated CD68-positive cells) and astrocytes (GFAP-positive cells) persisting til d14. ** $p < 0.01$.

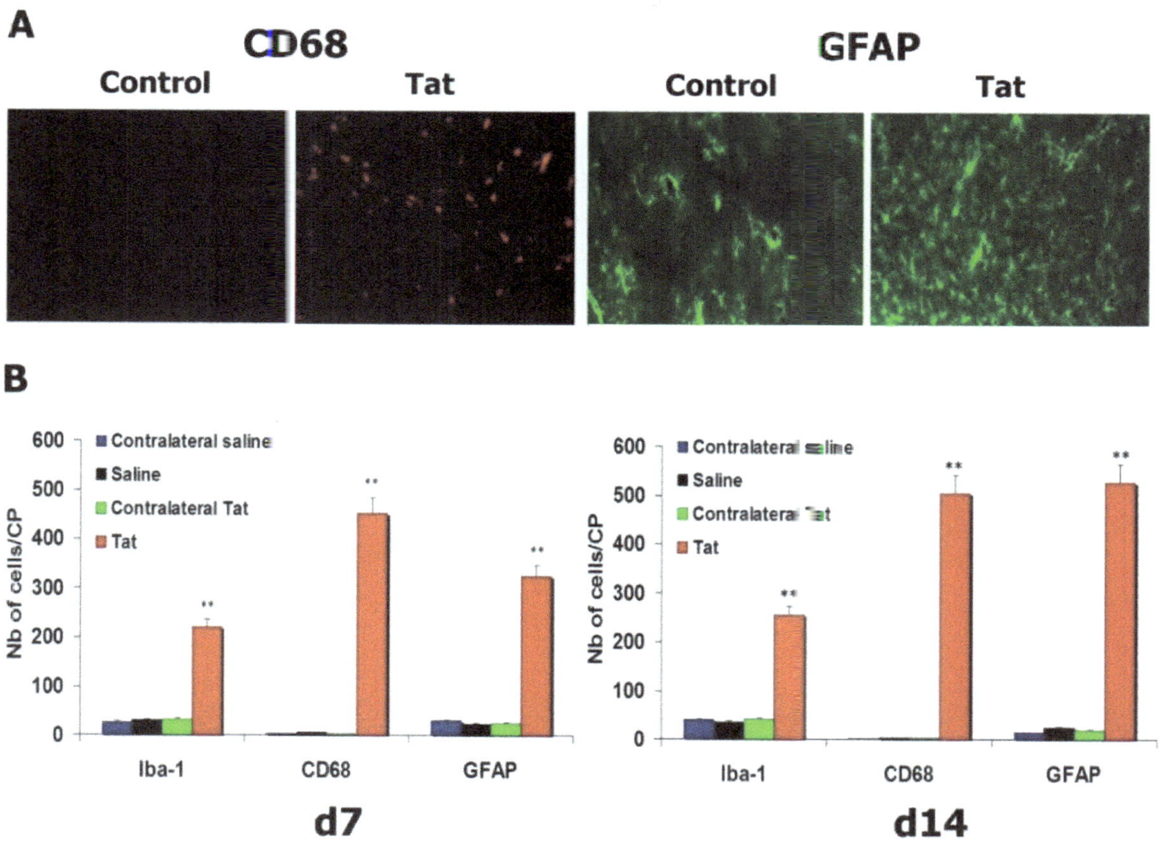

Apoptotic cells were detected at different times by TUNEL assay in SV(Tat) recipients. Rare TUNEL-positive cells were seen after injection of SV(BUGT) ($p < 0.001$). No apoptotic cells were detected on the contralateral uninjected side (not shown) (Table 1).

The neuronal loss, expressed as a percentage of NT-positive cells compared with the contralateral side, was between 26.7% and 34.3% after injection of SV(Tat) in the CP (7 and 28 days after Tat injection, respectively) and was significantly higher than after injection of SV(BUGT) in the same area ($p < 0.001$) (Table 1).

Lipid peroxidation, measured by calorimetric MDA assay, showed that injection of SV(Tat) induced significantly more MDA than was seen in the recipients of saline control (saline: 0.4 μM *vs.* SV(Tat): 1.4 μM; $p < 0.01$).

We enumerated Iba-1-, CD68-, and GFAP-positive cells in SV(Tat) recipients and controls (animals injected with SV(BUGT). Significant higher numbers of microglial cells and astrocytes were observed in the rats administered with SV(Tat), compared to controls (Figure 4), suggesting that continuing production of Tat is associated with neuroinflammation.

Figure 4. Injection of SV(Tat) in the caudate-putamen (CP) induces neuroinflammation. Brains were harvested one and two weeks after injection of SV(Tat) in the CP. Increased numbers of microglial cells (Iba-1- and CD68-positive cells) and astrocytes (GFAP-positive cells) were observed in the CPs injected with SV(Tat). No inflammation was seen in the CPs injected with the control vector, SV(BUGT).

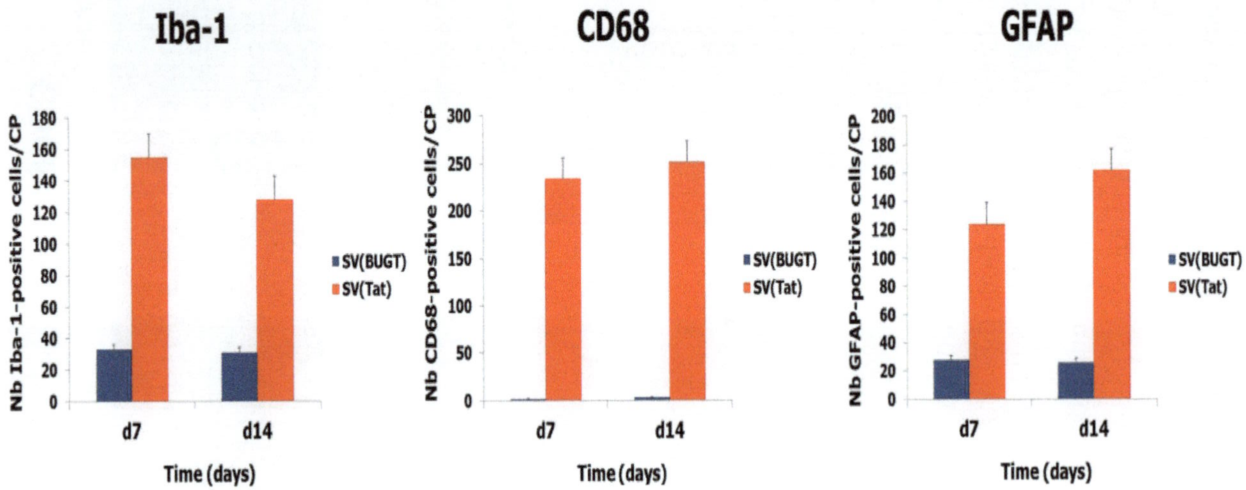

Table 1. Table showing the changes in the caudate-putamen (CP) of rat following injection of SV(Tat). More numerous Tat-positive cells and TUNEL-positive cells were seen one month after injection of SV(Tat) in the CP ($p < 0.01$: SV(Tat) *vs.* SV(BUGT)). Neuronal loss was observed ($p < 0.01$: SV(Tat) *vs.* SV(BUGT)). An increase in the level of MDA, suggesting of oxidative stress, was also detected ($p < 0.01$: SV(Tat) *vs.* SV(BUGT)). CPs injected with SV(BUGT), an unrelated vector, did not show any modifications.

Days/Tat-Induced	**Nb Tat-Positive Cells/Area**			**Nb TUNEL-Positive Cells/Area**			**Neuron Loss (% Compared to Contralateral Area)**			**MDA (µM)**		
Abnormalities	**SV(BUGT)**	**SV(Tat)**	***P***	**SV(BUGT)**	**SV(Tat)**	***P***	**SV(BUGT)**	**SV(Tat)**	***P***	**SV(BUGT)**	**SV(Tat)**	***P***
d7	-	39.4 ± 4.2	<0.01	2.1 ± 1.8	42.7 ± 4.8	<0.01	1.9 ± 0.1	26.7 ± 3.2	<0.01	NA	NA	-
d14	-	48.7 ± 3.8	<0.01	-	47.2 ± 4.5	<0.01	-	30.8 ± 2.9	<0.01	0.4 ± 0.03	1.4 ± 0.1	<0.01
d28	-	28.5 ± 3.4	<0.01	-	24.6 ± 3.1	<0.01	-	34.3 ± 3.6	<0.01	NA	NA	-

3.6. Overexpression of Antioxidant Enzymes Protects against Tat-Induced Lesions

To determine whether rSV40-delivered antioxidant enzymes Cu/Zn SOD1 and GPx1 could protect against Tat-induced CNS injury and its consequences, we administered SV(SOD1), SV(GPx1), and a mixture SV(SOD1)/SV(GPx1) to the CP 1 month before we injected Tat. We then assayed for apoptotic cells and oxidative stress 2 days after Tat inoculation. Prior SV40 delivery of antioxidant enzymes reduced Tat-induced lipid peroxidation (Table 2). The reduction in lipid peroxidation was seen in all antioxidant recipient groups, with animals receiving SV(GPx1), SV(SOD1), whether alone or together, this combination being the best protocol. Prior administration of SV(SOD1) and SV(GPx1) also protected the brains from the damage elicited by Tat. That is, there were fewer Tat-induced apoptotic cells in recipients of SV(SOD1) or SV(GPx1). However, the greatest protection from Tat-related neuronal apoptosis was seen when both vectors were administered into the CP together (Table 2). Finally, we harvested brains 2 weeks after Tat injection to assess neuroinflammation. Prior delivery of antioxidant enzymes mitigated Tat-induced neuroinflammation: numbers of Iba-1-, CD68-, and GFAP-positive cells were significantly reduced compared to controls [injection of SV(BUGT)] after injection of SV(SOD1) and/or (SV(GPx1) (Figure 5).

Thus, the injection of SV(Tat) induces substantial expression of Tat in neurons, lipid peroxidation, neuron death, and neuroinflammation.

4. Discussion

Advances in the treatment of HIV-1 have dramatically improved survival rates over the past 10 years, but HIV-associated neurocognitive disorder (HAND) remains highly prevalent and continues to represent a significant public health problem, partly because HIV-1 is largely impervious to HAART in the CNS. In the early 1990s, the neurologic complications of HIV-1 infection were classified into two levels of disturbance: (1) HIV-associated dementia (HAD) with motor, behavioral/psychosocial, or combined features; and (2) minor cognitive motor disorder (MCMD). HAD was considered as the most common cause of dementia in adults under 40 [54] and was estimated to affect as many as 30% of patients with advanced AIDS [54], but has become less common since HAART was introduced [55]. This reduction probably reflects better control of HIV in the periphery, since antiretroviral drugs penetrate the CNS poorly. Before the introduction of HAART, most neuroAIDS patients showed subcortical dementia, with predominant basal ganglia involvement, manifesting as psychomotor slowing, Parkinsonism, behavioral abnormalities and cognitive difficulties [56]. MCMD described a less severe presentation of HIV-associated neurocognitive impairment that did not meet criteria for HAD.

More recently, in light of the changing epidemiology of HIV infection, the need to update and further structure the diagnostic criteria for HAND has been recognized [57]. There are several reasons for this update. First, the applicability of the old criteria appears limited in the present age of HAART. Prior to the advent of HAART, a diagnosis of HAD was associated strongly with high viral loads, low T-cell counts, and opportunistic infections. With HAART limiting viral severity, patients with HIV typically live longer with milder medical symptoms. Secondly, guidelines regarding possible neurocognitive impairment due to comorbid conditions with CNS effects (e.g., substance use disorders) were not precisely described in the previous diagnostic scheme. This limitation is particularly important in the era of HAART as those infected with HIV-1 live longer with a host of CNS risk factors, including substance use disorders (e.g., methamphetamine dependence), medical conditions associated with HAART treatment (e.g., hyperlipidemia) and comorbid infectious diseases (e.g., hepatitis C virus) [58].

Table 2. Table showing the effect of gene delivery of antioxidant enzymes SOD1 and GPx1 on oxidative stress and apoptosis induced by Tat. Less apoptotic cells were observed in the caudate-putamen (CP) of rats administered with SV(SOD1) and/or SV(GPx1) in the CP before injection of Tat in the same location ($p < 0.05$: SV(SOD1) and SV(GPx1) *vs.* SV(BUGT); $p < 0.01$: SV(SOD1) + SV(GPx1) *vs.* SV(BUGT)). Gene delivery of antioxidant enzymes SOD1 and GPx1 mitigated Tat-induced oxidative stress assessed by MDA levels ($p < 0.05$: SV(SOD1) *vs.* SV(BUGT); $p < 0.01$: SV(GPx1) and SV((SOD1) + SV(GPx1) *vs.* SV(BUGT)).

Vector	Saline	SV(BUGT)	SV(SOD1)	SV(GPx1)	SV(SOD1) + SV(GPx1)
MDA level (μM)	0.38 ± 0.02	1.66 ± 1.5	0.83 ± 0.1	0.42 ± 0.05	0.38 ± 0.04
P value	0.01	-	0.05	0.01	0.01
Nb of TUNEL-positive cells/CP	2 ± 0.01	382 ± 41	232 ± 28	255 ± 28	52 ± 6
P value	0.01	-	0.05	0.05	0.01

Figure 5. Gene delivery of antioxidant enzymes mitigates Tat-induced neuroinflammation. SV(SOD1), SV(GPx1), or a mixture SV(SOD1)/SV(GPx1), were injected in the caudate-putamen (CP) one month before injection of Tat in the same structure. In the group administered with a control vector, SV(BUGT), increased numbers of microglial cells and astrocytes were seen 2 weeks after injection of Tat. CPs previously injected with SV(SOD1), SV(GPx1), or a mixture SV(SOD1)/SV(GPx1) exhibited significantly fewer microglial cells and astrocytes compared to the group injected with SV(BUGT) then Tat (* $p < 0.05$; ** $p < 0.01$). There were also less-apoptotic cells and no increase in MDA levels in the group injected with saline compared to the group injected with SV(BUGT) then Tat ($p < 0.01$).

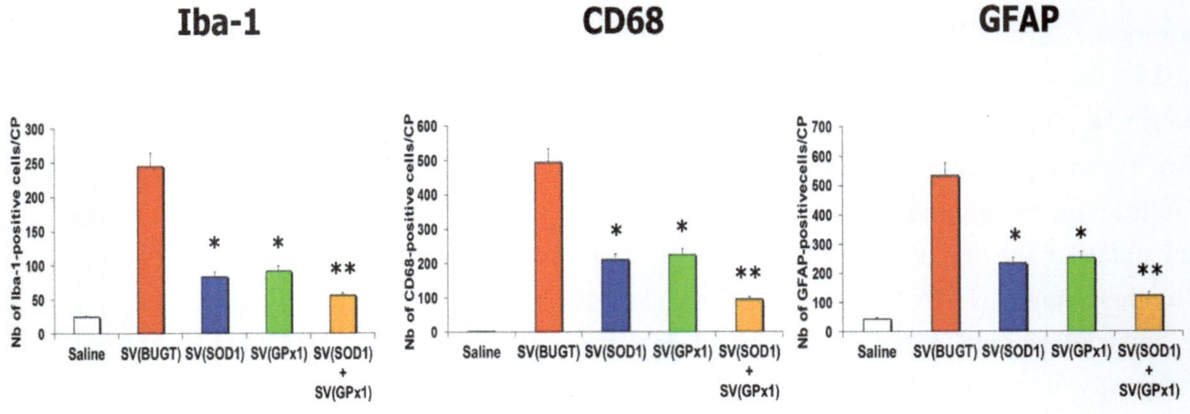

Thus, the newly redefined criteria allow for three possible research diagnoses: (1) asymptomatic neurocognitive impairment (ANI); (2) HIV-associated mild neurocognitive disorder (MND); and (3) HAD. In this classification, the diagnosis of HAND must be determined by assessing at least five areas of neurocognitive functioning known to be affected by HIV infection (e.g., attention/working memory, executive functions speed of information processing, episodic memory, motor skills, language, and sensoriperception) [57]. Considered as a mild neurocognitive impairment in the absence of declines in everyday functioning, ANI is now estimated to represent the majority of cases of HAND (*i.e.*, about 50% of diagnosed cases) and 21%–30% of the asymptomatic HIV-infected individuals. Detecting patients with mild, yet demonstrable, neurocognitive impairment may help in the effort to pre-identify those at risk for more significant cognitive as well as functional decline, before cognitive deficits contribute to a decline in everyday functioning with serious medical consequences [58]. As effective treatments for neurologic complications are developed, intervention at this earliest stage of HAND might offer the best opportunity to obtain remission, or at least, prevent progression. Formerly referred to as MCMD, mild neurocognitive disorder (MND) requires mild-to-moderate neurocognitive impairment in at least two cognitive domains in addition to mild everyday functioning impairment [57]. Approximately 30%–50% of persons with a HAND diagnosis experience some degree of functional impairment and it is estimated that 20%–40% of HAND diagnoses are of MND, which comprises 5%–20% of the HIV population overall [58]. The most severe form of HAND, HIV-associated dementia (HAD) is marked by at least moderate-to-severe cognitive impairment in at least two cognitive domains along with marked ADL declines that are not fully attributable to comorbidities or delirium [57,58]. Furthermore, HAD represents the most severe form of HAND in terms of its functional impact. After the advent of HAART in the late 1990s, estimates appeared to shift downward with approximately 4% to 7% of persons with AIDS, with more recent appraisals suggesting that as few as 1% to 2% of HIV+ patients meet criteria for HAD [58].

As survival with chronic HIV-1 infection improves, the number of people harboring the virus in their CNS increases, leading to new HIV-1-related neurological manifestations. The prevalence of HAND therefore continues to rise, and less fulminant forms of HAND have become more common than their more severe predecessors [57,58]. HAND remains a significant independent risk factor for AIDS mortality [17–20,55,57,58]. Incident cases of HAND are accelerating fastest among drug users, ethnic minorities, and women [17–20]. The number of HIV-infected individuals over 50 years of age is rapidly growing, including patients taking HAART [20]. It has been suggested that in 10 years, 50% of AIDS patients in the United States will be over the age of 50. Moreover, it is becoming clear that the brain is an important reservoir for the virus, and neurodegenerative and neuroinflammatory changes may continue despite HAART [19].

Oxidative stress plays a role in the development of HAND [59,60]. Oxidative stress in HIV-1 dementia has been documented by analyses of brain tissue, including increased levels of lipid peroxidation product (*i.e.*, by immunodetection of 4-hydroxynonenal (HNE) or measurement of malondialdehyde (MDA) levels) and the presence of oxidized proteins (*i.e.*, dinitrophenol (DNP)). Serum levels of GSH and GPx1 are decreased in HIV-1 patients while MDA levels are increased [61]. A characteristic of patients infected with HIV-1 in late stage disease is diffuse intracellular oxidation in the form of decreased availability of GSH, the main cellular antioxidant and redox buffer, and augmented lipid oxidation, which triggers a cascade of downstream signaling events.

Membrane-associated oxidative stress correlates with HIV-1 dementia pathogenesis and cognitive impairment [20]. HNE-positive neurons have been demonstrated in the brains of patients with HIV-1 encephalitis [60,62,63]. In the case of HIV-1 infection, Tat and gp120 can elicit such oxidative stress [20,38,64] which can induce apoptosis in cultured neurons [65]. It can also damage neurons and cause cognitive dysfunction *in vivo* [66]. Tat and gp120 induce ceramide production in cultured neurons by triggering sphingomyelinase activity via a mechanism that involves induction of oxidative stress by CXCR4 activation [20,67]. Oxidative stress can play a role in HAND in other ways as well. Circulating toxins in the CSF, derived from HIV-1-infected cells, may damage mitochondria, leading to release of cytochrome c and then to a cascade of events leading to apoptosis [59,60]. HIV-1 gp120 and Tat can cause free radical production, possibly as part of the signal-transduction pathways they activate [20,64].

It is still unclear whether oxidative stress is the primary initiating event associated with neurodegeneration. However, a growing body of evidence implicates it as being involved in at least the propagation of cellular injury that leads to neuron death [68]. Earlier reports support the hypothesis that oxidative modifications of macromolecular cell components (lipids, proteins and nucleic acids) may be an early step in the mechanism of Tat and gp120 neurotoxicity [36,37].

Microglial cells can proliferate in response to brain injury [69]. Following such insult, reactive microglial cells are mainly proliferating resident cells rather than infiltrating circulating cells [70]. Both populations are different. Infiltrating cells will undergo apoptosis while proliferating resident ones continue to expand [70]. Proliferating resident microglial cells can migrate towards the area of injury too (as infiltrating circulating cells could, but these ones are less numerous and are progressively disappearing because of apoptosis). If neuron loss [24,71–73] and astrogliosis [24] have been described in animals receiving gp120 directly into their brains, a temporal relationship between neuronal degeneration, astrocytic reaction and microglial proliferation remained to be established. Thus, we challenged rat CPs with 100–500 ng HIV-1BaL gp120, with or without prior rSV40-delivered superoxide dismutase or glutathione peroxidase [74]. CD11b-positive microglia were increased day 1 post-challenge, while Iba-1- and CD68-positive cells peaked at day 7 and day 14. Moreover, CD68-positive cells exhibited a shape that was close to reactive amoeboid microglial cells. Astrocyte infiltration was maximal at day 7–14. These sequential events were related to the expression of different chemokines and cytokines overtime. It is possible that different populations of microglial cells are recruited following gp120 injection, or that resident microglial cells can be stimulated by the different chemokines/cytokines expressed post-injury (in response to oxidative stress for example), leading to their proliferation and their migration towards the site of injury. SV(SOD1) or SV(GPx1) significantly limited neuroinflammation following gp120 administration into the CP. Thus, gp120 induces neuroinflammation when injected in the rat CP and gp120-induced neuroinflammation correlates with neuron loss [74]. An increase in ROS may play a role in this phenomenon, as evidenced by the protective effects of rSV40-delivered antioxidant enzymes. The results we observed here by injecting Tat in the CP are somehow comparable to those seen with gp120.

Free radical production may be accompanied by elevated expression of MIP-1 alpha contributing to microglial recruitment and delayed neuronal death in several models of CNS injury [75,76]. The radical scavengers, like vitamin E analogs, may inhibit free radicals and MIP-1 alpha production, and recruitment of microglia in the injured area [77]. In models of ischemia/reperfusion injury, transgenic mice that overexpressed antioxidant enzymes, such as SOD-1 and GPx1 showed less upregulation of MIP-1 alpha and MCP-1 and less neuron loss and inflammation [78]. Concerning HIV-1-related neurotoxicity, it has been recently shown that both gp120 and methamphetamine (MA) induce ROS production in concentration- and time dependant manners. Moreover, the involvement of cytochrome P 450 (CYP) and NADPH-oxidase (NOX) pathways in gp120/MA-induced oxidative stress and apoptotic cell death in astrocytes has been reported [79]. Tat can up-regulate cytokines (*i.e.*, IL-6, IL-8) expression in breast cancer cells [80], and can also increase the expression of the chemokine CCL5 in astrocytes [81]. Additionally, Tat-induced production of chemokine (MCP-1) and cytokines (TNF-α, IL-6) in astrocytes is increased by morphine, through NF-κB trafficking and transcription [82]. Our findings extend the principle of antioxidant protection from neuroinflammation to HIV-related injury, and suggest that rSV40 antioxidant gene delivery may be therapeutically applicable in the case of ongoing injury and neuroinflammation such as HAND.

A few antioxidants have been tried in small prospective controlled studies in HAND. However, the findings have all been relatively disappointing so far. Selegiline (L-deprenyl), which mechanism of action is speculative, albeit it might decrease the production of ROS and serve as an anti-apoptotic factor, was used in 2 double-blind controlled studies in the pre-HAART era. The first trial involving patients with minor cognitive and motor dysfunction (MCMD) showed improvement in verbal learning and trends for improvement in recall [83,84]. The second study was a smaller study in patients with MCMD and HIV dementia and showed significant improvement in delayed recall. However, other tests were not improved. A slight improvement was noted in patients treated with OPC-14117, a lipophilic compound structurally similar to vitamin E that acts as an antioxidant by scavenging superoxide radicals [85]. CPI-1189, a lipophilic antioxidant that scavenges superoxide anion radicals and block the neurotoxicity of gp120 and TNF-α [86], showed no effect on neurocognition in patients with MCMD and HIV dementia [87].

Upstream and downstream antioxidant therapeutic approaches in HAND have previously been discussed [88]. Upstream preventive treatment is based on prevention of free radical generation, regulation of neuronal protein interaction with redox metals (*i.e.*, Fe) and maintaining normal cellular metabolism. Our daily diet contains several natural antioxidants (lipoic acid, and vitamins E). Antioxidant therapy involving endogenous enzymes and some anti-inflammatory drugs constitute upstream therapy in ROS generation and can prevent downstream neurodegeneration. Vitamin E can block the neurotoxicity induced by CSF of patients with HIV dementia [60]. Flavinoids are a group of compounds made by plants that have antioxidant and neuroprotective properties. This class of molecules has weak estrogen-receptor-binding properties and thus, do not have the side effects of estradiol. It has been described that diosgenin, a plant-derived estrogen present in yam and fenugreek can prevent neurotoxicity by HIV-1 proteins and by CSF from patients with HIV dementia [60]. *N*-acetyl-L-cysteine (NAC) is a nutritional supplement precursor in the formation of the antioxidant glutathione in the body and its sulfhydryl group confers antioxidant effects and is able to reduce free radicals. NAC injected intraperitoneally into rodents increases glutathione levels in the brain and protects the CNS against the damaging effects of hydroxyl radicals and lipid peroxidation product acrolein [89]. However, NAC itself does not cross the BBB easily. *N*-acetylcysteine amide (NACA), a modified form of NAC, where the carboxyl group has been replaced by an amide group, has been found to be more effective in neurotoxic cases because of its ability to permeate cell membranes and the blood-brain barrier (BBB). Treatment of animals injected intravenously with gp120, Tat and methamphetamine METH by NACA significantly rescued the animals from oxidative stress. Further, NACA-treated animals had significantly less BBB permeability as compared to the group treated with gp120 + Tat + METH alone, indicating that NACA can protect the BBB from oxidative stress-induced damage in gp120, Tat and METH exposed animals [90].

The therapeutic coverage of post oxidative stress events can be done by downstream antioxidant therapy. Non steroidal anti-inflammatory drugs (NSAIDS) limit the infiltration of macrophages and can reduce the inflammatory cascade induced by oxidative stress. Minocycline is a tetracycline-derived compound that demonstrated neuroprotective profile in several models of neurodegeneration. The molecule has significant anti-inflammatory actions and can easily cross the BBB. Estradiol can protect against the neurotoxic effects of HIV-1 proteins in human neuronal cultures, probably by protecting the neuronal mitochondria in a receptor-independent manner [60]. However, estradiol has well known side effects in women (potential risk of developing breast or uterine cancer), and cannot be used in men or children because of feminizing effects. It has been shown that several novel antioxidants (ebselen, diosgenin) can protect *in vitro* against neurotoxicity induced by CSF from patients with HIV dementia [60].

It is likely that neuroprotective therapies should benefit from multiple and combination approaches targeting different aspects and pathways of the oxidative-stress insult. For example, coupling a potent antioxidant with a compound that modifies downstream signaling pathways (*i.e.*, minocycline) could provide a synergistic neuroprotective effects, at lower doses (and thus with less toxicity) that each molecule could achieve alone. The combination of HAART with an antioxidant compound and a molecule involved in downstream antioxidant therapy could be a promising avenue in the treatment of HAND. However, it should be reminded that one of the challenges in designing antioxidants to protect the CNS against ROS is the crossing of the BBB.

Experimental systems to study how gp120 and other HIV proteins affect the brain are limited to the acute effects of recombinant proteins *in vitro* or *in vivo*, or to Simian Immunodeficiency Virus (SIV)-infected monkeys. To circumvent these limitations, we have described an experimental rodent model of ongoing gp120-induced neurotoxicity in which HIV-1 Env is expressed in the brain using a SV40-derived gene delivery vector, SV(gp120) [53]. Inoculated stereotaxically into the rat CP, SV(gp120) causes a lesion in which neuron and other cell apoptosis continues for at least 12 weeks. HIV gp120 was expressed throughout this time. SV(gp120)-induced lipid peroxidation was documented by both MDA and HNE assays. Thus, *in vivo* inoculation of SV(gp120) into the rat CP causes ongoing oxidative stress and apoptosis in neurons and so may represent a useful animal model. We also tested the effect of SV(gp120) on neuroinflammation. Increase in microglia and astrocytes was seen following intra-CP SV(gp120) injection, suggesting that continuing gp120 production increased neuroinflammation, as well as microglia and astrocytes proliferation after injection of SV(gp120) in the striatum. However, SV(gp120)-induced inflammation was reduced by prior gene transfer of antioxidant enzymes. Thus, gp120-induced CNS injury, neuron loss and inflammation may be mitigated by antioxidant gene delivery. Similar results using SV(Tat) are shown in the present work.

We sought here to characterize Tat-induced neuroinflammation in different experimental settings and to test an ability to limit the extent of the inflammatory process by rSV40 gene delivery of antioxidant enzymes. The results presented here are somehow comparable to the ones observed with gp120. SV(Tat) induces protracted expression of Tat, mainly in neurons, oxidative stress, neuronal apoptosis, neuroinflammation. Further studies should be undertaken to dissect the role of Tat in oxidative stress; for example, it would be worth measuring free radicals (particularly hydrogen peroxide) after Tat injection.

5. Conclusions

HIV-1-associated neurocognitive disorder (HAND) is an increasingly common and progressive disease, characterized by progressively deteriorating CNS function. HIV-1 gene products, particularly gp120 and Tat, elicit ROS that lead to oxidant injury and causes neuron apoptosis, as well as subsequent consequences (e.g., neuroinflammation, abnormalities of the BBB). The understanding of, and developing therapies for HAND requires accessible models of the disease. We have devised experimental approaches to studying the acute and chronic effects of gp120 and Tat on the CNS. Even though HIV-1 gp120 and Tat cannot be solely responsible for the pathogenesis of HAND, the animal models used in the present study are able to recapitulate many aspects of HAND. These approaches to gp120 and Tat administration may therefore represent useful animal models for studying the pathogenesis and treatment of HIV-1 gp120- and Tat-related damage. Gene delivery of antioxidant enzymes by recombinant SV40-derived vectors protects against gp120 and Tat-induced oxidative stress and neuronal apoptosis, opening new avenues for potential therapeutics of HAND.

Acknowledgments

This work was supported by NIH grants MH70287, MH69122 and AH48244 to DS.

Author Contributions

JPL performed experiments and wrote the paper; LA and BE performed experiments; EVB supervised experiments; DS supervised experiments and wrote the paper.

Conflicts of Interest

The authors declare no conflict of interest.

References

1. Broughton, B.R.S.; Reutens, D.C.; Sobey, C.G. Apoptotic mechanisms after cerebral ischemia. *Stroke* **2009**, *11*, e331–e339.
2. Dexter, D.T.; Carter, C.J.; Wells, F.R.; Javoy-Agid, F.; Agid, Y.; Lees, A.; Jenner, P.; Marsden, C.D. Basal lipid peroxidation in substantia nigra is increased in Parkinson's disease. *J. Neurochem*. **1989**, *52*, 381–389.
3. Rosen, D.R.; Siddique, T.; Patterson, D.; Figlewicz, D.A.; Sapp, P.; Hentati, A.; Donaldson, D.; Goto, J.; O'Regan, J.P.; Deng, H.X.; *et al*. Mutations in Cu/Zn superoxide dismutase are associated with familial amyotrophic lateral sclerosis. *Nature* **1993**, *362*, 59–62.
4. Beal, M.F. Aging, energy, and oxidative stress in neurodegenerative diseases. *Ann. Neurol*. **1995**, *38*, 357–366.

5. Reddy, P.H.; Reddy, T.P. Mitochondria as a therapeutic target for aging and neurodegenerative diseases. *Curr. Alzheimer Res*. **2011**, *8*, 393–409.
6. Smith, M.A.; Sayre, L.M.; Monnier, V.M.; Perry, G. Radical ageing in Alzheimer's disease. *Trends Neurosci*. **1995**, *18*, 172–176.
7. Cao, W.; Carney, J.M.; Duchon, A.; Floyd, R.A.; Chevion, M. Oxygen free radicals involvement in ischemia and reperfusion of the brain injury to brain. *Neurosci. Lett.* **1998**, *88*, 233–238.
8. Montoliu, C.; Valles, S.; Renau-Piqueras, J.; Guerri, C. Ethanol-induced oxygen radical formation and lipid peroxidation in rat brain: Effect of chronic alcohol consumption. *J. Neurochem*. **1994**, *63*, 1855–1862.
9. Smith, C.D.; Carney, J.M.; Starke-Reed, P.E.; Oliver, C.N.; Stadtman, E.R.; Floyd, R.A.; Markesberry, W.R. Excess brain protein oxidation and enzyme dysfunction in normal aging and in Alzheimer's disease. *Proc. Natl. Acad. Sci. USA* **1991**, *88*, 10540–10543.
10. Nelson, P.T.; Soma, L.A.; Lavi, E. Microglia in diseases of the central nervous system. *Ann. Med.* **2002**, *34*, 491–500.
11. Liu, B.; Hong, J.S. Role of microglia in inflammation-mediated neurodegenerative diseases: Mechanisms and strategies for therapeutic intervention. *J. Pharmacol. Exp. Ther.* **2003**, *304*, 1–7.
12. Sheehan, J.J.; Zhou, C.; Gravanis, I.; Rogove, A.D.; Wu, Y.P.; Bogenhagen, D.F.; Tsirka, S.E. Proteolytic activation of monocyte chemoattractant protein-1 by plasmin underlies excitotoxic neurodegeneration in mice. *J. Neurosci.* **2007**, *27*, 1738–1745.
13. Ekdahl, C.T.; Claasen, J.H.; Bonde, S.; Kokaia, Z.; Lindvall, O. Inflammation is detrimental for neurogenesis in adult brain. *Proc. Natl. Acad. Sci. USA* **2003**, *100*, 13632–13637.
14. Cowell, R.M.; Xu, H.; Galasso, J.M.; Silverstein, F.S. Hypoxic-ischemic injury induces macrophage inflammatory protein-1 alpha expression in immature rat brain. *Stroke* **2002**, *33*, 795–801.
15. McGeer, P.L.; McGeer, E.G. Anti-inflammatory drugs in the fight against Alzheimer's disease. *Ann. N. Y. Acad. Sci.* **1996**, *777*, 213–220.
16. Perry, V.H.; Newwan, T.A.; Cunningham, C. The impact of systemic infection on the progression of neurodegenerative disease. *Nat. Rev. Neurosci.* **2003**, *4*, 103–112.
17. McArthur, J.C.; Brew, B.J.; Nath, A. Neurological complications of HIV infection. *Lancet Neurol.* **2005**, *4*, 543–555.
18. Nath, A.; Sacktor, N. Influence of highly active antiretroviral therapy on persistence of HIV in the central nervous system. *Curr. Opin. Neurol.* **2006**, *19*, 358–361.
19. Ances, B.M.; Ellis, R.J. Dementia and neurocognitive disorders due to HIV-1 infection. *Semin. Neurol.* **2007**, *27*, 86–92.
20. Mattson, M.P.; Haughey, N.J.; Nath, A. Cell death in HIV dementia. *Cell Death Diff.* **2005**, *12*, 893–904.
21. Kaul, M.; Lipton, S.A. Chemokines and activated macrophages in HIV gp120-induced neuronal apoptosis. *Proc. Natl. Acad. Sci. USA* **1999**, *96*, 8212–8216.
22. Kaul, M.; Garden, G.W.; Lipton, S.A. Pathways to neuronal injury and apoptosis in HIV-associated dementia. *Nature* **2001**, *19*, 988–994.

23. Van de Bovenkamp, M.; Nottet, H.S.; Pereira, C.F. Interactions of human immunodeficiencyvirus-1 proteins with neurons: Possible role in the development of human immunodeficiencyvirus-1 associated dementia. *Eur. J. Clin. Investig.* **2002**, *32*, 619–627.
24. Bansal, A.K.; Mactutus, C.F.; Nath, A.; Maragos, W.; Hauser, K.F.; Booze, R.M. Neurotoxicity of HIV-1 proteins gp120 and Tat in the rat striatum. *Brain Res.* **2000**, *879*, 42–49.
25. Agrawal, L.; Louboutin, J.P.; Reyes, B.A.S.; van Bockstaele, E.J.; Strayer, D.S. Antioxidant enzyme gene delivery to protect from HIV-1 gp120-induced neuronal apoptosis. *Gene Ther.* **2006**, *13*, 1645–1656.
26. Eugenin, E.A.; D'Aversa, T.G.; Lopez, L.; Calderon, T.M.; Berman, J.W. MCP-1 (CCL2) protects human neurons and astrocytes from NMDA or HIV-tat-induced apoptosis. *J. Neurochem.* **2003**, *85*, 1299–1311.
27. Ghezzi, S.; Noolan, D.M.; Aluigi, M.G.; Vallanti, G.; Cota, M.; Benelli, R.; Morini, M.; Reeves, J.D.; Vicenzi, E.; Poli, G.; *et al.* Inhibition of CXCR-3-dependent HIV-1 infection by extracellular HIV-1 Tat. *Biochem. Biophys. Res. Commun.* **2000**, *270*, 992–996.
28. Bonavia, R.; Bajetto, A.; Barbero, S.; Albini, A.; Noonan, D.M.; Schettini, G. HIV-1 Tat causes apoptosis death and calcium homeostasis alterations in rat neurons. *Biochem. Biophys. Res. Commun.* **2001**, *288*, 301–308.
29. Haughey, N.J.; Nath, A.; Mattson, M.P. HIV-1 tat through phosphorylation of NMDA receptors potentiates glutamate excitotoxicity. *J. Neurochem.* **2001**, *78*, 457–467.
30. Norman, J.P.; Perry, S.W.; Reynolds, H.M.; Kiebala, M.; de Mesy Bentley, K.L.; Trejo, M.; Volsky, D.J.; Maggirwar, S.B.; Dewhurst, S.; Masliah, E. HIV-1 Tat activates neuronal ryanodine receptors with rapid induction of the unfolded protein response and mitochondrial hyperpolarization. *PLoS One* **2008**, *3*, e3731.
31. Nath, A.; Haughey, N.J.; Jones, M.; Anderson, C.; Bell, J.E.; Geiger, J.D. Synergistic neurotoxicity by human immunodeficiency virus proteins Tat and gp120: Protection by memantine. *Ann. Neurol.* **2000**, *47*, 186–194.
32. Kruman, L.L.; Nath, A.; Mattson, M.P. HIV-1 protein Tat induces apoptosis of hippocampal neurons by a mechanism involving caspase activation, calcium overload, and oxidative stress. *Exp. Neurol.* **1998**, *154*, 276–288.
33. Magnuson, D.S.; Knudsen, B.E.; Geiger, J.D.; Brownstone, R.M.; Nath, A. Human immunodeficiency virus type 1 Tat activates non-*N*-methyl-o-aspartate excitatory amino receptors and causes neurotoxicity. *Ann. Neurol.* **1995**, *37*, 373–380.
34. Bonfoco, E.; Krainc, D.; Ankarcrona, M.; Nicotera, P.; Lipton, S.A. Apoptosis and necrosis: Two distinct events induced, respectively, by mild and intense insults with *N*-methyl-D-aspartate or nitric oxide/superoxide in cortical cell cultures. *Proc. Natl. Acad. Sci. USA* **1995**, *92*, 7162–7166.
35. Jones, M.; Olafson, K.; del Bigio, M.R.; Peeling, A.; Nath, A. Intraventricular injection of human immunodeficiency virus type 1 (HIV-1) tat protein causes inflammation, gliosis, apoptosis, and ventricular enlargment. *J. Neuropathol. Exp. Neurol.* **1998**, *57*, 563–570.
36. Askenov, M.Y.; Hasselrot, U.; Bansal, A.K.; Wu, G.; Nath, A.; Anderson, C.; Mactutus, C.F.; Booze, R.M. Oxidative damage induced by the injection of HIV-1 Tat protein in the rat striatum. *Neurosci. Lett.* **2001**, *305*, 5–8.

37. Askenov, M.Y.; Hasselrot, U.; Wu, G.; Nath, A.; Anderson, C.; Mactutus, C.F.; Booze, R.M. Temporal relationship between HIV-1 Tat-induced neuronal degeneration, OX-42 immunoreactivity, reactive astrocytosis, and protein oxidation in the rat striatum. *Brain Res.* **2003**, *987*, 1–9.
38. Agrawal, L.; Louboutin, J.P.; Strayer, D.S. Preventing HIV-1 Tat-induced neuronal apoptosis using antioxidant enzymes: Mechanistic and therapeutic implications. *Virology* **2007**, *363*, 462–472.
39. Strayer, D.S. Gene therapy using SV40-derived vectors: What does the future hold? *J. Cell. Physiol.* **1999**, *181*, 375–384.
40. McKee, H.J.; Strayer, D.S. Immune responses against SIV envelope glycoprotein, using recombinant SV40 as a vaccine delivery vector. *Vaccine* **2002**, *20*, 3613–3625.
41. Strayer, D.S.; Kondo, R.; Milano, J.; Duan, L.X. Use of SV40-based vectors to transduce foreign genes to normal human peripheral blood mononuclear cells. *Gene Ther.* **1997**, *4*, 219–225.
42. Strayer, D.S.; Lamothe, M.; Wei, D.; Milano, J.; Kondo, R. Generation of Recombinant SV40 Vectors for Gene Transfer. In *Methods in Molecular Biology*, *SV40 Protocols*; Raptis, L., Ed.; Humana Press: Totowa, NJ, USA, 2001; Volume 165, pp. 103–117.
43. Sauter, B.V.; Parashar, B.; Chowdhury, N.R.; Kadakol, A.; Ilan, Y.; Singh, H.; Milano, J.; Strayer, D.S.; Chowdhury, J.R. A replication-deficient rSV40 mediates liver-directed gene transfer and a long-term amelioration of jaundice in gunn rats. *Gastroenterology* **2000**, *119*, 1348–1357.
44. Theodore, S.; Cass, W.A.; Maragos, W.F. Methamphetamine and human immunodeficiency virus protein Tat synergize to destroy dopaminergic terminals in the rat striatum. *Neuroscience* **2006**, *137*, 925–935.
45. Paxinos, G.; Watson, C. *The Rat Brain in Stereotaxic Coordinates*, 2nd ed.; Academic Press: New York, NY, USA, 1986.
46. Rouger, K.; Louboutin, J.P.; Villanova, M.; Cherel, Y.; Fardeau, M. X-linked vacuolated myopathy: TNF-alpha and IFN-gamma expression in muscle fibers with MHC class I on sarcolemma. *Am. J. Pathol.* **2001**, *158*, 355–359.
47. Nikonov, A.A.; Finger, T.E.; Caprio, J. Beyond the olfactory bulb: An odotopic map in the forebrain. *Proc. Natl. Acad. Sci. USA* **2005**, *102*, 18688–18693.
48. Louboutin, J.P.; Liu, B.; Reyes, B.A.S.; van Bockstaele, E.J.; Strayer, D.S. Rat bone marrow progenitor cells transduced in situ by rSV40 vectors differentiate into multiple CNS cell lineages. *Stem Cells* **2006**, *24*, 2801–2809.
49. Louboutin, J.P.; Reyes, B.A.S.; Agrawal, L.; van Bockstaele, E.J.; Strayer, D.S. Strategies for CNS-directed gene delivery: *In vivo* gene transfer to the brain using SV40-derived vectors. *Gene Ther.* **2007**, *14*, 939–949.
50. Louboutin, J.P.; Chekmasova, A.; Marusich, E.; Agrawal, L.; Strayer, D.S. Role of CCR5 and its ligands in the control of vascular inflammation and leukocyte recruitment required for acute excitotoxic seizure induction and neural damage. *FASEB J.* **2011**, *25*, 737–753.
51. Louboutin, J.P.; Chekmasova, A.A.; Marusich, E.; Chowdury, D.; Strayer, D.S. Efficient CNS gene delivery by intravenous injection. *Nat. Meth.* **2010**, *7*, 905–907.

52. Mandel, R.J.; Rendahl, K.G.; Spratt, S.K.; Snyder, R.O.; Cohen, L.K.; Leff, S.E. Characterization of intrastriatal recombinant adeno-associated virus-mediated gene transfer of human tyrosine hydroxylase and human GTP-cyclohydrolase I in a rat model of Parkinson's disease. *J. Neurosci.* **1998**, *18*, 4271–4284.
53. Louboutin, J.P.; Agrawal, L.; Reyes, B.A.S.; van Bockstaele, E.J.; Strayer, D.S. A rat model of human immunodeficiency virus 1 encephalopathy using envelope glycoprotein gp120 expression delivered by SV40 vectors. *J. Neuropathol. Exp. Neurol.* **2009**, *68*, 456–473.
54. McArthur, J.C.; Hoover, D.R.; Bacellar, H.; Miller, E.N.; Cohen, B.A.; Becker, J.T.; Graham, N.M.; McArthur, J.H.; Selnes, O.A.; Jacobson, L.P.; *et al.* Dementia in AIDS patients: Incidence and risk factors. Multicenter AIDS cohort study. *Neurology* **1993**, *43*, 2245–2252.
55. Major, E.O.; Rausch, D.; Marra, C.; Clifford, D. HIV-associated dementia. *Science* **2000**, *288*, 440–442.
56. Koutsilieri, E.; Sopper, S.; Scheller, C.; ter Meulen, V.; Riederer, P. Parkinsonism in HIV dementia. *J. Neural Transm.* **2002**, *109*, 767–775.
57. Antinori, A.; Arendt, G.; Becker, J.T.; Brew, B.J.; Byrd, D.A.; Cherner, M.; Clifford, D.B.; Cinque, P.; Epstein, L.G.; Gookin, K.; *et al.* Updated research nosology for HIV-associated neurocognitive disorders. *Neurology* **2007**, *69*, 1789–1799.
58. Woods, S.P.; Moore, D.J.; Weber, E.; Grant, I. Cognitive neuropsychology of HIV-associated neurocognitive disorders. *Neuropsychol. Rev.* **2009**, *19*, 152–168.
59. Mollace, V.; Nottet, H.S.; Clayette, P.; Turco, M.C.; Muscoli, C.; Salvemini, D.; Perno, C.F. Oxidative stress and neuroAIDS: Triggers, modulators and novel antioxidants. *Trends Neurosci.* **2001**, *24*, 411–416.
60. Turchan, J.; Pocernich, C.B.; Gairola, C.; Chauhan, A.; Schifitto, G.; Butterfield, D.A.; Buch, S.; Naravan, O.; Sinai, A.; Geiger, J.; *et al.* Oxidative stress in HIV demented patients and protection *ex vivo* with novel antioxidants. *Neurology* **2003**, *60*, 307–314.
61. Steiner, J.; Haughey, N.; Li, W.; Venkatesan, A.; Anderson, C.; Reid, R.; Malpica, T.; Pocernich, C.; Butterfield, D.A.; Nath, A. Oxidative stress and therapeutic approaches in HIV dementia. *Antioxid. Redox Signal* **2006**, *8*, 2089–2100.
62. Haughey, N.J.; Cutler, R.G.; Tamara, A.; McArthur, J.C.; Vargas, D.L.; Pardo, C.A.; Turchan, J.; Nath, A.; Mattson, M.P. Perturbation of sphingolipid metabolism and ceramide production in HIV-dementia. *Ann. Neurol.* **2004**, *5*, 257–267.
63. Cutler, R.G.; Haughey, N.J.; Tammara, A.; McArthur, J.C.; Nath, A.; Reid, R.; Vargas, D.L.; Pardo, C.A.; Mattson, M.P. Dysregulation of sphingolipids and sterol metabolism by ApoE4 in HIV dementia. *Neurology* **2004**, *63*, 626–630.
64. Agrawal, L.; Louboutin, J.P.; Reyes, B.A.S.; van Bockstaele, E.J.; Strayer, D.S. HIV-1 Tat neurotoxicity: A model of acute and chronic exposure, and neuroprotection by gene delivery by antioxidant enzymes. *Neurobiol. Dis.* **2012**, *45*, 657–670.
65. Kruman, I.; Bruce-Keller, A.J.; Bredesen, D.; Waq, G.; Mattson, M.P. Evidence that 4-hydroxynonenal mediates oxidative stress-induced neuronal apoptosis. *J. Neurosci.* **1997**, *17*, 5089–5100.

66. Bruce-Keller, A.J.; Li, Y.J.; Lovell, M.A.; Kraemer, P.J.; Gary, D.S.; Brown, R.R.; Markesbery, W.R.; Mattson, M.P. 4-Hydroxynonenal, a product of lipid peroxidation, damages cholinergic neurons and impairs visuospatial memory in rats. *J. Neuropathol. Exp. Neurol.* **1998**, *57*, 257–267.
67. Bruce-Keller, A.J.; Barger, S.W.; Moss, N.I.; Pham, J.T.; Keller, J.N.; Nath, A. Proinflammatory and pro-oxidant properties of Tat in a microglial cell line: Attenuation by 17β-estradiol. *J. Neurochem.* **2001**, *78*, 1315–1324.
68. Uttara, B.; Singh, A.V.; Zamboni, P.; Mahajan, R.T. Oxidative stress and neurodegenerative diseases: A review of upstream and downstream antioxidant therapeutic options. *Curr. Neuropharmacol.* **2009**, *7*, 65–74.
69. Gomez-Nicola, D.; Fransen, N.L.; Suzzi, S.; Perry, V.H. Regulation of microglial proliferation during chronic degeneration. *J. Neurosci.* **2013**, *33*, 2481–2493.
70. Li, T.; Pang, S.; Yu, Y.; Wu, X.; Guo, J.; Zhang, S. Proliferation of parenchymal microglia is the main source of microgliosis after ischaemic stroke. *Brain* **2013**, *136*, 3578–3588.
71. Nosheny, R.L.; Bachis, A.; Acquas, E.; Mocchetti, I. Human immunodeficiency virus type 1 glycoprotein gp120 reduces the levels of brain-derived neurotrophic factor *in vivo*: Potential implication for neuronal cell death. *Eur. J. Neurosci.* **2004**, *20*, 2857–2864.
72. Louboutin, J.P.; Agrawal, L.; Reyes, B.A.S.; van Bockstaele, E.J.; Strayer, D.S. Protecting neurons from HIV-1 gp120 induced oxidant stress using both localized intracerebral and generalized intraventricular administration of antioxidant enzymes delivered by SV40 derived vectors. *Gene Ther.* **2007**, *14*, 1650–1661.
73. Louboutin, J.P.; Agrawal, L.; Reyes, B.A.S.; van Bockstaele, E.J.; Strayer, D.S. HIV-1 gp120 neurotoxicity proximally and at a distance from the point of exposure: Protection by rSV40 delivery of antioxidant enzymes. *Neurobiol. Dis.* **2009**, *34*, 462–476.
74. Louboutin, J.P.; Reyes, B.A.S.; Agrawal, L.; van Bockstaele, E.J.; Strayer, D.S. HIV-1 gp120-induced neuroinflammation: Relationship to neuron loss and protection by rSV40-delivered antioxidant enzymes. *Exp. Neurol.* **2010**, *221*, 231–245.
75. Chan, P.H.; Schmidley, J.W.; Fishman, R.A.; Longar, S.M. Brain injury, edema, and vascular permeability changes induced by oxygen-derived free radicals. *Neurology* **1984**, *34*, 315–320.
76. Chan, P.H.; Yang, G.Y.; Carlson, E.; Epstein, C.J. Cold-induced brain edema and infarction are reduced in transgenic mice overexpressing CuZn-superoxide dismutase. *Ann. Neurol.* **1991**, *29*, 482–486.
77. Wang, H.K.; Park, U.J.; Kim, S.Y.; Lee, J.H.; Kim, S.U.; Gwaq, B.J.; Lee, Y.B. Free radical production in CA1 neurons induces MIP-1alpha expression, microglial recruitment, and delayed neuronal death after transient forebrain ischemia. *J. Neurosci.* **2008**, *28*, 1721–1727.
78. Nishi, T.; Maier, C.M.; Hayashi, T.; Saito, A.; Chan, P.H. Superoxide dismutase 1 overexpression reduces MCP-1 and MIP-1 alpha expression after transient focal cerebral ischemia. *J. Cereb. Blood Flow Metab.* **2005**, *25*, 1312–1324.
79. Shah, A.; Kumar, S.; Simon, S.D.; Singh, D.P.; Kumar, A. HIV gp120- and methamphetamine-mediated oxidative stress induces astrocyte apoptosis via cytochrome P450 2E1. *Cell Death Dis.* **2013**, *4*, e850.

80. Lee, Y.W.; Hirani, A.A.; Kyprianou, N.; Toborek, M. Human immunodeficiency virus-1Tat protein up-regulates interleukin-6 and interleukin-8 expression in human breast cancer cells. *Inflamm. Res.* **2005**, *54* 380–389.

81. Nookala, A.R.; Shah, A.; Noel, R.J.; Kumar, A. HIV-1 Tat-mediated induction of CCL5 in astrocytes involves NF κB, AP-1, C/EBPα and C/EBPγ transcription factors and JAK, PI3K/Akt and p38 MAPK signaling pathways. *PLoS One* **2013**, *8*, e78855.

82. El-Hage, N.; Bruce-Keller, A.J.; Yakovleva, T.; Bazov, I.; Bakalkin, G.; Knapp, P.E.; Hauser, K.F. Morphine exacerbates HIV1 Tat-induced cytokine production in astrocytes through convergent effets on ([Ca^{2+}]$_i$, NF-κB trafficking and transcription. *PLoS One* **2008**, *3*, e4093.

83. Consortium, D. A randomized, double-blind, placebo-controlled trial of deprenyl and thioctic acid in human immunodeficiency virus-associated cognitive impairment: Dana Consortium on the therapy of HIV dementia and related cognitive disorders. *Neurology* **1998**, *50*, 645–651.

84. Sacktor, N.; Schifitto G.; McDermott, M.P.; Marder, K.; McArthur, J.C.; Kieburtz, K. Transdermal seleginine in HIV-associated cognitive impairment: Pilot, placebo-controlled study. *Neurology* **2000**, *54*, 233–235.

85. Consortium, D. Safety and tolerability of the antioxidant OPC-14117 in HIV-associated cognitive impairment: The Dana Consortium on the therapy of HIV dementia and related cognitive disorders. *Neurology* **1997**, *49*, 142–146.

86. Pulliam, L.; Irwin, I.; Kusdra, L.; Rempel, H.; Flitter, W.D.; Garland, W.A. CPI-1189 attenuates effects of suspected neurotoxins associated with AIDS dementia: A possible role for ERK activation. *Brain Res.* **2001**, *893*, 95–103.

87. Clifford, D.B.; McArthur, J.C.; Schifitto, G.; Kieburtz, K.; McDermott, M.P.; Letendre, S.; Cohen, B.A.; Marder, K.; Ellis, R.J.; Marra, C.M. Neurologic AIDS Research Consortium. A randomized clinical trial of CPI-1189 for HIV-associated cognitive-motor impairment. *Neurology* **2002**, *59*, 1568–1573.

88. Louboutin, J.P.; Strayer, D.S. HIV-1-Associated Neurocognitive Disorder: Role of Oxidative Stress and Protection by Gene Delivery of Antioxidant Enzymes. In *Encephalitis, Encephalomyelitis, Encephalopathies: Symptoms, Causes and Potential Complications*; Ruiz, A., Fleming, D., Eds.; Nova Science Publishers: Hauppauge, NY, USA, 2013.

89. Pocernich, C.B.; la Fontaine, M.; Butterfield, D.A. *In-vivo* glutathione elevation protects against hydroxyl free radical-induced protein oxidation in rat brain. *Neurochem. Int.* **2000**, *36*, 185–191.

90. Banerjee, A.; Zhanq, X.; Manda, K.R.; Banks, W.A.; Ercal, N. HIV proteins (gp120 and Tat) and methamphetamine in oxidative stress induced damage in the brain: Potential role of the thiol antioxidant *N*-acetylcysteine amide. *Free Radic. Biol. Med.* **2010**, *48*, 1388–1398.

2

Oxidative Stress and the Use of Antioxidants in Stroke

Rachel Shirley [†]**, Emily N. J. Ord** [†] **and Lorraine M. Work** *

Institute of Cardiovascular & Medical Sciences, College of Medical, Veterinary & Life Sciences, University of Glasgow, BHF GCRC, 126 University Place, Glasgow G12 8TA, UK;
E-Mails: Rachel.Shirley@glasgow.ac.uk (R.S.); Emily.Ord@glasgow.ac.uk (E.N.J.O.)

† These authors contributed equally to this work.

* Author to whom correspondence should be addressed; E-Mail: Lorraine.Work@glasgow.ac.uk

---

Abstract: Transient or permanent interruption of cerebral blood flow by occlusion of a cerebral artery gives rise to an ischaemic stroke leading to irreversible damage or dysfunction to the cells within the affected tissue along with permanent or reversible neurological deficit. Extensive research has identified excitotoxicity, oxidative stress, inflammation and cell death as key contributory pathways underlying lesion progression. The cornerstone of treatment for acute ischaemic stroke remains reperfusion therapy with recombinant tissue plasminogen activator (rt-PA). The downstream sequelae of events resulting from spontaneous or pharmacological reperfusion lead to an imbalance in the production of harmful reactive oxygen species (ROS) over endogenous anti-oxidant protection strategies. As such, anti-oxidant therapy has long been investigated as a means to reduce the extent of injury resulting from ischaemic stroke with varying degrees of success. Here we discuss the production and source of these ROS and the various strategies employed to modulate levels. These strategies broadly attempt to inhibit ROS production or increase scavenging or degradation of ROS. While early clinical studies have failed to translate success from bench to bedside, the combination of anti-oxidants with existing thrombolytics or novel neuroprotectants may represent an avenue worthy of clinical investigation. Clearly, there is a pressing need to identify new therapeutic alternatives for the vast majority of patients who are not eligible to receive rt-PA for this debilitating and devastating disease.

Keywords: anti-oxidant; stroke; oxidative stress

1. Introduction

In addition to being the second leading cause of death worldwide [1], stroke is also the leading cause of acquired adult disability [2]. Stroke therefore has a very large socioeconomic impact with one third of all stroke patients requiring permanent residential care, costing the NHS in the UK £3.8 billion per annum [3]. The only approved pharmacological intervention for stroke is intravenous administration of the thrombolytic, recombinant tissue plasminogen activator (rtPA), within 4.5 h of the onset of ischaemia [4]. This short therapeutic window results in only 2%–5% of all stroke patients receiving this intervention with successful reperfusion of the brain occurring in only 50% of that cohort [5], as such this is a disease with largely unmet clinical needs. Ischaemic stroke (as opposed to haemorrhagic stroke) results from an atherothrombotic or embolic blockage to a cerebral artery and accounts for ~80% of all stroke cases. Finding a new pharmacological treatment for stroke is incredibly complex for a number of reasons. The brain is a highly metabolically active organ that relies on constant oxygen and glucose supply from the circulation. The brain accounts for 2% of the total body but requires 20% O_2 and 2% of the entire body's glucose consumption, although it performs no mechanical work or external secretory activity [6]. Storage of energy and metabolites within the brain is extremely low and as such the brain is exceptionally sensitive to interruptions in blood flow [7]. Although the brain is protected from systemic toxins under normal physiological conditions by the blood-brain barrier (BBB), this is broken down during cerebral ischaemia allowing infiltration of inflammatory mediators and other potentially toxic molecules. Following the onset of ischaemia numerous pathways contribute to brain injury, there is extensive crosstalk between these deleterious pathways with them also, in the main, existing as positive feedback loops serving to amplify insult. In what is the most significant challenge of stroke treatment, the majority of damage occurs within minutes and the acute hours following cerebral ischaemia and as such, stroke treatment at present remains mainly preventative. Here, we will discuss the source and consequence of reactive oxygen species (ROS) imbalance following cerebral ischaemia/reperfusion before considering anti-oxidant strategies attempted clinically based on the pre-clinical evidence for each. What is clear is that while the contributory role of ROS in stroke cannot be disputed, the relative merit of anti-oxidant therapy alone has yet to be established and combined therapy may be where agents modulating the balance of ROS prove beneficial.

2. Sources of Reactive Oxygen Species (ROS)

Oxidative stress as a result of excess production of ROS and/or impaired metabolism is a fundamental mechanism of cell damage following cerebral ischaemia, where ROS refers to molecular oxygen ($\bullet O_2^-$) or its derivatives. Although oxidative stress has been implicated in numerous pathologies including cancer, atherosclerosis and neurodegenerative diseases, the brain is particularly sensitive to oxidative damage (reviewed in [8]). There are several reasons for this; the high consumption of oxygen under basal conditions, high concentrations of peroxidisable lipids, and high levels of iron that act as a pro-oxidant during stress. The primary sources of ROS in the brain are the mitochondrial respiratory chain (MRC), NAPDH oxidases, and xanthine oxidase [9–11] (Figure 1). Under normal cellular conditions, mitochondria produce superoxide as a by-product of their primary function—ATP generation by oxidative phosphorylation through the MRC. Superoxide produced in this way gets converted to hydrogen peroxide (H_2O_2) by superoxide dismutase (SOD) before leaving the mitochondria to act as an intracellular messenger, functioning in neuronal signalling in both the peripheral nervous system (PNS) and the central nervous system (CNS) [12]. In the ischaemic cell, O_2 levels are depleted before glucose, favouring a switch to the glycolytic pathway of anaerobic ATP production [13]. The switch to glycolysis in the O_2-depleted cell results in lactate acid and H^+ build-up in the mitochondria and the subsequent reversal of the H^+ uniporter on the mitochondrial membrane which causes excess cytosolic H^+ accumulation and acidosis [14]. Acidosis contributes to oxidative stress by providing H^+ for the conversion of $\bullet O_2^-$ into H_2O_2 or the more reactive hydroxyl radical (•OH). In addition, in the O_2-depleted cell the potent protein and lipid oxidant peroxynitrite ($ONOO^-$) is formed by the reaction of nitric oxide (NO) and $\bullet O_2^-$, rapidly exhausting the NO bioavailability. Activation of NMDA receptors (NMDARs) by glutamate also increases intracellular NO and subsequent $ONOO^-$ production in the ATP depleted post-synaptic cell. Neuronal nitric oxide synthase (nNOS) is physically anchored to NMDARs and following activation and influx of Ca^{2+}, Ca^{2+} binds calmodulin and rapidly activates nNOS generating NO [15]. NO reacts with superoxide anions ($\bullet O_2^-$), produced by anaerobic metabolism of the energy-depleted mitochondria, forming $ONOO^-$. $ONOO^-$ mediates apoptosis through classic oxidative stress pathways described in a later section of this review (Section 3.1). In what is a well-documented paradigm of stroke, reperfusion of the previously ischaemic brain has severely deleterious cellular effects, including a large increase in ROS production [16,17]. The recovery of the MRC following return of cerebral blood flow causes a spike in the production of mitochondrial ROS. The reversal of complex I of the MRC and the subsequent overproduction of $\bullet O_2^-$ is believed to be a significant contributor [18]. More recent studies have further demonstrated the importance of complex I, the entry point for electrons from NADH in the MRC, following ischaemic injury [19,20]. Pretreatment of neonatal mice with pyridaben to inhibit complex I resulted in reduced infarct volume determined 7 days after cerebral hypoxic-ischaemic injury [19]. Similarly, inhibition of complex I reactivation by *S*-nitrosation of a cysteine residue decreased ROS production, oxidative damage and tissue necrosis following cardiac ischaemia/reperfusion [20].

In addition to mitochondrial ROS production, nicotinamide adenine dinucleotide phosphate-oxidases (NOXs) are a significant source of ROS production following cerebral ischaemia and specifically during reperfusion injury [21]. The NOX family has seven members (NOX1, NOX2, NOX3, NOX4, NOX5, DUOX1, and DUOX2) with the isoforms NOX2, NOX3 and NOX4 predominantly expressed in the CNS. Under normal physiological conditions NOX enzymes function as membrane bound enzymes which generate ROS for biological functions such as blood pressure regulation, microbial killing and otoconia formation [22]. The catalysis of $\bullet O_2^-$ occurs by one electron reduction of O_2 using NADPH as an electron donor: $2O_2 + NADPH \rightarrow 2O_2^-$ NAPD + H^+. Under pathological conditions however, NOXs are significant contributors to pathological damage by oxidative stress from $\bullet O_2^-$ overproduction and ROS imbalance. Although all seven NOX isoforms catalyse the reduction of molecular oxygen their mechanism of activation differs between isoforms. NOX2 is activated and simulated by phosphorylation-activated p47phox and by p67phox, in conjunction with activated Rac. NOX3 is activated by NOXO1 but is insensitive to additional stimulation by NOXA1 or activated Rac [23]. Activation of NOX4 has not been fully elucidated however it is thought to be controlled by transcriptional factors [24].

Figure 1. Sources of reactive oxygen species (ROS) and consequences of imbalance. Several sources of ROS exist endogenously which are balanced by natural anti-oxidant systems. In times of excess ROS production, such as following cerebral ischaemia/reperfusion, the balance of oxidants exceeds anti-oxidant protection. Excess ROS, in turn, result in apoptosis, inflammation, DNA damage, lipid peroxidation and protein denaturation—all of which contribute to and amplify signals leading to damage following stroke.

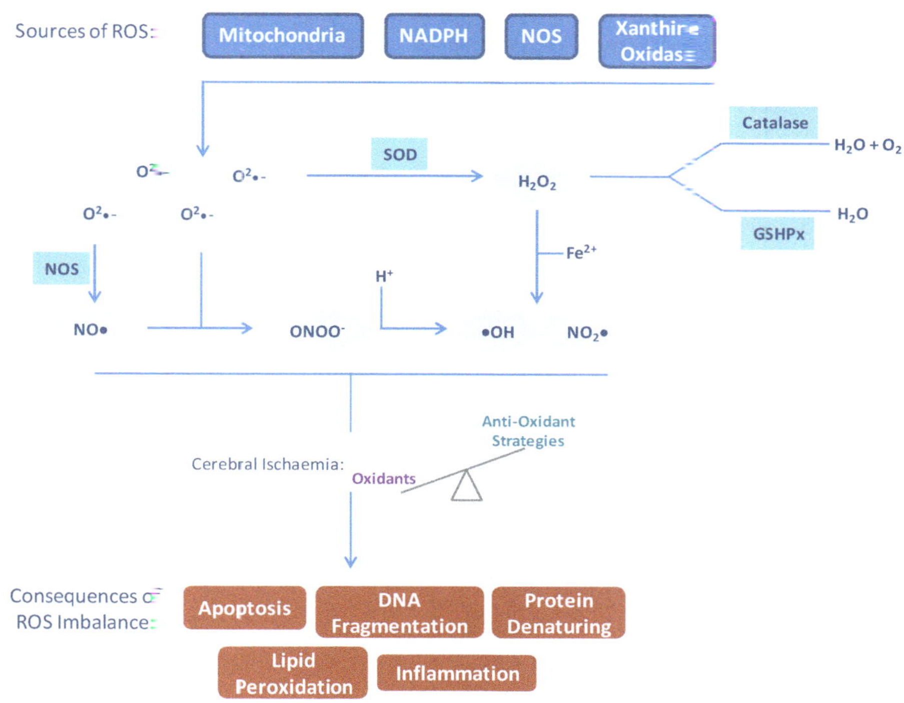

Xanthine oxidase (XO) functions to catalyse the oxidation of hypoxanthine to xanthine and oxidation of xanthine to uric acid. Under normoxic conditions XO exists as in interchangeable form of xanthine hydrogenase (XDH) [25]. During ischaemia cellular adenosine triphosphate (ATP) is catabolised to hypoxanthine which accumulates in the ischaemic tissue, and XDH is cleaved to the active XO. During the reperfusion phase, XO can then oxidise the reaction of hypoxanthine to xanthine and xanthine to uric acid, producing $\bullet O_2^-$ and H_2O_2 [26].

3. Consequences of ROS Imbalance

The results of ROS imbalance are considerable and affect many processes within the brain parenchyma and all cells of the neurovascular unit (Figure 1). These events should not be considered as distinct from one another as considerable crosstalk and amplification occurs.

3.1. Apoptosis

ROS have a number of direct detrimental effects which result in cell damage and tissue destruction, such as: lipid peroxidation, protein denaturing, disruption of DNA and multiple cell signalling effects resulting in initiation of apoptosis [27–29]. Lipid peroxidation is the main mechanism by which ROS cause damage within the brain. Initiation of lipid peroxidation results in a positive-feedback loop of damage. The •OH initiates removal of one H^+ from a polyunsaturated fatty acid resulting in formation of a lipid radical that reacts readily with O_2 to form a lipid peroxyl radical and another lipid radical. The lipid radical by-product will further react with oxygen causing a positive feedback reaction. As an example of the positive-feedback loop of lipid peroxidation: excess ROS can activate phospholipase A_2 (PLA_2) which in turn releases and activates arachidonic acid (AA) and a by-product of the activation of AA is ROS. ROS act directly on lipids to ultimately produce aldehydes, dienals or alkanes, such as malondialdehyde (MDA) and 4-hydroxynonenal (4-HNE). The latter, 4-HNE induces apoptosis following cerebral ischaemia in neurons [30] and has been shown to be upregulated in a time-dependent manner in the ipsilateral striatum following focal ischaemia in rats [31]. Direct oxidative damage of DNA by ROS differs to endonuclease-mediated DNA fragmentation in that it occurs at earlier time-points following cerebral ischaemia and is potentially reversible. Oxidative damage to DNA occurs from direct attack of ROS on DNA, resulting in primarily DNA base damage and single-strand breaks (SSBs), observed in rodent models of cerebral ischaemia [32–34]. Although oxidative damage is potentially reversible, in cerebral ischaemia the multiple mechanisms that induce ROS ultimately generate fatal DNA damage to neuronal cells due to the ROS/antioxidant imbalance [33,35].

As aforementioned, a primary site for ROS generation following cerebral ischaemia is the mitochondria, where they exert their most detrimental role in initiation of cell death via cytochrome C (CytC) release [36,37]. Mitochondrial CytC release is in part controlled by the Bcl-2 family of proteins which are vitally involved in neuronal survival and programmed cell death. This gene family contains both pro-apoptotic and anti-apoptotic proteins and the anti-apoptotic members of the Bcl-2 family act by inhibiting the pro-apoptotic members. High $[Ca^{2+}]_i$ caused by excitotoxicty activates release of pro-apoptotic mediators from the mitochondria through activation of calpains [38] causing mitochondrial transition pore (MTP) opening. ROS can also mediate mitochondrial permeabilisation through activation of cytosolic phospholipase A_2 ($cPLA_2$). Activated $cPLA_2$ triggers AA release by freeing it from an inhibiting phospholipid molecule through an enzymatic process. Activated AA has been shown to directly act on the MTP on mitochondria [39]. Release of pro-apoptotic CytC from the mitochondria results in initiation of the mitochondrial caspase-dependant intrinsic pathway of cell death. Following release, CytC forms a complex with cytosolic adapter protein (APAF-1) and caspase-9, known as the apoptosome, to mediate the activation of pro-caspase-9 in the presence of deoxy-ATP (dATP). Activated caspase-9 cleaves and activates caspase-3, which initiates apoptosis through DNA fragmentation by releasing the endonuclease caspase-activated DNase (CAD) from inhibition by cleaving its inhibitor ICAD [40,41]. CAD is a deoxyribose- and double-strand-specific enzyme [42] which preferentially cleaves the internucleosomal linker regions in chromatin [43].

ROS also mediate apoptosis through a direct interaction with nuclear factor κB (NF-κB) and subsequent activation of the MAPK/JNK pathway of cell death. NF-κB is known to be activated by the redox state of the cell in a number of disease pathologies and activation can be inhibited through use of antioxidants [44]. Additional downstream gene targets of NF-κB also include, NOS [45], cyclooxygenase-2 (COX-2) [46], matrix metalloproteinase-9 (MMP-9) [47], intracellular adhesion molecules (ICAMs) and cytokines [48] which are involved in a number of detrimental pathways of cerebral ischaemia such as, apoptosis, BBB breakdown, and inflammation. JNK activates mitochondrial-mediated apoptosis by direct action on Bcl-2 [49]. Following translocation to the nucleus, JNK activates the transcription factor c-Jun and ATF-2, leading to the formation of Jun-ATF-2 complex activator protein-1 (AP-1). The AP-1 pathway is involved in regulation of pro-apoptotic genes such as TNF-α, Fas-L and Bak [50]. ROS also increase JNK activation through their direct interaction with the upstream mediator of JNK, ASK1 [51]. Under normal conditions, ASK1 remains inactive through binding with thioredoxin (Trx), a ubiquitously expressed protein with a reduction/oxidation active site sequence.

3.2. Blood-Brain Barrier (BBB) Disruption

The BBB is a highly selective permeability barrier that separates the circulating blood from the brain extracellular fluid (BECF) in the CNS. Capillary endothelial cells, connected by tight junctions and surrounded by the basal lamina and astrocytic end feet, form the BBB [52]. The BBB allows the selective passage of H_2O, some gases, and lipid soluble molecules by passive diffusion, and selective transport of molecules such as glucose and amino acids that are crucial to neuronal function whilst protecting the brain by prevention of passage of potential neurotoxins [53].

Following cerebral ischaemia ± reperfusion, generation of ROS (by previously described mechanisms) results in the breakdown of the BBB. Proteases, partly responsible for the breakdown of the BBB by digestion of the basil lamina, are generated within the ischaemic cells of the vasculature and are also released by adhered leukocytes within the lumen [54]. Matrix metalloproteinases (MMPs) expressed in microvascular endothelial cells are a family of proteolytic enzymes, of this family MMP-2 and -9 play key roles in the degradation of the vascular matrix as they digest type IV collagen and laminin, major components of vascular basement membranes [55]. ROS generated within the endothelium during ischaemia cause MMP activation, both directly through oxidation or nitrosylation of MMPs or indirectly through action on the redox-sensitive element of transcription factors (such as NF-κB and AP-1) that are known to be an integral part of the binding sites for MMP transcription [56]. In addition to basal lamina breakdown, expression of the tight and adherent junction proteins responsible for the tight cell-to-cell interactions in the cerebral microvasculature are downregulated following ischaemia by changes in both intra- and extracellular Ca^{2+} ion concentrations, [57–59]. Low $[Ca^{2+}]_i$ results in removal of calcium from binding sites on E-cadherin extracellular domains of adherent junctions, causing a conformational change which interrupts cell-to-cell adhesion inducing BBB breakdown [60]. Within the perivascular space degranulated mast cells release vasoactive mediators such as histamine and proteases, promoting breakdown of the basal lamina from the side of the brain parenchyma. Stress-activated macrophages in the perivascular space release proinflammatory mediators which promote further expression of adhesion molecules on endothelial cells, resulting in more leukocyte adhesion, protease release and subsequent infiltration through the now permeable BBB [61–63].

3.3. Immune Response

During cerebral ischaemia the inflammatory process is initiated within the occluded vessel. Within the neurovascular unit, the onset of ischaemia results in an initial production of ROS which activates platelets and endothelial cells [64,65]. Within minutes following the onset of ischaemia, pro-inflammatory signals are rapidly generated by translocation of adhesion molecule *p*-selectin to the membrane of the ROS-activated platelets and endothelial cells within the neurovascular unit [66]. Within endothelial cells, the decrease in NO bioavailability (as discussed earlier in this review) results in vasoconstriction, further reducing blood flow to the ischaemic territory and contributing to platelet-leukocyte aggregation. In addition to endothelial derived NO mediated vasoconstriction, oxidative stress within the contractile cells of the capillaries (the pericytes) results in further constriction of the microvasculature [67]. Thrombin generated by ROS-activated platelets causes conversion of fibrinogen to fibrin, the resultant build up of fibrin traps platelets and leukocytes forming clots leading to further microvascular occlusions, and exacerbating the ischaemic insult [68].

In the brain parenchyma microglia, as the innate immune cells of the CNS, are the source of production and release of inflammatory mediators. In the minutes following cerebral ischaemia, there is increased accumulation of ATP or UTP in the extracellular space of the brain parenchyma as a result of excitotoxicity, oedema and subsequent neuronal membrane breakdown [69]. Increased extracellular ATP activates the P2X7 receptors of the microglia, leading to release of pro-inflammatory mediators, such as cytokines, ROS and NO [70].

Under normal conditions, cell-to-cell interaction between neurons and microglia maintains the polarisation and quiescence of the microglia. For example, the membrane protein CD200 expressed on neurons interacts with the CD200R on microglia and enforces the resting phenotype [71]. During ischaemia, expression of this protein is reduced leading to activation of the microglia. In a similar fashion, the cell-surface bound neuronal chemokine, CX3CL1, acts on the microglial CX3CL1 receptor promoting quiescence during normal respiration [72]. Thus, during cerebral ischaemia loss of these interactions by matrix breakdown, releases microglia from suppression and promotes the inflammatory response.

In the later stages following cerebral ischaemia molecular signals are released from the intracellular compartment of dead/dying cells and are produced from the digestion of matrix proteins, known as danger-associated molecular pattern molecules (DAMPs) [73]. DAMPs act on the Toll-like receptors and scavenger receptors of the microglia, perivascular macrophages and brain endothelial cells to stimulate further release of pro-inflammatory mediators such as IL-6 and TNF through NF-κB activation [74]. In addition to this, DAMPs prime dendritic cells for antigen presentation; this interaction demonstrates the main cross over between innate and adaptive immunity following cerebral ischaemia. Although the immune response following stroke is classically thought of in the direction of infiltration from the circulation to the brain parenchyma, it is likely that in the highly vascularised brain the inflammatory mediators released from the brain parenchyma would feed back onto the perivascular unit and the vasculature, reinforcing infiltration of the circulating inflammatory mediators.

4. Antioxidant Strategies

In normal brain tissue, ROS are continuously produced during physiological processes but are balanced by endogenous antioxidant defence mechanisms. After cerebral ischaemic injury, free radical production is greatly increased and causes redox disequilibrium in the natural endogenous antioxidant system; detoxification mechanisms are inactivated and oxidants are overproduced. An increase in ROS levels after cerebral ischaemia results in overt oxidative stress and subsequent neuronal injury [75] making free radicals a valid therapeutic target, and much research has focused on assessing the therapeutic effects of antioxidants. There are three main strategies by which antioxidants work; (i) inhibition of free radical production; (ii) scavenging of free radical production; or (iii) increasing free radical degradation [76]. Antioxidant strategies can either focus on the upregulation of endogenous antioxidants or on the delivery of exogenous antioxidants.

4.1. Inhibition of Free Radical Production

In this approach, the source of disease promoting ROS generation is targeted by specific inhibitors of ROS generating enzymes. One main source of ROS production in cerebral ischaemia/reperfusion injury is the NADPH oxidases (NOXs). Inhibition of NADPH oxidase complexes with the pharmacological agent apocynin prior to reperfusion has demonstrated an attenuation in cerebral ischaemia in rat models of experimental stroke [77,78] highlighting the contributory role of NOX in brain injury. There are seven homologues of NOX, with NOX2 and NOX4 both shown to be upregulated following I/R injury [79,80]. NOX2 is known to facilitate the production of superoxide, whilst NOX4 produces hydrogen peroxide [81]. NOX2 knockout (KO) mice were found to have decreased lesion volume and improved neurological outcome at 24 h and 72 h post-ischaemic injury with an observed decrease in products of oxidative stress compared to their wild-type (WT) controls [21,82,83]. NOX4 deficient mice have shown protective effects in both transient and permanent models of occlusion at 24 h post-stroke [84]. Furthermore, pharmacological inhibition of TLR4-NOX4 signalling led to reduced expression of NOX4 and a subsequent decrease in volume and area of cerebral infarction of 40% [85]. There are conflicting reports regarding the role of NOX1 in experimental stroke. Studies have shown NOX1 to have a protective role in ischaemic injury in experimental stroke with NOX1 KO mice displaying a four-fold greater cortical infarct volume than WT mice [86]. Similarly, no protection (although no worsening) from experimental stroke was described following tMCAO in NOX1 KO mice in a further study [84]. In contrast, Kahles *et al.* (2010) demonstrated a 55% attenuation in lesion size after 1 h of ischaemia in NOX1 KO mice and a corresponding improvement in neurological improvement compared to WT mice [87]. Interestingly, no difference in lesion volume between WT and NOX1 KO mice was observed when occlusion time was lengthened to 2 h and beyond [87]. Taken together, these data suggest a functional importance for the NOXs in I/R injury and as such represent a novel therapeutic target, especially as apart from their role in ROS production, they have no other essential function [88]. NOX inhibitors are known to be non-specific and not isoform selective; whilst this may not ultimately be important for the treatment of stroke, the development of selective NOX inhibitors would help to validate the role of the various NOX isoforms in stroke [89].

Xanthine Oxidase (XO) is another enzyme that is involved in redox signalling pathways and is an important source of ROS in the setting of brain injury. Inhibition of XO is a potential therapeutic approach for the treatment of cerebral ischaemia that has received little attention. Allopurinol is a commonly used XO inhibitor that not only reduces levels of uric acid, but also reduces the level of superoxide anion formation. Initial trials with this drug are promising; patients treated with allopurinol showed an improvement in vascular [90] and beneficial effects on inflammatory indices compared to placebo [91]. However, in a randomised double-blind trial to investigate the effects of allopurinol in patients with recent subcortical stroke, no improvement in cerebrovascular function was observed [92].

4.2. Free Radical Scavengers

Compounds capable of scavenging free radicals have been developed for the treatment of cerebral ischaemic stroke although translation from pre-clinical to clinical trials has largely been disappointing. One of these compounds is Tirilazad mesylate (U-74006F), an inhibitor of lipid peroxidation that was studied extensively in pre-clinical models in the mid-1990s and was shown to reduce infarct size in rats following transient focal ischaemia but not permanent occlusion [93,94]. A meta-analysis of the previously published data was released in 2007 [95], where an overall improvement in both lesion size and neurological recovery was reported. Across 19 publications, tirilazad was demonstrated to reduce lesion size by an average of 29% and improve neurological score by 48% [95]. Maximum efficiency of tirilazad treatment was observed when administered prior to focal ischaemia, with a decreasing efficiency in action with administration time from ischaemic onset thereafter. The largest clinical trial of tirilazad comprised 660 patients, in which tirilazad was administered within 6 h of the onset of cerebral ischaemia [96]. Primary outcome of disability measured by the Glasgow Outcome Scale and Barthel index at 3 months showed no change between groups at an independent interim analysis of 556 patients, and the trial was subsequently terminated. It was later determined that women metabolise tirilazad up to 60% more efficiently than men, and therefore had perhaps not been administered a high enough dose to mediate neuroprotection, reducing the efficacy across the whole trial [97]. These studies highlight the need to more tightly regulate the consistency of methodologies from pre-clinical to clinical studies.

NXY-059 is another example of a drug that showed promising results pre-clinically but failed to show clinical efficacy. A number of pre-clinical studies confirmed the neuroprotective action of the spin trap, NXY-059, in infarct reduction and neurological recovery across a variety of stroke models in both rodents [98–100] and non-human primates [101,102]. Spin-trapping is a technique that allows scavenging of free radicals. It involves the addition of a free radical, to a nitrone spin trap resulting in the formation of a spin adduct, without the formation of further free radicals and as such can terminate radical chain reactions. Following extensive and successful pre-clinical studies, NXY-059 was studied in two large randomised and double-blinded trials. The initial trial (SAINT I) involved 1722 patients [103], and the following year SAINT II enrolled 3306 subjects [104]. In both trials, patients were assigned to receive either a 72 h infusion of NXY-059 or placebo, starting within 6 h of the onset of cerebral ischaemia. SAINT I showed a significant improvement in NXY-059 treated patients assessed by the modified Rankin score, but not by the NIHSS scale or Barthel index. However, the subsequent SAINT II trial published entirely negative results in primary and secondary endpoints. The difference in the outcomes of these trials have been attributed to statistical weakness of the SAINT I trial [105,106] and the poor BBB permeability of NXY-059 [107].

Edaravone is a free radical scavenger that has been approved for use in Japan since 2001 [108] and is widely in use in clinics in Japan for the treatment of cerebral infarctions [109]. It is known to scavenge peroxyl, hydroxyl and superoxide radicals [110]. Although free radicals are known to be a major contributor to lesion progression, the effectiveness of edaravone is still unclear. Pre-clinical studies show promising results with decreased infarct sizes in rodent models [111–114]. In human clinical trials, the results are less clear however. In a multicentre, randomized, placebo-controlled double-blind study on acute ischaemic stroke patients, significant clinical improvements in all patients receiving edaravone and at all time points were described [115]. Conversely, in patients with cardioembolic stroke treatment with edaravone showed minimal improvements [116]. In a further study to assess the effects of edaravone in both acute and chronic stages of cerebral ischaemia, infarct size was significantly reduced in small-vessel occlusion stroke patients within one year; however associated observed neurological improvements were not significantly sustained at one year [117]. Drug dose and therapeutic window for treatment is not consistent between all these trials and so a trial that addresses these issues is warranted to fully assess the efficacy profile of edaravone in stroke patients [109].

4.3. Free Radical Degradation

Strategies aimed at reducing oxidative stress by increasing levels of the antioxidant SOD in experimental models of stroke have demonstrated the integral role of ROS in lesion progression. SOD catalyses the conversion of O_2^- to less reactive H_2O_2 and O_2. Catalase (CAT) and glutathione peroxidase (GPx) help to eliminate the by-product of H_2O_2, thus increasing the overall efficacy of SOD [118]. Overexpression of CAT by adenoviral vectors [119] and transduction with PEP-1-CAT fusion protein [120] have both demonstrated neuroprotection in neuronal cells *in vitro* against I/R injury. Furthermore, catalase overexpression was shown to be protective when delivered prior to ischaemic injury in rats; however protection was lost when delivery was after the ischaemic insult [121]. Transgenic mice overexpressing GPx showed significant reduction in infarct volume compared to non-transgenic mice following I/R damage [122,123] whilst Gpx-1 knockout (KO) mice demonstrated a three-fold increase in infarct volume [124].

Of the three SOD enzyme isoforms, SOD1 has been studied most in relation to experimental models of stroke. Approaches to overexpress SOD1 using transgenic mice [125] and rats [37] demonstrated reduced apoptosis in transient focal ischaemia stroke models. Conversely, deficient SOD1 expression in knockout mice resulted in mortality within 24 h of MCAO in $SOD1^{-/-}$ mice and increased infarct volume and oedema in $SOD1^{+/-}$ heterozygotes compared to WT controls [126]. Using gene therapy to overexpress SOD1 locally before and 2 h post-transient MCAO a significant improvement in neuronal survival was seen [127]. Furthermore, transient MCAO in transgenic mice overexpressing SOD3 resulted in reduced infarct size compared to wild type mice [128]. SOD2 (or manganese-containing superoxide dismutase, Mn-SOD) is a mitochondrial antioxidant enzyme. Whilst homozygous SOD2 KO mice ($SOD2^{-/-}$) die within 10 days of birth [129], heterozygotes ($SOD2^{+/-}$) have increased levels of superoxide and show an increase in infarct volume after cerebral ischaemia compared to WT [130] suggesting that SOD2 protects against oxidative stress-induced damage. Transgenic mice overexpressing SOD2 displayed neuroprotective effects following transient focal ischaemia [131]. SOD2 was revealed to be a gene that is a specific target of STAT3 with the loss of STAT3 activity by ischemic reperfusion resulting in a reduction of SOD2 expression [132]. Injections of interleukin-6 (IL-6) before and after middle cerebral artery occlusion in mice restored activity of STAT3 and additionally restored the transcriptional activity of the Mn-SOD promoter through recovery of the recruitment of STAT3 to the Mn-SOD promoter; a resulting reduction in infarct volume was observed [133]. Thus targeting these pathways may have therapeutic potential against oxidative stress in cerebral infarction.

Ebselen is an inhibitor of glutathione peroxidase-like activity, and also reacts with and subsequently scavenges $ONOO^-$. In pre-clinical rodent models of focal ischaemia pre-treatment with ebselen [134] or administration at point of reperfusion [135] in transient occlusion models improved ischaemic damage and neurological deficit, respectively. Post-treatment at 30 min following onset of ischaemia in a rodent model of permanent occlusion resulted in modest protection [136]. However, a randomised and blinded trial of 302 ischaemic stroke patients who were administered ebselen at 48 h post ischaemia for 2 weeks failed to replicate the protective effects seen in the pre-clinical models at 3 months, although improvements in the ebselen treated groups were observed prior to this at 1 month [137].

A novel antioxidant approach is the inhalation of gases during or after ischaemia. The use of inhaled hydrogen gas to selectively reduce the hydroxyl radical in a transient model of MCAO demonstrated a marked reduction in infarct volume 1 day post-occlusion and an improvement in neurological scores assessed after 7 days [138]. Importantly, gas administration during reperfusion was adequate to elicit the beneficial effect. Normobaric oxygen (NBO) has been shown in several studies to reduce infarct volume and neurological deficits in rat models of focal ischaemia [139–141] and to extend the time window of successful reperfusion in rats [142]. Furthermore, combination therapy with NBO and ethanol was shown to have neuroprotective effects after I/R injury in rats [143,144]. A similar approach to the treatment of ischaemic injury is the induction of a natural cell protection molecule NO. NO is a vasoactive molecule that is produced by either endothelial NO synthase (eNOS), inducible NO synthase (iNOS) or neuronal NO synthase (nNOS) with NO playing a dual contradictory role in focal cerebral ischaemia [145,146]. NO derived from eNOS has neuroprotective effects [67] and can terminate chain reactions during lipid peroxidation, whilst NO derived from iNOS acts as a pro-oxidant and reacts with superoxide O_2^- to form the strongly oxidative/nitrative molecule $ONOO^-$ and ultimately exacerbates cell death [147]. In a recent study, it was shown that inhalation of NO could significantly decrease ischaemic brain damage and improve neurological outcome in rat neonatal stroke models [148], murine models of cerebral ischaemia and a large animal model of ischaemic stroke [149]. Gaseous treatment may have several therapeutic advantages including the ability of gases to rapidly penetrate biomembranes and diffuse into the cytosol, mitochondria and nucleus [138].

Lubeluzole acts to reduce NO levels and subsequent $ONOO^-$ production in hypoxic cells through inhibition of the glutamate-mediated nitric oxide synthase pathway [150]. Proof-of-concept was confirmed *in vitro*, lubeluzole protected both hippocampal slices [151] and primary neurons [152] from both membrane depolarisations and nitric oxide toxicity, respectively. In addition, in a pre-clinical model of photochemical parietal sensorimotor cortical stroke in rats, lubeluzole rescued hindlimb placing when administered 5 min following ischaemic onset in all rats and 60% of rats when administered at 6 h [153]. In a transient middle cerebral artery occlusion (MCAO) model lubeluzole treatment 15 minutes after the onset of stroke rescued infarct by 50% [154]. When treatment of lubeluzole was administered 3 h following the onset of permanent MCA, infarct was reduced by 33% [154]. Primary clinical safety studies of lubeluzole in 193 patients were terminated early as a result of a mortality imbalance in the higher dose group (20 mg/day) which was not noted in the lower dose group (10 mg/day) [155]. The following year a multicentre randomised and double-blinded trial of 721 patients was carried out in the US and Canada, where patients were randomised to lubeluzole or placebo administration within 6 h following ischaemic onset. Mortality was not improved at 12 weeks, improvement was demonstrated in the lubeluzole groups across the NIHSS scale and Barthel index at the same timepoint [156]. These results were confirmed in a similar study of comparable candidate number the following year [157]. In light of these positive trials, a large clinical study of 1786 patients was initiated, however unfortunately no difference was observed between lubeluzole or placebo groups in either the primary or secondary outcome measures [158]. A meta-analysis of all five clinical trials of lubeluzole reported no improvement of mortality or dependency between groups, but did report a significant increase in the heart-conduction disorder, Q-T prolongation, in lubeluzole treated subjects [159].

4.4. Mitochondrial Targeted Anti-Oxidants

The mitochondrial matrix is an important site of free radical generation [160]. Mitochondria have been reported to act as major sources of ROS in ischaemia and particularly in reperfusion injury. Oxidative damage to the mitochondria can result in a decrease in essential ATP production, an increase in mitochondrial generated ROS production and in the release of pro-apoptotic signals. The MRC, which is made up of four membrane-bound complexes (I-IV), has been identified as one potential source of ROS production [161]. Inhibition of the mitochondrial complex I was found to inhibit both ischaemic and reperfusion-mediated oxidative damage protecting the mouse brain from hypoxic/ischaemic (HI) injury [19].

A lack of efficacy in the use of antioxidants can in part be explained by a difficulty in achieving high concentrations in the necessary intracellular location [162]. Mitochondrial targeted antioxidants could specifically target the interior of the mitochondrion and potentially ameliorate oxidative damage. Targeting antioxidants to the mitochondria generally involves conjugating an antioxidant to a lipophilic cation to promote diffusion and accumulation within the mitochondria. A number of antioxidants have been targeted to the mitochondria in an attempt to improve efficacy. Mitochondrial targeted vitamin E was shown to protect cerebellar granule cells *in vitro* from ethanol-induced oxidative damage [163]. Additionally, supplementation of bovine aortic endothelial cells with mitochondrial targeted vitamin E mitigates peroxide-mediated oxidative stress and inhibits apotosis [164].

Mitoquinone (mitoQ) is a derivative of ubiquinone and has a high affinity for the mitochondria [165]. $MitoQ_{10}$ is reduced to ubiquinol and has been found to be an effective antioxidant protecting mitochondria from oxidative damage and apoptosis caused by H_2O_2 [166]. It has been shown to be therapeutic in several animal models of disease and in humans (reviewed in [167]). Pretreatment of rats for 2 weeks prior to *ex vivo* cardiac ischaemia/reperfusion demonstrated cardiac protection [168]. Furthermore, administration of $MitoQ_{10}$ prevented hypertension, cardiac hypertrophy and improved endothelial function after oral administration in young spontaneously hypertensive stroke prone rats (SHRSP) [169,170]. Administration of $MitoQ_{10}$ reduced levels of oxidative stress and cell death in rat brain induced by chemical treatment with the organophosphate pesticide dichlorvos [171]. However, in a rat model of neonatal HI no such protection was described for MitoQ [172]. Thus mitochondrial targeted antioxidants represent an important developing therapeutic strategy in the treatment of stroke.

4.5. Upregulation of Endogenous Antioxidants

Antioxidant vitamins are one of the body's main natural defence mechanisms against oxidative stress. Vitamin E and C are two of the most studied natural antioxidants. Dietary vitamin C is mostly provided through the consumption of fruit and vegetables and has a biological role as a hydrogen donor to reverse oxidation. One form of vitamin C, ascorbic acid, was found to protect newborn rat brain from HI injury [173]. In a large animal stroke model, the administration of dehydroascorbic acid did not significantly decrease infarct volume or improve neurological outcome and the study was terminated early [174]. In a recent study however, it was found that 4 weeks of pre-treatment of stroke-prone spontaneously hypertensive rats with vitamins C and E lowered levels of lipid peroxidation and significantly lowered infarct volume following MCAO [175]. In large human observational studies, it was determined that an increase in vitamin C plasma levels correlated with a lowered incidence of stroke [176–178]. However, in randomised control trials, patients receiving antioxidant vitamin supplementation displayed no difference in incidence of stroke compared to those receiving placebo [179–181]. Similar results were found for vitamin E supplementation with meta-analysis of randomised control trials showing no benefit on the incidence of stroke in patients receiving supplementation compared to those taking placebo [182,183]. These data would suggest that the use of antioxidant vitamin supplementation in stroke is not therapeutically viable.

Hypoxia-inducible factor 1 (HIF-1) is an important mediator in stroke and is responsible for the inductions of genes that are involved in the cell's survival response to hypoxia [184]. The neuroprotective effects of HIF-1 have been well documented in pre-clinical models. Pre-conditioning of the brain 24 h prior to ischaemic insult has been shown to reduce infarct volume by up to 30% [185] through the increase in expression of HIF-1 and its target genes [186]. Additionally, pre-treatment of rats with deferoxamine, a known inducer of HIF-1, demonstrated significant protection against ischaemic injury [187,188]. This effect may also be attributed to the ability of deferoxamine to chelate Fe^{2+} and inhibit the formation of the damaging •OH radical through the Fenton reaction.

The exact function and mechanism of neuroglobin (Ngb), a member of the globin superfamily, remains elusive but its upregulation has been shown to be neuroprotective in a number of studies of *in vivo* brain ischaemia models. Transgenic mice overexpressing Ngb showed neuroprotective effects in the form of reduced infarct volume and reduced lipid peroxidation levels following both focal [189] and global ischaemia [190]. Adeno-associated viral mediated Ngb expression also reduced infarct size and improved neurological outcome 24 h post-stroke in rats [191]. The use of cell-penetrating peptides to deliver Ngb across the blood brain barrier in mice resulted in significantly reduced lesion size and improved neurological recovery when given as a pre-treatment [192]. No improvement was seen when delivered post stroke, however. In a recent combination study to assess the effects of targeting both oxidative stress and apoptotic pathways using a combination of the antiapoptotic c-Jun *N*-terminal kinase (JNK) inhibitor and the antioxidant neuroglobin (Ngb), combined treatment reduced infarct and improved neurological outcome more than single therapy after *in vivo* experimental stroke in hypertensive rats [193]. This demonstrates how targeting multiple physiological pathways can be beneficial.

4.6. Combination Therapy

No single antioxidant has advanced beyond clinical trials in the UK and the only approved treatment remains tissue-plasminogen activator (tPA). Few patients receive this treatment, as a result of its narrow treatment window of 4.5 h post-stroke [194], making stroke a vastly undertreated disease. A promising strategy in the treatment of stroke is the identification of agents that when used in combination may have increased efficacy in stroke treatment compared to single-agent therapy. This approach has proven successful in other pathologies of CVD. As many neuroprotective trials have failed due to dose-limiting toxicity, combination therapy may decrease the dose required for each agent so reducing adverse events. It has been shown that combination with activated protein C reduces tPA associated neurovascular toxicity thus improving efficacy in the treatment of stroke [195]. Although complicating study design, multimodal therapy would allow the targeting of multiple pathophysiological mechanisms. Indeed, our own studies in stroke combining stem cell therapy and targeting oxidative stress and matrix metalloproteinases found that triple therapy was more effective than single or double combinations [196]. Furthermore, our previously discussed study combining the antioxidant Ngb with the antiapoptotic JNK inhibitor demonstrated improved outcome following ischaemia with combination therapy compared to either single therapy alone [193].

Indeed, the majority of pre-clinical studies indicate that treatment with thrombolytics is suboptimal if not in combination with neuroprotective agents. At least additive but also synergistic effects have been demonstrated by combination of thrombolytics with neuroprotectants in pre-clinical models including the free radical spin trap α-Phenyl-*tert*-butyl-nitrone (PBN) [197]. In this experiment, tPA-induced haemorrhage volumes were reduced by 40% with alpha-PBN, and infarction and neurological deficits were also decreased. PBN has also been used in combination with NMDA receptor antagonist (MK-801) in an *in vitro* model of OGD and demonstrated substantial synergistic effects in combination [198]. The use of tPA in combination with the free radical scavenger edaravone prevented the reduction in levels of protein factors relating to neurorepair and neuroregeneration and decreased infarct volume when both were delivered during stroke surgery in rats [199]. However, disappointingly, NBO administration in combination with tPA showed no additional beneficial neuroprotective effects in a rat model of thromboembolic stroke [200]. The volume of ischaemic brain damage and swelling in these animals was equivalent to that of control animals and greater than that of tPA- and NBO- treated animals suggesting this may not be a safe strategy. Synergistic effects have been observed with two different antioxidants, U-74389G and U-101033E. Sprague-Dawley rats were subjected to 90 min tMCAO, and treatment was administered 15 min prior to ischaemia, during ischaemia 15 min prior to reperfusion and 45 min following reperfusion. Synergistic improvement was observed in functional recovery but no improvement with combined therapy was noted regarding lesion size at 7 days [201].

A meta-analysis of combination therapy used in stroke research found that of the 126 treatments tested, single treatments reduced infarct size by 20% and improved neurological score by 12% compared with control; whilst a second therapy improved efficacy by an additional 18% and 25%, respectively [202]. When used in combination with thrombolytics, combined therapies can increase the therapeutic time window up to 8.8 h in animal models [202]. Combinations of neuroprotective agents thus represent a relatively new field of stroke therapy, with incredibly large potential.

4.7. Reasons for Failure?

Despite advancement in the understanding of the pathophysiology of stroke and a vast effort in therapeutic research, many clinical trials have failed regardless of their success at the pre-clinical stage [203]. The reason behind this is unclear but a number of factors may play a part in this anomaly, for example factors such as, the animal model, physiological monitoring and outcome measures; the majority of pre-clinical experiments are carried out on young, male animals without comorbidities [202]. For this reason, and in order to address these issues, a conference of academics and industry representatives was convened to suggest a set of guidelines for the evaluation of pre-clinical therapies known as the Stroke Therapy Academic Industry Roundtable (STAIR) initially in 1999 [204], and reviewed in 2009 [205]. A systematic review by O'Collins *et al.* in 2006 [206] of ~3500 articles published addressing various neuroprotective strategies between 1957 and 2003 showed that only five out of 550 of the drugs reported to be effective fully met the standards set by the STAIR guidelines [206]. One of the main findings within the review was a lack of randomisation and blinding, resulting in an overestimated efficacy of therapies. In fact, although there has been an overall trend towards improvement in stroke study design, only 36% of studies report randomisation, 11% report concealment, 29% report blinded assessment of outcome, and 3% reported use of power calculations in generation of sample size [207]. To increase the chance of successful translation of pre-clinical to clinical, it is essential to improve study design and to test across a range of models as no single model is likely to represent the heterogenic nature of stroke [208].

5. Conclusions

While there is no disputing the deleterious effects and detrimental contribution of ROS to lesion progression following ischaemic stroke there remains doubt over the clinical efficacy of anti-oxidants in this setting. Many strategies have proved therapeutic in the pre-clinical setting with translation to the clinic failing to replicate benefit. Efforts to improve the validity of existing animal models through the revised STAIR [205], pre-clinical stroke [209] and ARRIVE [210] guidelines along with the potential implementation of international multicentre pre-clinical stroke studies [211] will, undoubtedly, result in improved clinical translation for stroke therapeutics. However, many potentially beneficial antioxidant strategies with proven efficacy from robust animal studies remain worthy of clinical investigation. Advances in knowledge of the source and nature of these ROS will lead to further new directions to interrogate. Finally, the potential to combine anti-oxidant protection with existing thrombolytics and novel neuroprotectants has yet to be fully established and may represent a powerful means to improve outcome after this devastating and debilitating ischaemic event.

Acknowledgments

The authors thank the MRC (G1100562) and The Wellcome Trust Institutional Strategic Support Fund (ISSF) for funding.

Author Contributions

E.N.J.O., R.S. and L.M.W. prepared the manuscript.

Conflicts of Interest

The authors declare no conflict of interest.

References

1. Lozano, R.; Naghavi, M.; Foreman, K.; Lim, S.; Shibuya, K.; Aboyans, V.; Abraham, J.; Adair, T.; Aggarwal, R.; Ahn, S.Y.; *et al.* Global and regional mortality from 235 causes of death for 20 age groups in 1990 and 2010: A systematic analysis for the global burden of disease study 2010. *Lancet* **2012**, *380*, 2095–2128.
2. Murray, C.J.L.; Vos, T.; Lozano, R.; Naghavi, M.; Flaxman, A.D.; Michaud, C.; Ezzati, M.; Shibuya, K.; Salomon, J.A.; Abdalla, S.; *et al.* Disability-adjusted life years (dalys) for 291 diseases and injuries in 21 regions, 1990–2010: A systematic analysis for the global burden of disease study 2010. *Lancet* **2012**, *380*, 2197–2223.
3. Townsend, N.; Wickramasinghe, K.; Bhatnagar, P.; Smolina, K.; Nichols, M.; Leal, J.; Luengo-Fernandez, R.; Rayner, M. *Coronary Heart Disease Statistics*; British Heart Foundation: London, UK, 2012; pp. 1–206.
4. Li, B.-H.; Ding, X.; Yin, Y.-W.; Liu, Y.; Gao, C.-Y.; Zhang, L.-L.; Li, J.-C. Meta-analysis of clinical outcomes of intravenous recombinant tissue plasminogen activator for acute ischemic stroke: Within 3 h *versus* 3–4.5 h. *Curr. Med. Res. Opin.* **2013**, *29*, 1105–1114.
5. Adeoye, O.; Hornung, R.; Khatri, P.; Kleindorfer, D. Recombinant tissue-type plasminogen activator use for ischemic stroke in the united states: A doubling of treatment rates over the course of 5 years. *Stroke* **2011**, *42*, 1952–1955.
6. Herculano-Houzel, S. Scaling of brain metabolism with a fixed energy budget per neuron: Implications for neuronal activity, plasticity and evolution. *PLoS One* **2011**, *6*, e17514.
7. Pauwels, P.J.; Opperdoes, F.R.; Trouet, A. Effects of antimycin, glucose deprivation, and serum on cultures of neurons, astrocytes, and neuroblastoma cells. *J. Neurochem.* **1985**, *44*, 143–148.
8. Uttara, B.; Singh, A.V.; Zamboni, P.; Mahajan, R.T. Oxidative stress and neurodegenerative diseases: A review of upstream and downstream antioxidant therapeutic options. *Curr. Neuropharmacol.* **2009**, *7*, 65–74.
9. Kahles, T.; Brandes, R.P. NADPH oxidases as therapeutic targets in ischemic stroke. *Cell. Mol. Life Sci.* **2012**, *69*, 2345–2363.

10. Sanderson, T.H.; Reynolds, C.A.; Kumar, R.; Przyklenk, K.; Huttemann, M. Molecular mechanisms of ischemia-reperfusion injury in brain: Pivotal role of the mitochondrial membrane potential in reactive oxygen species generation. *Mol. Neurobiol.* **2013**, *47*, 9–23.
11. Vergeade, A.; Mulder, P.; Vendeville, C.; Ventura-Clapier, R.; Thuillez, C.; Monteil, C. Xanthine oxidase contributes to mitochondrial ros generation in an experimental model of cocaine-induced diastolic dysfunction. *J. Cardiovasc. Pharmacol.* **2012**, *60*, 538–543.
12. Rice, M.E. H2O2: A dynamic neuromodulator. *Neuroscientist* **2011**, *17*, 389–406.
13. Liu, S.; Shi, H.; Liu, W.; Furuichi, T.; Timmins, G.S.; Liu, K.J. Interstitial pO2 in ischemic penumbra and core are differentially affected following transient focal cerebral ischemia in rats. *J. Cereb. Blood Flow Metab.* **2004**, *24*, 343–349.
14. Ying, W.; Han, S.K.; Miller, J.W.; Swanson, R.A. Acidosis potentiates oxidative neuronal death by multiple mechanisms. *J. Neurochem.* **1999**, *73*, 1549–1556.
15. Stanika, R.I.; Villanueva, I.; Kazanina, G.; Andrews, S.B.; Pivovarova, N.B. Comparative impact of voltage-gated calcium channels and nmda receptors on mitochondria-mediated neuronal injury. *J. Neurosci.* **2012**, *32*, 6642–6650.
16. Yamato, M.; Egashira, T.; Utsumi, H. Application of *in vivo* ESR spectroscopy to measurement of cerebrovascular ROS generation in stroke. *Free Radic. Biol. Med.* **2003**, *35*, 1619–1631.
17. Peters, O.; Back, T.; Lindauer, U.; Busch, C.; Megow, D.; Dreier, J.; Dirnagl, U. Increased formation of reactive oxygen species after permanent and reversible middle cerebral artery occlusion in the rat. *J. Cereb. Blood Flow Metab.* **1998**, *18*, 196–205.
18. Chen, Q.; Moghaddas, S.; Hoppel, C.L.; Lesnefsky, E.J. Ischemic defects in the electron transport chain increase the production of reactive oxygen species from isolated rat heart mitochondria. *Am. J. Physiol. Cell. Physiol.* **2008**, *294*, C460–C466.
19. Niatsetskaya, Z.V.; Sosunov, S.A.; Matsiukevich, D.; Utkina-Sosunova, I.V.; Ratner, V.I.; Starkov, A.A.; Ten, V.S. The oxygen free radicals originating from mitochondrial complex I contribute to oxidative brain injury following hypoxia-ischemia in neonatal mice. *J. Neurosci.* **2012**, *32*, 3235–3244.
20. Chouchani, E.T.; Methner, C.; Nadtochiy, S.M.; Logan, A.; Pell, V.R.; Ding, S.; James, A.M.; Cocheme, H.M.; Reinhold, J.; Lilley, K.S.; *et al*. Cardioprotection by *S*-nitrosation of a cysteine switch on mitochondrial complex I. *Nat. Med.* **2013**, *19*, 753–759.
21. Chen, H.; Song, Y.S.; Chan, P.H. Inhibition of NADPH oxidase is neuroprotective after ischemia-reperfusion. *J. Cereb. Blood Flow Metab.* **2009**, *29*, 1262–1272.
22. Bokoch, G.M.; Knaus, U.G. NADPH oxidases: Not just for leukocytes anymore! *Trends Biochem. Sci.* **2003**, *28*, 502–508.
23. Cheng, G.; Ritsick, D.; Lambeth, J.D. Nox3 regulation by NOXO1, p47phox, and p67phox. *J. Biol. Chem.* **2004**, *279*, 34250–34255.
24. Matsushima, S.; Kuroda, J.; Ago, T.; Zhai, P.; Park, J.Y.; Xie, L.H.; Tian, B.; Sadoshima, J. Increased oxidative stress in the nucleus caused by Nox4 mediates oxidation of HDAC4 and cardiac hypertrophy. *Circ. Res.* **2013**, *112*, 651–663.
25. Granger, D.N.; Rutili, G.; McCord, J.M. Superoxide radicals in feline intestinal ischemia. *Gastroenterology* **1981**, *81*, 22–29.

26. Parks, D.A.; Granger, D.N. Xanthine oxidase: Biochemistry, distribution and physiology. *Acta Physiol. Scand. Suppl.* **1986**, *548*, 87–99.
27. Crack, P.J.; Taylor, J.M. Reactive oxygen species and the modulation of stroke. *Free Radic. Biol. Med.* **2005**, *38*, 1433–1444.
28. Gursoy-Ozdemir, Y.; Can, A.; Dalkara, T. Reperfusion-induced oxidative/nitrative injury to neurovascular unit after focal cerebral ischemia. *Stroke* **2004**, *35*, 1449–1453.
29. Nelson, C.W.; Wei, E.P.; Povlishock, J.T.; Kontos, H.A.; Moskowitz, M.A. Oxygen radicals in cerebral ischemia. *Am. J. Physiol.* **1992**, *263*, H1356–H1362.
30. McCracken, E.; Valeriani, V.; Simpson, C.; Jover, T.; McCulloch, J.; Dewar, D. The lipid peroxidation by-product 4-hydroxynonenal is toxic to axons and oligodendrocytes. *J. Cereb. Blood Flow Metab.* **2000**, *20*, 1529–1536.
31. Matsuda, S.; Umeda, M.; Uchida, H.; Kato, H.; Araki, T. Alterations of oxidative stress markers and apoptosis markers in the striatum after transient focal cerebral ischemia in rats. *J. Neural Transm.* **2009**, *116*, 395–404.
32. Liu, P.K.; Hsu, C.Y.; Dizdaroglu, M.; Floyd, R.A.; Kow, Y.W.; Karakaya, A.; Rabow, L.E.; Cui, J.K. Damage, repair, and mutagenesis in nuclear genes after mouse forebrain ischemia-reperfusion. *J. Neurosci.* **1996**, *16*, 6795–6806.
33. Chen, J.; Jin, K.; Chen, M.; Pei, W.; Kawaguchi, K.; Greenberg, D.A.; Simon, R.P. Early detection of DNA strand breaks in the brain after transient focal ischemia: Implications for the role of DNA damage in apoptosis and neuronal cell death. *J. Neurochem.* **1997**, *69*, 232–245.
34. Nagayama, T.; Simon, R.P.; Chen, D.; Henshall, D.C.; Pei, W.; Stetler, R.A.; Chen, J. Activation of poly(adp-ribose) polymerase in the rat hippocampus may contribute to cellular recovery following sublethal transient global ischemia. *J. Neurochem.* **2000**, *74*, 1636–1645.
35. Kawase, M.; Fujimura, M.; Morita-Fujimura, Y.; Chan, P.H. Reduction of apurinic/apyrimidinic endonuclease expression after transient global cerebral ischemia in rats: Implication of the failure of DNA repair in neuronal apoptosis. *Stroke* **1999**, *30*, 441–449.
36. Kirkland, R.A.; Windelborn, J.A.; Kasprzak, J.M.; Franklin, J.L. A bax-induced pro-oxidant state is critical for cytochrome c release during programmed neuronal death. *J. Neurosci.* **2002**, *22*, 6480–6490.
37. Sugawara, T.; Lewen, A.; Gasche, Y.; Yu, F.; Chan, P.H. Overexpression of SOD1 protects vulnerable motor neurons after spinal cord injury by attenuating mitochondrial cytochrome c release. *FASEB J.* **2002**, *16*, 1997–1999.
38. Croall, D.E.; DeMartino, G.N. Calcium-activated neutral protease (calpain) system: Structure, function, and regulation. *Physiol. Rev.* **1991**, *71*, 813–847.
39. Scorrano, L.; Penzo, D.; Petronilli, V.; Pagano, F.; Bernardi, P. Arachidonic acid causes cell death through the mitochondrial permeability transition. Implications for tumor necrosis factor-alpha aopototic signaling. *J. Biol. Chem.* **2001**, *276*, 12035–12040.
40. Enari, M.; Sakahira, H.; Yokoyama, H.; Okawa, K.; Iwamatsu, A.; Nagata, S. A caspase-activated dnase that degrades DNA during apoptosis, and its inhibitor icad. *Nature* **1998**, *391*, 43–50.
41. Jänicke, R.U.; Sprengart, M.L.; Wati, M.R.; Porter, A.G. Caspase-3 is required for DNA fragmentation and morphological changes associated with apoptosis. *J. Biol. Chem.* **1998**, *273*, 9357–9360.

42. Hanus, J.; Kalinowska-Herok, M.; Widlak, P. The major apoptotic endonuclease DFF40/CAD is a deoxyribose-specific and double-strand-specific enzyme. *Apoptosis* **2008**, *13*, 377–382.
43. Widlak, P.; Li, P.; Wang, X.; Garrard, W.T. Cleavage preferences of the apoptotic endonuclease DFF40 (caspase-activated dnase or nuclease) on naked DNA and chromatin substrates. *J. Biol. Chem.* **2000**, *275*, 8226–8232.
44. Dalton, T.P.; Shertzer, H.G.; Puga, A. Regulation of gene expression by reactive oxygen. *Annu. Rev. Pharmacol. Toxicol.* **1999**, *39*, 67–101.
45. Pautz, A.; Art, J.; Hahn, S.; Nowag, S.; Voss, C.; Kleinert, H. Regulation of the expression of inducible nitric oxide synthase. *Nitric Oxide* **2010**, *23*, 75–93.
46. Kim, E.J.; Raval, A.P.; Hirsch, N.; Perez-Pinzon, M.A. Ischemic preconditioning mediates cyclooxygenase-2 expression via nuclear factor-kappa B activation in mixed cortical neuronal cultures. *Transl. Stroke Res.* **2010**, *1*, 40–47.
47. Hsieh, H.L.; Wang, H.H.; Wu, W.B.; Chu, P.J.; Yang, C.M. Transforming growth factor-beta1 induces matrix metalloproteinase-9 and cell migration in astrocytes: Roles of ros-dependent ERK- and JNK-NF-kappaB pathways. *J. Neuroinflamm.* **2010**, *7*, 88.
48. Park, T.Y.; Baik, E.J.; Lee, S.H. Prostaglandin e(2)-induced intercellular adhesion molecule-1 expression is mediated by cAMP/Epac signalling modules in bEnd.3 brain endothelial cells. *Br. J. Pharmacol.* **2013**, *169*, 604–618.
49. Deng, X.; Xiao, L.; Lang, W.; Gao, F.; Ruvolo, P.; May, W.S., Jr. Novel role for JNK as a stress-activated Bcl2 kinase. *J. Biol. Chem.* **2001**, *276*, 23681–23688.
50. Fan, M.; Chambers, T.C. Role of mitogen-activated protein kinases in the response of tumor cells to chemotherapy. *Drug Resist. Updat* **2001**, *4*, 253–267.
51. Soberanes, S.; Urich, D.; Baker, C.M.; Burgess, Z.; Chiarella, S.E.; Bell, E.L.; Ghio, A.J.; de Vizcaya-Ruiz, A.; Liu, J.; Ridge, K.M.; *et al.* Mitochondrial complex III-generated oxidants activate ASK1 and JNK to induce alveolar epithelial cell death following exposure to particulate matter air pollution. *J. Biol. Chem.* **2009**, *284*, 2176–2186.
52. De Vries, H.E.; Kuiper, J.; de Boer, A.G.; van Berkel, T.J.; Breimer, D.D. The blood-brain barrier in neuroinflammatory diseases. *Pharmacol. Rev.* **1997**, *49*, 143–155.
53. Grieb, P.; Forster, R.E.; Strome, D.; Goodwin, C.W.; Pape, P.C. O_2 exchange between blood and brain tissues studied with $^{18}O_2$ indicator-dilution technique. *J. Appl. Physiol.* **1985**, *58*, 1929–1941.
54. Neumann-Haefelin, T.; Kastrup, A.; de Crespigny, A.; Yenari, M.A.; Ringer, T.; Sun, G.H.; Moseley, M.E. Serial mri after transient focal cerebral ischemia in rats: Dynamics of tissue injury, blood-brain barrier damage, and edema formation. *Stroke* **2000**, *31*, 1965–1973.
55. Rosell, A.; Cuadrado, E.; Ortega-Aznar, A.; Hernández-Guillamon, M.; Lo, E.H.; Montaner, J. Mmp-9-positive neutrophil infiltration is associated to blood-brain barrier breakdown and basal lamina type IV collagen degradation during hemorrhagic transformation after human ischemic stroke. *Stroke* **2008**, *39*, 1121–1126.
56. Cortez, D.M.; Feldman, M.D.; Mummidi, S.; Valente, A.J.; Steffensen, B.; Vincenti, M.; Barnes, J.L.; Chandrasekar, B. Il-17 stimulates MMP-1 expression in primary human cardiac fibroblasts via p38 MAPK- and ERK1/2-dependent C/EBP-β, NF-κB, and AP-1 activation. *Am. J. Physiol. Heart Circ. Physiol.* **2007**, *293*, H3356–H3365.

57. Mark, K.S.; Davis, T.P. Cerebral microvascular changes in permeability and tight junctions induced by hypoxia-reoxygenation. *Am. J. Physiol. Heart Circ. Physiol.* **2002**, *282*, H1485–H1494.

58. Huber, J.D.; Witt, K.A.; Hom, S.; Egleton, R.D.; Mark, K.S.; Davis, T.P. Inflammatory pain alters blood-brain barrier permeability and tight junctional protein expression. *Am. J. Physiol. Heart Circ. Physiol.* **2001**, *280*, H1241–H1248.

59. Yamagata, K.; Tagami, M.; Takenaga, F.; Yamori, Y.; Itoh, S. Hypoxia-induced changes in tight junction permeability of brain capillary endothelial cells are associated with IL-1beta and nitric oxide. *Neurobiol. Dis.* **2004**, *17*, 491–499.

60. Pokutta, S.; Herrenknecht, K.; Kemler, R.; Engel, J. Conformational changes of the recombinant extracellular domain of E-cadherin upon calcium binding. *Eur. J. Biochem.* **1994**, *223*, 1019–1026.

61. Cipolla, M.J.; Crete, R.; Vitullo, L.; Rix, R.D. Transcellular transport as a mechanism of blood-brain barrier disruption during stroke. *Front. Biosci.* **2004**, *9*, 777–785.

62. Xu, H.; Dawson, R.; Crane, I.J.; Liversidge, J. Leukocyte diapedesis *in vivo* induces transient loss of tight junction protein at the blood-retina barrier. *Investig. Ophthalmol. Vis. Sci.* **2005**, *46*, 2487–2494.

63. Konsman, J.P.; Drukarch, B.; van Dam, A.M. (Peri)vascular production and action of pro-inflammatory cytokines in brain pathology. *Clin. Sci.* **2007**, *112*, 1–25.

64. Peerschke, E.I.; Yin, W.; Ghebrehiwet, B. Complement activation on platelets: Implications for vascular inflammation and thrombosis. *Mol. Immunol.* **2010**, *47*, 2170–2175.

65. Pinsky, D.J.; Naka, Y.; Liao, H.; Oz, M.C.; Wagner, D.D.; Mayadas, T.N.; Johnson, R.C.; Hynes, R.O.; Heath, M.; Lawson, C.A.; *et al.* Hypoxia-induced exocytosis of endothelial cell weibel-palade bodies. A mechanism for rapid neutrophil recruitment after cardiac preservation. *J. Clin. Investig.* **1996**, *97*, 493–500.

66. Yilmaz, G.; Granger, D.N. Leukocyte recruitment and ischemic brain injury. *Neuromol. Med.* **2010**, *12*, 193–204.

67. Atochin, D.N.; Wang, A.; Liu, V.W.; Critchlow, J.D.; Dantas, A.P.; Looft-Wilson, R.; Murata, T.; Salomone, S.; Shin, H.K.; Ayata, C.; *et al.* The phosphorylation state of enos modulates vascular reactivity and outcome of cerebral ischemia *in vivo*. *J. Clin. Investig.* **2007**, *117*, 1961–1967.

68. Del Zoppo, G.J.; Schmid-Schonbein, G.W.; Mori, E.; Copeland, B.R.; Chang, C.M. Polymorphonuclear leukocytes occlude capillaries following middle cerebral artery occlusion and reperfusion in baboons. *Stroke* **1991**, *22*, 1276–1283.

69. Melani, A.; Turchi, D.; Vannucchi, M.G.; Cipriani, S.; Gianfriddo, M.; Pedata, F. ATP extracellular concentrations are increased in the rat striatum during *in vivo* ischemia. *Neurochem. Int.* **2005**, *47*, 442–448.

70. Korcok, J.; Raimundo, L.N.; Ke, H.Z.; Sims, S.M.; Dixon, S.J. Extracellular nucleotides act through P2X7 receptors to activate NF-kappaB in osteoclasts. *J. Bone Miner. Res.* **2004**, *19*, 642–651.

71. Lyons, A.; Downer, E.J.; Crotty, S.; Nolan, Y.M.; Mills, K.H.; Lynch, M.A. CD200 ligand receptor interaction modulates microglial activation *in vivo* and *in vitro*: A role for IL-4. *J. Neurosci.* **2007**, *27*, 8309–8313.
72. Denes, A.; Ferenczi, S.; Halasz, J.; Kornyei, Z.; Kovacs, K.J. Role of CX3CR1 (fractalkine receptor) in brain damage and inflammation induced by focal cerebral ischemia in mouse. *J. Cereb. Blood Flow Metab.* **2008**, *28*, 1707–1721.
73. Chen, G.Y.; Nunez, G. Sterile inflammation: Sensing and reacting to damage. *Nat. Rev. Immunol.* **2010**, *10*, 826–837.
74. Marsh, B.J.; Williams-Karnesky, R.L.; Stenzel-Poore, M.P. Toll-like receptor signaling in endogenous neuroprotection and stroke. *Neuroscience* **2009**, *158*, 1007–1020.
75. Facchinetti, F.; Dawson, V.L.; Dawson, T.M. Free radicals as mediators of neuronal injury. *Cell. Mol. Neurobiol.* **1998**, *18*, 667–682.
76. Margaill, I.; Plotkine, M.; Lerouet, D. Antioxidant strategies in the treatment of stroke. *Free Radic. Biol. Med.* **2005**, *39*, 429–443.
77. Tang, L.L.; Ye, K.; Yang, X.F.; Zheng, J.S. Apocynin attenuates cerebral infarction after transient focal ischaemia in rats. *J. Int. Med. Res.* **2007**, *35*, 517–522.
78. Genovese, T.; Mazzon, E.; Paterniti, I.; Esposito, E.; Bramanti, P.; Cuzzocrea, S. Modulation of NADPH oxidase activation in cerebral ischemia/reperfusion injury in rats. *Brain Res.* **2011**, *1372*, 92–102.
79. McCann, S.K.; Dusting, G.J.; Roulston, C.L. Early increase of NOX4 NADPH oxidase and superoxide generation following endothelin-1-induced stroke in conscious rats. *J. Neurosci. Res.* **2008**, *86*, 2524–2534.
80. Yoshioka, H.; Niizuma, K.; Katsu, M.; Okami, N.; Sakata, H.; Kim, G.S.; Narasimhan, P.; Chan, P.H. NADPH oxidase mediates striatal neuronal injury after transient global cerebral ischemia. *J. Cereb. Blood Flow Metab.* **2011**, *31*, 868–880.
81. Serrander, L.; Cartier, L.; Bedard, K.; Banfi, B.; Lardy, B.; Plastre, O.; Sienkiewicz, A.; Forro, L.; Schlegel, W.; Krause, K.H. NOX4 activity is determined by MRNA levels and reveals a unique pattern of ros generation. *Biochem. J.* **2007**, *406*, 105–114.
82. Chen, H.; Kim, G.S.; Okami, N.; Narasimhan, P.; Chan, P.H. NADPH oxidase is involved in post-ischemic brain inflammation. *Neurobiol. Dis.* **2011**, *42*, 341–348.
83. De Silva, T.M.; Brait, V.H.; Drummond, G.R.; Sobey, C.G.; Miller, A.A. NOX2 oxidase activity accounts for the oxidative stress and vasomotor dysfunction in mouse cerebral arteries following ischemic stroke. *PLoS One* **2011**, *6*, e0028393.
84. Kleinschnitz, C.; Grund, H.; Wingler, K.; Armitage, M.E.; Jones, E.; Mittal, M.; Barit, D.; Schwarz, T.; Geis, C.; Kraft, P.; *et al.* Post-stroke inhibition of induced NADPH oxidase type 4 prevents oxidative stress and neurodegeneration. *PLoS Biol.* **2010**, *8*, e1000479.
85. Suzuki, Y.; Hattori, K.; Hamanaka, J.; Murase, T.; Egashira, Y.; Mishiro, K.; Ishiguro, M.; Tsuruma, K.; Hirose, Y.; Tanaka, H.; *et al.* Pharmacological inhibition of TLR4-NOX4 signal protects against neuronal death in transient focal ischemia. *Sci. Rep.* **2012**, *2*, doi:10.1038/srep00896.

86. Jackman, K.A.; Miller, A.A.; Drummond, G.R.; Sobey, C.G. Importance of NOX1 for angiotensin II-induced cerebrovascular superoxide production and cortical infarct volume following ischemic stroke. *Brain Res.* **2009**, *1286*, 215–220.
87. Kahles, T.; Kohnen, A.; Heumueller, S.; Rappert, A.; Bechmann, I.; Liebner, S.; Wittko, I.M.; Neumann-Haefelin, T.; Steinmetz, H.; Schroeder, K.; *et al.* NADPH oxidase NOX1 contributes to ischemic injury in experimental stroke in mice. *Neurobiol. Dis.* **2010**, *40*, 185–192.
88. Radermacher, K.A.; Wingler, K.; Kleikers, P.; Altenhofer, S., Jr.; Hermans, J.; Kleinschnitz, C.; Hhw Schmidt, H. The 1027th target candidate in stroke: Will NADPH oxidase hold up? *Exp. Transl. Stroke Med.* **2012**, *4*, 11.
89. Altenhofer, S.; Radermacher, K.A.; Kleikers, P.; Wingler, K.; Schmidt, H.H. Evolution of NADPH oxidase inhibitors: Selectivity and mechanisms for target engagement. *Antioxid. Redox Signal.* **2014**, in press.
90. Khan, F.; George, J.; Wong, K.; McSwiggan, S.; Struthers, A.D.; Belch, J.J. Allopurinol treatment reduces arterial wave reflection in stroke survivors. *Cardiovasc. Ther.* **2008**, *26*, 247–252.
91. Muir, K.W. Glutamate-based therapeutic approaches: Clinical trials with nmda antagonists. *Curr. Opin. Pharmacol.* **2006**, *6*, 53–60.
92. Dawson, J.; Quinn, T.J.; Harrow, C.; Lees, K.R.; Walters, M.R. The effect of allopurinol on the cerebral vasculature of patients with subcortical stroke; a randomized trial. *Br. J. Clin. Pharmacol.* **2009**, *68*, 662–668.
93. Park, C.K.; Hall, E.D. Dose-response analysis of the effect of 21-aminosteroid tirilazad mesylate (U-74006F) upon neurological outcome and ischemic brain damage in permanent focal cerebral ischemia. *Brain Res.* **1994**, *645*, 157–163.
94. Xue, D.; Slivka, A.; Buchan, A.M. Tirilazad reduces cortical infarction after transient but not permanent focal cerebral ischemia in rats. *Stroke* **1992**, *23*, 894–899.
95. Sena, E.; Wheble, P.; Sandercock, P.; Macleod, M. Systematic review and meta-analysis of the efficacy of tirilazad in experimental stroke. *Stroke* **2007**, *38*, 388–394.
96. RANTTAS. A randomized trial of tirilazad mesylate in patients with acute stroke (ranttas). The ranttas investigators. *Stroke* **1996**, *27*, 1453–1458.
97. Fleishaker, J.C.; Hulst-Pearson, L.K.; Peters, G.R. Effect of gender and menopausal status on the pharmacokinetics of tirilazad mesylate in healthy subjects. *Am. J. Ther.* **1995**, *2*, 553–560.
98. Kuroda, S.; Tsuchidate, R.; Smith, M.L.; Maples, K.R.; Siesjo, B.K. Neuroprotective effects of a novel nitrone, NXY-059, after transient focal cerebral ischemia in the rat. *J. Cereb. Blood Flow Metab.* **1999**, *19*, 778–787.
99. Zhao, Z.; Cheng, M.; Maples, K.R.; Ma, J.Y.; Buchan, A.M. NXY-059, a novel free radical trapping compound, reduces cortical infarction after permanent focal cerebral ischemia in the rat. *Brain Res.* **2001**, *909*, 46–50.
100. Sydserff, S.G.; Borelli, A.R.; Green, A.R.; Cross, A.J. Effect of NXY-059 on infarct volume after transient or permanent middle cerebral artery occlusion in the rat; studies on dose, plasma concentration and therapeutic time window. *Br. J. Pharmacol.* **2002**, *135*, 103–112.

101. Marshall, J.W.; Duffin, K.J.; Green, A.R.; Ridley, R.M. NXY-059, a free radical—Trapping agent, substantially lessens the functional disability resulting from cerebral ischemia in a primate species. *Stroke* **2001**, *32*, 190–198.

102. Marshall, J.W.; Cummings, R.M.; Bowes, L.J.; Ridley, R.M.; Green, A.R. Functional and histological evidence for the protective effect of NXY-059 in a primate model of stroke when given 4 h after occlusion. *Stroke* **2003**, *34*, 2228–2233.

103. Lees, K.R.; Davalos, A.; Davis, S.M.; Diener, H.C.; Grotta, J.; Lyden, P.; Shuaib, A.; Ashwood, T.; Hardemark, H.G.; Wasiewski, W.; *et al.* Additional outcomes and subgroup analyses of NXY-059 for acute ischemic stroke in the SAINT I trial. *Stroke* **2006**, *37*, 2970–2978.

104. Shuaib, A.; Lees, K.R.; Lyden, P.; Grotta, J.; Davalos, A.; Davis, S.M.; Diener, H.C.; Ashwood, T.; Wasiewski, W.W.; Emeribe, U. NXY-059 for the treatment of acute ischemic stroke. *N. Engl. J. Med.* **2007**, *357*, 562–571.

105. Koziol, J.A.; Feng, A.C. On the analysis and interpretation of outcome measures in stroke clinical trials: Lessons from the saint i study of NXY-059 for acute ischemic stroke. *Stroke* **2006**, *37*, 2644–2647.

106. Saver, J.L. Clinical impact of NXY-059 demonstrated in the saint I trial: Derivation of number needed to treat for benefit over entire range of functional disability. *Stroke* **2007**, *38*, 1515–1518.

107. Fisher, M.; Lees, K.; Papadakis, M.; Buchan, A.M. NXY-059: Brain or vessel protection. *Stroke* **2006**, *37*, 2189–2190.

108. Watanabe, T.; Tanaka, M.; Watanabe, K.; Takamatsu, Y.; Tobe, A. Research and development of the free radical scavenger edaravone as a neuroprotectant. *Yakugaku Zasshi* **2004**, *124*, 99–111.

109. Lapchak, P.A. A critical assessment of edaravone acute ischemic stroke efficacy trials: Is edaravone an effective neuroprotective therapy? *Exp. Opin. Pharmacother.* **2010**, *11*, 1753–1763.

110. Higashi, Y. Edaravone for the treatment of acute cerebral infarction: Role of endothelium-derived nitric oxide and oxidative stress. *Exp. Opin. Pharmacother.* **2009**, *10*, 323–331.

111. Watanabe, T.; Yuki, S.; Egawa, M.; Nishi, H. Protective effects of MCI-186 on cerebral-ischemia—Possible involvement of free-radical scavenging and antioxidant actions. *J. Pharmacol. Exp. Ther.* **1994**, *268*, 1597–1604.

112. Wu, T.W.; Zeng, L.H.; Wu, J.; Fung, K.P. MCI-186: Further histochemical and biochemical evidence of neuroprotection. *Life Sci.* **2000**, *67*, 2387–2392.

113. Jin, Y.J.; Mima, T.; Raicu, V.; Park, K.C.; Shimizu, K. Combined argatroban and edaravone caused additive neuroprotection against 15 min of forebrain ischemia in gerbils. *Neurosci. Res.* **2002**, *43*, 75–79.

114. Ikeda, S.; Harada, K.; Ohwatashi, A.; Kamikawa, Y. Effects of edaravone, a free radical scavenger, on photochemically induced cerebral infarction in a rat hemiplegic model. *Sci. World J.* **2013**, *2013*, 175280.

115. Otomo, E.; Tohgi, H.; Kogure, K.; Hirai, S.; Takakura, K.; Terashi, A.; Gotoh, F.; Maruyama, S.; Tazaki, Y.; Shinohara, Y.; *et al.* Effect of a novel free radical scavenger, edaravone (MCI-186), on acute brain infarction—Randomized, placebo-controlled, double-blind study at multicenters. *Cerebrovas. Dis.* **2003**, *15*, 222–229.

116. Inatomi, Y.; Takita, T.; Yonehara, T.; Fujioka, S.; Hashimoto, Y.; Hirano, T.; Uchino, M. Efficacy of edaravone in cardioembolic stroke. *Int. Med.* **2006**, *45*, 253–257.

117. Nakase, T.; Yoshioka, S.; Suzuki, A. Free radical scavenger, edaravone, reduces the lesion size of lacunar infarction in human brain ischemic stroke. *BMC Neurol.* **2011**, *11*, 39.

118. Warner, D.S.; Sheng, H.; Batinic-Haberle, I. Oxidants, antioxidants and the ischemic brain. *J. Exp. Biol.* **2004**, *207*, 3221–3231.

119. Gaspar, T.; Domoki, F.; Lenti, L.; Institoris, A.; Snipes, J.A.; Bari, F.; Busija, D.W. Neuroprotective effect of adenoviral catalase gene transfer in cortical neuronal cultures. *Brain Res.* **2009**, *1270*, 1–9.

120. Kim, D.W.; Jeong, H.J.; Kang, H.W.; Shin, M.J.; Sohn, E.J.; Kim, M.J.; Ahn, E.H.; An, J.J.; Jang, S.H.; Yoo, K.Y.; *et al.* Transduced human PEP-1-catalase fusion protein attenuates ischemic neuronal damage. *Free Radic. Biol. Med.* **2009**, *47*, 941–952.

121. Gu, W.; Zhao, H.; Yenari, M.A.; Sapolsky, R.M.; Steinberg, G.K. Catalase over-expression protects striatal neurons from transient focal cerebral ischemia. *Neuroreport* **2004**, *15*, 413–416.

122. Weisbrot-Lefkowitz, M.; Reuhl, K.; Perry, B.; Chan, P.H.; Inouye, M.; Mirochnitchenko, O. Overexpression of human glutathione peroxidase protects transgenic mice against focal cerebral ischemia/reperfusion damage. *Brain Res. Mol. Brain Res.* **1998**, *53*, 333–338.

123. Ishibashi, N.; Prokopenko, O.; Weisbrot-Lefkowitz, M.; Reuhl, K.R.; Mirochnitchenko, O. Glutathione peroxidase inhibits cell death and glial activation following experimental stroke. *Brain Res. Mol. Brain Res.* **2002**, *109*, 34–44.

124. Crack, P.J.; Taylor, J.M.; Flentjar, N.J.; de Haan, J.; Hertzog, P.; Iannello, R.C.; Kola, I. Increased infarct size and exacerbated apoptosis in the glutathione peroxidase-1 (GPX-1) knockout mouse brain in response to ischemia/reperfusion injury. *J. Neurochem.* **2001**, *78*, 1389–1399.

125. Fujimura, M.; Morita-Fujimura, Y.; Noshita, N.; Sugawara, T.; Kawase, M.; Chan, P.H. The cytosolic antioxidant copper/zinc-superoxide dismutase prevents the early release of mitochondrial cytochrome c in ischemic brain after transient focal cerebral ischemia in mice. *J. Neurosci.* **2000**, *20*, 2817–2824.

126. Kondo, T.; Reaume, A.G.; Huang, T.T.; Murakami, K.; Carlson, E.; Chen, S.; Scott, R.W.; Epstein, C.J.; Chan, P.H. Edema formation exacerbates neurological and histological outcomes after focal cerebral ischemia in cuzn-superoxide dismutase gene knockout mutant mice. *Brain Edema X* **1997**, *70*, 62–64.

127. Davis, A.S.; Zhao, H.; Sun, G.H.; Sapolsky, R.M.; Steinberg, G.K. Gene therapy using SOD1 protects striatal neurons from experimental stroke. *Neurosci. Lett.* **2007**, *411*, 32–36.

128. Sheng, H.; Bart, R.D.; Oury, T.D.; Pearlstein, R.D.; Crapo, J.D.; Warner, D.S. Mice overexpressing extracellular superoxide dismutase have increased resistance to focal cerebral ischemia. *Neuroscience* **1999**, *88*, 185–191.

129. Li, P.F. Oxidative modification of cupro-zinc superoxide dismutase by reactive oxygen species. *Sheng Li Ke Xue Jin Zhan* **1995**, *26*, 50–52.
130. Kim, G.W.; Chan, P.H. Involvement of superoxide in excitotoxicity and DNA fragmentation in striatal vulnerability in mice after treatment with the mitochondrial toxin, 3-nitropropionic acid. *J. Cereb. Blood Flow Metab.* **2002**, *22*, 798–809.
131. Maier, C.M.; Hsieh, L.; Crandall, T.; Narasinnhan, P.; Chan, P.H. A new approach for the investigation of reperfusion-related brain injury. *Biochem. Soc. Trans.* **2006**, *34*, 1366–1369.
132. Jung, J.E.; Kim, G.S.; Narasimhan, P.; Chan, P.H. STAT3 regulates the transcription of the mouse Mn-SOD gene as a neuroprotectant in cerebral ischemic reperfusion. *J. Cereb. Blood Flow Metab.* **2009**, *29*, S565–S566.
133. Jung, J.E.; Kim, G.S.; Chan, P.H. Neuroprotection by interleukin-6 is mediated by signal transducer and activator of transcription 3 and antioxidative signaling in ischemic stroke. *Stroke* **2011**, *42*, 3574–3579.
134. Namura, S.; Nagata, I.; Takami, S.; Masayasu, H.; Kikuchi, H. Ebselen reduces cytochrome c release from mitochondria and subsequent DNA fragmentation after transient focal cerebral ischemia in mice. *Stroke* **2001**, *32*, 1906–1911.
135. Imai, H.; Masayasu, H.; Dewar, D.; Graham, D.I.; Macrae, I.M. Ebselen protects both gray and white matter in a rodent model of focal cerebral ischemia. *Stroke* **2001**, *32*, 2149–2154.
136. Takasago, T.; Peters, E.E.; Graham, D.I.; Masayasu, H.; Macrae, I.M. Neuroprotective efficacy of ebselen, an anti-oxidant with anti-inflammatory actions, in a rodent model of permanent middle cerebral artery occlusion. *Br. J. Pharmacol.* **1997**, *122*, 1251–1256.
137. Yamaguchi, T.; Sano, K.; Takakura, K.; Saito, I.; Shinohara, Y.; Asano, T.; Yasuhara, H. Ebselen in acute ischemic stroke: A placebo-controlled, double-blind clinical trial. Ebselen study group. *Stroke* **1998**, *29*, 12–17.
138. Ohsawa, I.; Ishikawa, M.; Takahashi, K.; Watanabe, M.; Nishimaki, K.; Yamagata, K.; Katsura, K.-I.; Katayama, Y.; Asoh, S.; Ohta, S. Hydrogen acts as a therapeutic antioxidant by selectively reducing cytotoxic oxygen radicals. *Nat. Med.* **2007**, *13*, 688–694.
139. Singhal, A.B.; Wang, X.; Sumii, T.; Mori, T.; Lo, E.H. Effects of normobaric hyperoxia in a rat model of focal cerebral ischemia-reperfusion. *J. Cereb. Blood Flow Metab.* **2002**, *22*, 861–868.
140. Singhal, A.B.; Dijkhuizen, R.M.; Rosen, B.R.; Lo, E.H. Normobaric hyperoxia reduces MRI diffusion abnormalities and infarct size in experimental stroke. *Neurology* **2002**, *58*, 945–952.
141. Esposito, E.; Mandeville, E.T.; Hayakawa, K.; Singhal, A.B.; Lo, E.H. Effects of normobaric oxygen on the progression of focal cerebral ischemia in rats. *Exp. Neurol.* **2013**, *249*, 33–38.
142. Kim, H.Y.; Singhal, A.B.; Lo, E.H. Normobaric hyperoxia extends the reperfusion window in focal cerebral ischemia. *Ann. Neurol.* **2005**, *57*, 571–575.
143. Geng, X.; Fu, P.; Ji, X.; Peng, C.; Fredrickson, V.; Sy, C.; Meng, R.; Ling, F.; Du, H.; Tan, X.; *et al.* Synergetic neuroprotection of normobaric oxygenation and ethanol in ischemic stroke through improved oxidative mechanism. *Stroke* **2013**, *44*, 1418–1425.
144. Geng, X.; Parmar, S.; Li, X.; Peng, C.; Ji, X.; Chakraborty, T.; Li, W.A.; Du, H.; Tan, X.; Ling, F.; *et al.* Reduced apoptosis by combining normobaric oxygenation with ethanol in transient ischemic stroke. *Brain Res.* **2013**, *1531*, 17–24.

145. Dalkara, T.; Moskowitz, M.A. The complex role of nitric oxide in the pathophysiology of focal cerebral ischemia. *Brain Pathol.* **1994**, *4*, 49–57.

146. Dalkara, T.; Yoshida, T.; Irikura, K.; Moskowitz, M.A. Dual role of nitric oxide in focal cerebral ischemia. *Neuropharmacology* **1994**, *33*, 1447–1452.

147. Huang, Y.; McNamara, J.O. Ischemic stroke: Acidotoxicity is a perpetrator. *Cell* **2004**, *118*, 665–666.

148. Charriaut-Marlangue, C.; Bonnin, P.; Gharib, A.; Leger, P.-L.; Villapol, S.; Pocard, M.; Gressens, P.; Renolleau, S.; Baud, O. Inhaled nitric oxide reduces brain damage by collateral recruitment in a neonatal stroke model. *Stroke* **2012**, *43*, 3078–3084.

149. Terpolilli, N.A.; Kim, S.-W.; Thal, S.C.; Kataoka, H.; Zeisig, V.; Nitzsche, B.; Klaesner, B.; Zhu, C.; Schwarzmaier, S.; Meissner, L.; *et al.* Inhalation of nitric oxide prevents ischemic brain damage in experimental stroke by selective dilatation of collateral arterioles. *Circ. Res.* **2012**, *110*, 727–738.

150. Lesage, A.S.; Peeters, L.; Leysen, J.E. Lubeluzole, a novel long-term neuroprotectant, inhibits the glutamate-activated nitric oxide synthase pathway. *J. Pharmacol. Exp. Ther.* **1996**, *279*, 759–766.

151. Ashton, D.; Willems, R.; Wynants, J.; van Reempts, J.; Marrannes, R.; Clincke, G. Altered Na^+-channel function as an *in vitro* model of the ischemic penumbra: Action of lubeluzole and other neuroprotective drugs. *Brain Res.* **1997**, *745*, 210–221.

152. Maiese, K.; TenBroeke, M.; Kue, I. Neuroprotection of lubeluzole is mediated through the signal transduction pathways of nitric oxide. *J. Neurochem.* **1997**, *68*, 710–714.

153. De Ryck, M.; Keersmaekers, R.; Duytschaever, H.; Claes, C.; Clincke, G.; Janssen, M.; van Reet, G. Lubeluzole protects sensorimotor function and reduces infarct size in a photochemical stroke model in rats. *J. Pharmacol. Exp. Ther.* **1996**, *279*, 748–758.

154. Aronowski, J.; Strong, R.; Grotta, J.C. Treatment of experimental focal ischemia in rats with lubeluzole. *Neuropharmacology* **1996**, *35*, 689–693.

155. Diener, H.C.; Hacke, W.; Hennerici, M.; Radberg, J.; Hantson, L.; de Keyser, J. Lubeluzole in acute ischemic stroke. A double-blind, placebo-controlled phase II trial. Lubeluzole international study group. *Stroke* **1996**, *27*, 76–81.

156. Grotta, J. Lubeluzole treatment of acute ischemic stroke. The US and Canadian lubeluzole ischemic stroke study group. *Stroke* **1997**, *28*, 2338–2346.

157. Diener, H.C. Multinational randomised controlled trial of lubeluzole in acute ischaemic stroke. European and Australian lubeluzole ischaemic stroke study group. *Cerebrovasc. Dis* **1998**, *8*, 172–181.

158. Diener, H.C.; Cortens, M.; Ford, G.; Grotta, J.; Hacke, W.; Kaste, M.; Koudstaal, P.J.; Wessel, T. Lubeluzole in acute ischemic stroke treatment: A double-blind study with an 8-h inclusion window comparing a 10-mg daily dose of lubeluzole with placebo. *Stroke* **2000**, *31*, 2543–2551.

159. Gandolfo, C.; Sandercock, P.; Conti, M. Lubeluzole for acute ischaemic stroke. *Cochrane Database Syst. Rev.* **2002**, doi:10.1002/14651858.CD001924.

160. Weisiger, R.A.; Fridovich, I. Mitochondrial superoxide dismutase. Site of synthesis and intramitochondrial localization. *J. Biol. Chem.* **1973**, *248*, 4793–4796.

161. Abramov, A.Y.; Scorziello, A.; Duchen, M.R. Three distinct mechanisms generate oxygen free radicals in neurons and contribute to cell death during anoxia and reoxygenation. *J. Neurosci.* **2007**, *27*, 1129–1138.
162. Murphy, M.P. Antioxidants as therapies: Can we improve on nature? *Free Radic. Biol. Med.* **2014**, *66*, 20–23.
163. Siler-Marsiglio, K.I.; Pan, Q.; Paiva, M.; Madorsky, F.; Khurana, N.C.; Heaton, M.B. Mitochondrially targeted vitamin E and vitamin E mitigate ethanol-mediated effects on cerebellar granule cell antioxidant defense systems. *Brain Res.* **2005**, *1052*, 202–211.
164. Dhanasekaran, A.; Kotamraju, S.; Kalivendi, S.V.; Matsunaga, T.; Shang, T.; Keszler, A.; Joseph, J.; Kalyanaraman, B. Supplementation of endothelial cells with mitochondria-targeted antioxidants inhibit peroxide-induced mitochondrial iron uptake, oxidative damage, and apoptosis. *J. Biol. Chem.* **2004**, *279*, 37575–37587.
165. Murphy, M.P.; Smith, R.A. Targeting antioxidants to mitochondria by conjugation to lipophilic cations. *Annu. Rev. Pharmacol. Toxicol.* **2007**, *47*, 629–656.
166. Kelso, G.F.; Porteous, C.M.; Hughes, G.; Ledgerwood, E.C.; Gane, A.M.; Smith, R.A.J.; Murphy, M.P. Prevention of mitochondrial oxidative damage using targeted antioxidants. *Increasing Healthy Life Span* **2002**, *959*, 263–274.
167. Smith, R.A.; Murphy, M.P. Animal and human studies with the mitochondria-targeted antioxidant mitoq. *Ann. N. Y. Acad.Sci.* **2010**, *1201*, 96–103.
168. Adlam, V.J.; Harrison, J.C.; Porteous, C.M.; James, A.M.; Smith, R.A.; Murphy, M.P.; Sammut, I.A. Targeting an antioxidant to mitochondria decreases cardiac ischemia-reperfusion injury. *FASEB J.* **2005**, *19*, 1088–1095.
169. Graham, D.; Huynh, N.N.; Hamilton, C.A.; Beattie, E.; Smith, R.A.; Cocheme, H.M.; Murphy, M.P.; Dominiczak, A.F. Mitochondria-targeted antioxidant MitoQ10 improves endothelial function and attenuates cardiac hypertrophy. *Hypertension* **2009**, *54*, 322–328.
170. McLachlan, J.; Beattie, E.; Murphy, M.P.; Koh-Tan, C.H.; Olson, E.; Beattie, W.; Dominiczak, A.F.; Nicklin, S.A.; Graham, D. Combined therapeutic benefit of mitochondria-targeted antioxidant, MitoQ10, and angiotensin receptor blocker, losartan, on cardiovascular function. *J. Hypertens.* **2014**, *32*, 555–564.
171. Wani, W.Y.; Gudup, S.; Sunkaria, A.; Bal, A.; Singh, P.P.; Kandimalla, R.J.; Sharma, D.R.; Gill, K.D. Protective efficacy of mitochondrial targeted antioxidant mitoq against dichlorvos induced oxidative stress and cell death in rat brain. *Neuropharmacology* **2011**, *61*, 1193–1201.
172. Hobbs, C.E.; Murphy, M.P.; Smith, R.A.; Oorschot, D.E. Neonatal rat hypoxia-ischemia: Effect of the anti-oxidant mitoquinol, and S-PBN. *Pediatr. Int.* **2008**, *50*, 481–488.
173. Miura, S.; Ishida-Nakajima, W.; Ishida, A.; Kawamura, M.; Ohmura, A.; Oguma, R.; Sato, Y.; Takahashi, T. Ascorbic acid protects the newborn rat brain from hypoxic-ischemia. *Brain Dev.* **2009**, *31*, 307–317.
174. Ducruet, A.F.; Mack, W.J.; Mocco, J.; Hoh, D.J.; Coon, A.L.; D'Ambrosio, A.L.; Winfree, C.J.; Pinsky, D.J.; Connolly, E.S., Jr. Preclinical evaluation of postischemic dehydroascorbic acid administration in a large-animal stroke model. *Transl. Stroke Res.* **2011**, *2*, 399–403.

175. Zhang, X.H.; Lei, H.; Liu, A.J.; Zou, Y.X.; Shen, F.M.; Su, D.F. Increased oxidative stress is responsible for severer cerebral infarction in stroke-prone spontaneously hypertensive rats. *CNS Neurosci. Ther.* **2011**, *17*, 590–598.
176. Yokoyama, T.; Date, C.; Kokubo, Y.; Yoshiike, N.; Matsumura, Y.; Tanaka, H. Serum vitamin C concentration was inversely associated with subsequent 20-year incidence of stroke in a japanese rural community. The shibata study. *Stroke* **2000**, *31*, 2287–2294.
177. Myint, P.K.; Luben, R.N.; Welch, A.A.; Bingham, S.A.; Wareham, N.J.; Khaw, K.T. Plasma vitamin C concentrations predict risk of incident stroke over 10 year in 20,649 participants of the european prospective investigation into cancer norfolk prospective population study. *Am. J. Clin. Nutr.* **2008**, *87*, 64–69.
178. Kubota, Y.; Iso, H.; Date, C.; Kikuchi, S.; Watanabe, Y.; Wada, Y.; Inaba, Y.; Tamakoshi, A. Dietary intakes of antioxidant vitamins and mortality from cardiovascular disease: The Japan collaborative cohort study (JACC) study. *Stroke* **2011**, *42*, 1665–1672.
179. Heart Protection Study Collaborative Group. MRC/BHF heart protection study of antioxidant vitamin supplementation in 20,536 high-risk individuals: A randomised placebo-controlled trial. *Lancet* **2002**, *360*, 23–33.
180. Cook, N.R.; Albert, C.M.; Gaziano, J.M.; Zaharris, E.; MacFadyen, J.; Danielson, E.; Buring, J.E.; Manson, J.E. A randomized factorial trial of vitamins C and E and beta carotene in the secondary prevention of cardiovascular events in women: Results from the women's antioxidant cardiovascular study. *Arch. Intern. Med.* **2007**, *167*, 1610–1618.
181. Sesso, H.D.; Buring, J.E.; Christen, W.G.; Kurth, T.; Belanger, C.; MacFadyen, J.; Bubes, V.; Manson, J.E.; Glynn, R.J.; Gaziano, J.M. Vitamins E and C in the prevention of cardiovascular disease in men: The physicians' health study II randomized controlled trial. *JAMA* **2008**, *300*, 2123–2133.
182. Schurks, M.; Glynn, R.J.; Rist, P.M.; Tzourio, C.; Kurth, T. Effects of vitamin E on stroke subtypes: Meta-analysis of randomised controlled trials. *Br. Med. J.* **2010**, doi:10.1136/bmj.c5702.
183. Bin, Q.; Hu, X.Y.; Cao, Y.; Gao, F. The role of vitamin E (tocopherol) supplementation in the prevention of stroke a meta-analysis of 13 randomised controlled trials. *Thromb. Haemost.* **2011**, *105*, 579–585.
184. Wang, G.L.; Semenza, G.L. Purification and characterization of hypoxia-inducible factor 1. *J. Biol. Chem.* **1995**, *270*, 1230–1237.
185. Bernaudin, M.; Nedelec, A.S.; Divoux, D.; MacKenzie, E.T.; Petit, E.; Schumann-Bard, P. Normobaric hypoxia induces tolerance to focal permanent cerebral ischemia in association with an increased expression of hypoxia-inducible factor-1 and its target genes, erythropoietin and VEGF, in the adult mouse brain. *J. Cereb. Blood Flow Metab.* **2002**, *22*, 393–403.
186. Jones, N.M.; Bergeron, M. Hypoxic preconditioning induces changes in HIF-1 target genes in neonatal rat brain. *J. Cereb. Blood Flow Metab.* **2001**, *21*, 1105–1114.
187. Prass, K.; Ruscher, K.; Karsch, M.; Isaev, N.; Megow, D.; Priller, J.; Scharff, A.; Dirnagl, U.; Meisel, A. Desferrioxamine induces delayed tolerance against cerebral ischemia *in vivo* and *in vitro*. *J. Cereb. Blood Flow Metab.* **2002**, *22*, 520–525.

188. Freret, T.; Valable, S.; Chazalviel, L.; Saulnier, R.; Mackenzie, E.T.; Petit, E.; Bernaudin, M.; Boulouard, M.; Schumann-Bard, P. Delayed administration of deferoxamine reduces brain damage and promotes functional recovery after transient focal cerebral ischemia in the rat. *Eur. J. Neurosci.* **2006**, *23*, 1757–1765.
189. Wang, X.; Liu, J.; Zhu, H.; Tejima, E.; Tsuji, K.; Murata, Y.; Atochin, D.N.; Huang, P.L.; Zhang, C.; Lo, E.H. Effects of neuroglobin overexpression on acute brain injury and long-term outcomes after focal cerebral ischemia. *Stroke* **2008**, *39*, 1869–1874.
190. Li, R.C.; Guo, S.Z.; Lee, S.K.; Gozal, D. Neuroglobin protects neurons against oxidative stress in global ischemia. *J. Cereb. Blood Flow Metab.* **2010**, *30*, 1874–1882.
191. Sun, Y.; Jin, K.; Peel, A.; Mao, X.O.; Xie, L.; Greenberg, D.A. Neuroglobin protects the brain from experimental stroke *in vivo*. *Proc. Natl. Acad. Sci. USA* **2003**, *100*, 3497–3500.
192. Cai, B.; Lin, Y.; Xue, X.H.; Fang, L.; Wang, N.; Wu, Z.Y. Tat-mediated delivery of neuroglobin protects against focal cerebral ischemia in mice. *Exp. Neurol.* **2011**, *227*, 224–231.
193. Ord, E.N.; Shirley, R.; McClure, J.D.; McCabe, C.; Kremer, E.J.; Macrae, I.M.; Work, L.M. Combined antiapoptotic and antioxidant approach to acute neuroprotection for stroke in hypertensive rats. *J. Cereb. Blood Flow Metab.* **2013**, *33*, 1215–1224.
194. Hacke, W.; Kaste, M.; Bluhmki, E.; Brozman, M.; Davalos, A.; Guidetti, D.; Larrue, V.; Lees, K.R.; Medeghri, Z.; Machnig, T.; *et al.* Thrombolysis with alteplase 3 to 4.5 h after acute ischemic stroke. *N. Engl. J. Med.* **2008**, *359*, 1317–1329.
195. Liu, D.; Cheng, T.; Guo, H.; Fernandez, J.A.; Griffin, J.H.; Song, X.; Zlokovic, B.V. Tissue plasminogen activator neurovascular toxicity is controlled by activated protein c. *Nat. Med.* **2004**, *10*, 1379–1383.
196. Baker, A.H.; Sica, V.; Work, L.M.; Williams-Ignarro, S.; de Nigris, F.; Lerman, L.O.; Casamassimi, A.; Lanza, A.; Schiano, C.; Rienzo, M.; *et al.* Brain protection using autologous bone marrow cell, metalloproteinase inhibitors, and metabolic treatment in cerebral ischemia. *Proc. Natl. Acad. Sci. USA* **2007**, *104*, 3597–3602.
197. Asahi, M.; Asahi, K.; Wang, X.; Lo, E.H. Reduction of tissue plasminogen activator-induced hemorrhage and brain injury by free radical spin trapping after embolic focal cerebral ischemia in rats. *J. Cereb. Blood Flow Metab.* **2000**, *20*, 452–457.
198. Barth, A.; Barth, L.; Newell, D.W. Combination therapy with MK-801 and alpha-phenyl-tert-butyl-nitrone enhances protection against ischemic neuronal damage in organotypic hippocampal slice cultures. *Exp. Neurol.* **1996**, *141*, 330–336.
199. Deguchi, K.; Miyazaki, K.; Tian, F.; Liu, N.; Liu, W.; Kawai, H.; Omote, Y.; Kono, S.; Yunoki, T.; Deguchi, S.; *et al.* Modifying neurorepair and neuroregenerative factors with TPA and edaravone after transient middle cerebral artery occlusion in rat brain. *Brain Res.* **2012**, *1436*, 168–177.
200. David, H.N.; Haelewyn, B.; Degoulet, M.; Colomb, D.G., Jr.; Risso, J.J.; Abraini, J.H. Prothrombolytic action of normobaric oxygen given alone or in combination with recombinant tissue-plasminogen activator in a rat model of thromboembolic stroke. *J. Appl. Physiol.* **2012**, *112*, 2068–2076.

201. Schmid-Elsaesser, R.; Hungerhuber, E.; Zausinger, S.; Baethmann, A.; Reulen, H.J. Neuroprotective efficacy of combination therapy with two different antioxidants in rats subjected to transient focal ischemia. *Brain Res.* **1999**, *816*, 471–479.
202. O'Collins, V.E.; Macleod, M.R.; Donnan, G.A.; Howells, D.W. Evaluation of combination therapy in animal models of cerebral ischemia. *J. Cereb. Blood Flow Metab.* **2012**, *32*, 585–597.
203. Dirnagl, U. Bench to bedside: The quest for quality in experimental stroke research. *J. Cereb. Blood Flow Metab.* **2006**, *26*, 1465–1478.
204. Stroke Therapy Academic Industry Roundtable (STAIR). Recommendations for standards regarding preclinical neuroprotective and restorative drug development. *Stroke* **1999**, *30*, 2752–2758.
205. Fisher, M.; Feuerstein, G.; Howells, D.W.; Hurn, P.D.; Kent, T.A.; Savitz, S.I.; Lo, E.H.; Group, F.T.S. Update of the stroke therapy academic industry roundtable preclinical recommendations. *Stroke* **2009**, *40*, 2244–2250.
206. O'Collins, V.E.; Macleod, M.R.; Donnan, G.A.; Horky, L.L.; van der Worp, B.H.; Howells, D.W. 1026 Experimental treatments in acute stroke. *Ann. Neurol.* **2006**, *59*, 467–477.
207. Sena, E.S.; van der Worp, H.B.; Howells, D.; Macleod, M. How can we improve the pre-clinical development of drugs for stroke? *Trends Neurosci.* **2007**, *30*, 433–439.
208. O'Collins, V.E.; Donnan, G.A.; Macleod, M.R.; Howells, D.W. Scope of preclinical testing *versus* quality control within experiments. *Stroke* **2009**, *40*, e497.
209. Macleod, M.R.; Fisher, M.; O'Collins, V.; Sena, E.S.; Dirnagl, U.; Bath, P.M.W.; Buchan, A.; van der Worp, H.B.; Traystman, R.; Minematsu, K.; *et al*. Good laboratory practice: Preventing introduction of bias at the bench. *Stroke* **2009**, *40*, e50–e52.
210. Kilkenny, C.; Browne, W.J.; Cuthill, I.C.; Emerson, M.; Altman, D.G. Improving bioscience research reporting: The arrive guidelines for reporting animal research. *PLoS Biol.* **2010**, *8*, e1000412.
211. Dirnagl, U.; Hakim, A.; Macleod, M.; Fisher, M.; Howells, D.; Alan, S.M.; Steinberg, G.; Planas, A.; Boltze, J.; Savitz, S.; *et al*. A concerted appeal for international cooperation in preclinical stroke research. *Stroke* **2013**, *44*, 1754–1760.

3

Investigation of the Antioxidant and Hepatoprotective Potential of *Hypericum mysorense*

Raghu C. Hariharapura [1,*], Ramamurthy Srinivasan [2], Godavarthi Ashok [3], Santoshkumar H. Dongre [4], Hitesh V. Jagani [1] and Pottekkad Vijayan [5]

[1] Department of Pharmaceutical Biotechnology, Manipal College of Pharmaceutical Sciences, Manipal University, Manipal 576 201, India; E-Mail: hiteshjagani@gmail.com

[2] School of Pharmacy, International Medical University, Kuala Lumpur 57000, Malaysia; E-Mail: rsriniv@gmail.com

[3] Radiant Research Services Pvt. Ltd., Bangalore 560 050, India; E-Mail: surya.ashok@gmail.com

[4] Department of Chemical Technology, Dr. Babasaheb Ambedkar Marathwada University, Aurangabad 431001, India. E-Mail: santoshdongre@gmail.com

[5] Department of Pharmaceutical Biotechnology, Jagadguru Sri Shivarathreeshwara (JSS) College of Pharmacy, Ooty 643 001, India; E-Mail: vijayanp4@rediffmail.com

* Author to whom correspondence should be addressed; E-Mail: raghushekhar@gmail.com

---

Abstract: Background: *Hypericum* is a well-known plant genus in herbal medicine. *Hypericum mysorense* (Family: *Hypericaceae*), a plant belonging to the same genus, is well known in folklore medicine for its varied therapeutic potential. **Objective:** The aim of the present study was to investigate the different parts of the plant for antioxidant and hepatoprotective properties. **Materials and Methods:** The methanol extracts of *Hypericum mysorense* prepared from various parts of the plant were tested *in vitro* for their free radical scavenging activity against $ABTS^{\bullet}$ (diammonium salt), $DPPH^{\bullet}$ (1,1-diphenyl-2-picrylhydrazyl), $NO^{\bullet}$, $O_2^{\bullet-}$ and $^{\bullet}OH$ radicals, using standard systems of assays. The total antioxidant capacity, total phenolic and total flavonoid content of the extracts were analyzed. Further, the leaf and flowering top extracts were tested for their *in vivo* antioxidant and hepatoprotective activities on Wistar rats using a carbon tetrachloride-induced hepatic injury model. Results: The leaf and flowering top extract showed potent antioxidant activity and also possessed highest total phenolic and flavonoid content. The antioxidant activity and the total phenolic and flavonoid content present in these extracts showed a good correlation. The leaf and flowering top extracts at 200 mg/kg restored aspartate amino transferase (ASAT), alanine amino transferase (ALAT), alkaline phosphatase (ALP), total bilirubin and protein levels significantly in CCl_4-intoxicated rats. The tested extracts also showed a significant ($p < 0.001$) reduction in 2-thiobarbituric acid reactive substance (TBARS) levels with an increase in SOD and CAT levels. The histopathology of liver did not show any toxicity after the treatment with the extracts. The active extracts were standardized using two marker compounds, hyperoside and rutin, which were isolated from the plant by HPLC. HPLC studies revealed that the maximum concentration of hyperoside and rutin is present in the flowering top extract.

Keywords: *Hypericum mysorense*; antioxidant; free radical; hepatoprotective activity

---

1. Introduction

Reactive oxygen species (ROS) and reactive nitrogen species (RNS) generated in our body are quite reactive and harmful to the cells. If generated ROS and RNS are not scavenged, they can damage important molecules, such as proteins, DNA and lipids, which lead to the development of a variety of diseases, including aging, mutagenesis, carcinogenesis, coronary heart disease, diabetes and neuro-degeneration [1–3]. There is an increasing interest in natural antioxidants, namely phenols and flavonoids, present in medicinal and dietary plants, as they might help to prevent oxidative damage to critical cellular constituents. Flavonoids represent a large group of plant polyphenols possessing a wide range of biological activities, *viz.*, vasoprotective, anti-inflammatory, anti-hepatotoxic and anti-carcinogenic action [4–6]. Besides their biological activity, they are also known to scavenge free radicals, such as ROS and RNS, through electron transfer from flavonoids/phenols towards these oxygen radicals [7,8]. Flavonoids can also prevent the formation of highly reactive •OH radicals through the Fenton reaction by forming chelates with metals, like iron and copper [9].

Hypericum (Guttiferae) is a large genus of herbaceous plants, which grows widely in temperate regions and is being used in traditional medicine in various parts of the world [10]. In recent years, the antidepressant activity of *Hypericum perforatum* L., known as St. John's wort, has caused wide-spread interest in the study of *Hypericum* genus [11]. Compounds isolated from this genus have shown antifungal [12], antibacterial [13], antiviral [14] and anticancer [15] properties. Flavonoids isolated from the *Hypericum* genus have been shown to have several biological activities, such as antidepressant [16], nitric oxide synthesis inhibition [17], antiproliferative [18] and antioxidant activity [19].

Hypericum mysorense (HM) is an ornamental bush found in the Konkan and Palani hills at a height of 900–1500 meters. *Hypericum mysorense* is well known in folklore medicine for its varied therapeutic potential, including spasmolytic, hypotensive and antibacterial activities [20,21]. Earlier studies in our laboratory have shown the significant antiviral [22], cytotoxic and antitumor [23] properties of this plant. We compared the antioxidant activities of the methanolic leaf extract from different *Hypericum* species such as *H. mysorense*, *H. perforatum*, *H. japonicum* and *H. patulum*, were compared. HM with the highest phenol content (24.72 mg/g) showed the highest activity, followed by

H. perforatum [24]. In continuation of our work in the present study, we investigated the *in vitro* and *in vivo* antioxidant potential and hepatoprotective effect of HM and compared its activity among different parts of the plant.

2. Materials and Methods

2.1. Collection and Identification of Plant Material

HM was collected from, in and around Ooty, a famous hill station in southern India, belonging to the Nilgiris, a district of Tamil Nadu state. The plant was identified and authenticated by Medicinal Plants Survey and Collection Unit, Ooty, Tamil Nadu, India, where a voucher specimen was preserved for further reference (voucher specimen No. 8570).

2.2. Preparation of Extracts

The aerial parts, flowering tops, leaves, root and stem were separated and dried in the shade. Each of these was then separately powdered, sieved (No. 20), weighed and extracted with a Soxhlet extractor (Borosil, Mumbai, India), using methanol. The extracts were concentrated to dryness under reduced pressure and controlled temperature. All extracts were preserved in a refrigerator at 4 °C till further use.

2.3. Preparation of Test and Standard Solutions

Extracts of the aerial parts (HMA), flowering tops (HMF), leaves (HML), root (HMR) and stem (HMS) and the standard antioxidants (ascorbic acid, rutin, butylated hydroxy anisole and α-tocopherol) were dissolved in dimethyl sulfoxide (DMSO) and used for the *in vitro* antioxidant assays using seven different methods, except the hydrogen peroxide method. For the hydrogen peroxide method (where DMSO interferes with the method), the extracts and standards were dissolved in distilled methanol and used. The stock solutions were appropriately diluted with the respective solvents to obtain lower dilutions.

2.4. Chemicals

1,1-Diphenyl-2-picrylhydrazyl (DPPH), 2,2′-azino-bis (3-ethylbenzo-thiazoline-6-sulfonic acid) diammonium salt (ABTS), butylated hydroxy anisole (BHA) *tert*-butyl hydroperoxide, chlorpromazine, guanosine, tryptophan, ascorbic acid, silymarin and hyperoside were obtained from Sigma-Aldrich Co., St. Louis, MO, USA. Rutin and *p*-nitroso dimethyl aniline (*p*-NDA) was from Acros Organics, Morris Plains, NJ, USA. Naphthyl ethylenediamine dihydrochloride (NEDD) was from Roch-Light Ltd., Suffolk, UK. Nitro blue tetrazolium (NBT) was from SD Fine Chemicals Ltd., Mumbai, India, and 2-deoxy-D-ribose was from Hi-Media Laboratories Pvt. Ltd., Mumbai, India. Sodium nitroprusside was from Ranbaxy Laboratories Ltd., Mohali, India. Sodium carboxy methyl cellulose (CMC), sulfanilic acid and α-tocopherol were from Merck (India) Ltd., Delhi, India. Cupric chloride, ferric chloride, ferrous ammonium sulfate and all other chemicals were of analytical or equivalent grade. All chemicals were used without further purification. The water used for the preparation of solutions was purified through a Milli-Q water purification system (Millipore, Billerica, MA, USA; Specific conductivity <0.1 μs·cm^{-1}), and the sample solutions were prepared just prior to carrying out the experiments.

2.5. Selection and Maintenance of Animals

Healthy male albino rats of the Wister strain (180–220 g) were obtained from the animals house, J.S.S. College of Pharmacy, Ooty, India, and were maintained under standard environmental conditions (22–28 °C, 60%–70% relative humidity 12 h dark/light cycle) and fed with standard rat feed (Amrut Rat Feed, Nav Maharasthra Chakan Oil Mill Ltd., Pune, India) and water *ad libitum*. The experiments were conducted as per the guidelines of Committee for the Purpose of Control and Supervision of Experiments on Animals (CPCSEA), Chennai, India. The protocol was approved by the institutional animal ethics committee (Approval No. JSSCP/IAEC/PhD/PH.BIOTECH/01/2005-06).

2.6. In Vitro Antioxidant Activity

Methanolic extracts of different parts of HM and different standards were assessed for *in vitro* antioxidant activity on the basis of the radical scavenging effects of the stable ABTS [25] and DPPH [26] free radicals, hydroxyl radical by deoxyribose [27] and the *p*-NDA method [28], hydrogen peroxide [29], lipid peroxide inhibition using the standard 2-thiobarbituric acid (TBA) colorimetric method [30,31], nitric oxide [32,33] and super oxide radical by the alkaline DMSO method [34]. In all these methods, a particular concentration of the extract or standard solution was used, which, after the addition of all the reagents, gave a final concentration of 1000 μg/mL to 0.45 μg/mL. Absorbance was measured against an appropriate reagent blank. A control test was performed without adding extracts or standards. The results were expressed in IC_{50} values (concentration of test or standard required to inhibit 50% of free radicals). Measurement of total antioxidant capacity [35] and the total phenol [36] and flavonol [37] content of the methanolic extracts of different parts of HM were carried out. The phytochemical screening of methanolic extracts of different parts of HM was performed using standard methods [38,39].

2.7. In Vivo Antioxidant and Hepatoprotective Studies

Carbon tetrachloride (CCl_4)-induced hepatic injury is the model used for *in vivo* antioxidant and hepatoprotective drug screening [40]. The principle causes of CCl_4-induced hepatic damage are free radical-mediated lipid peroxidation, leading to the disruption of the biomembrane, dysfunction of cells and tissues, decreased levels of antioxidant enzymes and the generation of free radicals [41]. The antioxidant activity involving the inhibition of the generation of free radicals is important in providing protection against hepatic damage.

2.7.1. Preparation of Extracts and Standard

One hundred and 200 mg/mL of HMF and HML were prepared in 0.5% sodium CMC. One hundred milligrams per milliliter of standard silymarin were prepared in 0.5% sodium CMC.

2.7.2. Experimental Design

The animals were divided into seven groups with six animals in each group. Group I served as the normal control, and Group II served as the toxicant control. Both Groups I and II received 1 mL of 0.5% sodium CMC. Group III received standard silymarin at a dose of 100 mg/kg p.o. Groups IV and V received HMF at a dose of 100 and 200 mg/kg p.o. body weight, respectively. Group VI and VII animals received HML at a dose of 100 and 200 mg/kg p.o. body weight, respectively. Silymarin and extracts were administered orally for 7 days. On the eighth day, all groups received 1 mL/kg body weight of CCl_4, intraperitoneally, except Group I. On the ninth day, the rats were anesthetized using anesthetic ether, and blood was collected from retro-orbital plexus. After collection, the blood was kept at 37 °C for 30 min. Later, it was centrifuged at 2500 rpm for 10 min to separate serum, which was used for biochemical estimations. Later, all of the animals were sacrificed by decapitation. The liver was removed, weighed and homogenized immediately with Elvenjan homogenizer fitted with a Teflon plunger, in ice-chilled 10% KCl solution (10 mg/g of tissue). The suspension was centrifuged at 2000 rpm at 4 °C for 10 min, and the clear supernatant was used for the biochemical estimations. The levels of antioxidant enzymes, *viz.*, catalase (CAT), superoxide dismutase (SOD) and lipid peroxidation (LPO or 2-thiobarbituric acid reactive substances (TBARS)) were measured. Marker enzymes, such as alanine amino transferase (ALAT), aspartate amino transferase (ASAT), alkaline phosphatase (ALP), total bilirubin (TB) and total protein (TP) were measured spectrophotometrically in serum and liver samples using commercially available Ecoline diagnostic kits (Merck, Mumbai, India) [42,43].

2.8. Histopathological Studies

On the ninth day of the experiment, all the animals were sacrificed by decapitation, and the liver was dissected out, the surrounding tissues removed and kept in 10% buffered neutral formalin. The materials were processed by standard methods [44]. Paraffin blocks were made and sections were cut. These sections were stained with hematoxylin and eosin and mounted on glass slides. The histopathological changes were observed and recorded.

2.9. HPLC Quantitation

Different biological activities of HM have been reported in recent years [22,45,46], but no method for quantitation has been reported so far. It is important to standardize the different parts of HM, because of its widespread availability in various geographic regions and to detect its adulteration with other materials. Hence, the quantitation of HMF and HML was carried out by using two marker compounds, hyperoside and rutin. The extracts were dissolved in methanol (1 mg/mL) and filtered through Whatman filter paper, and the filtrate was used for HPLC analysis. Ten milligrams of standards hyperoside and rutin were dissolved separately in 5 mL of methanol in 10 mL volumetric flasks, and the volume was made up to 10 mL with the same solvent. Various concentrations were prepared from the stock solution and used for HPLC analysis. Chromatographic separation was performed on a Shimadzu® liquid chromatographic system (Shimadzu, Kyoto, Japan), equipped with a LC-10AT-vp solvent delivery system, an Shimadzu® SPD M-10AVP photo diode array detector

(Shimadzu, Kyoto, Japan) and a Rheodyne 7725i injector (Sigma-Aldrich, St. Louis, MO, USA), with a 5-μL loop. A Phenomenex GEMINI C18 column (Phenomenex, Torrance, CA, USA) (25 cm × 4.6 mm i.d., 5 μm) was used for the separation. A mixture (75:25 v/v) of phosphate buffer (25 mM %) and acetonitrile was used as the mobile phase. It was delivered at a flow rate of 1.0 mL per min with detection at 360 nm. The retention time of hyperoside was found to be 5.80 min. The injection volume of the HMF and HML extracts was 50 μL. Analysis was performed at ambient temperature. Based on the peak area of standard and sample solution, the amount of hyperoside and rutin (%) was calculated.

2.10. Statistical Analysis

The experimental results were expressed as means ± S.E.M. The significance of the *in vivo* results was analyzed by one-way analysis of variance (ANOVA) followed by Tukey–Kramer multiple comparison tests, and $p < 0.05$ was considered as statistically significant.

3. Results and Discussion

3.1. Preparation of Extracts

The yield of dried methanolic extracts after Soxhlet extraction was 12.5% ± 0.25%, 10.33% ± 0.29%, 9.25% ± 0.11%, 4.21% ± 0.06% and 4.1% ± 0.02%, respectively for HMA, HMF, HML, HMR and HMS of HM. Phytochemical studies of these extracts showed the presence of saponins, flavonoids and tannins in all the parts of HM.

3.2. Estimation of Total Phenolic and Flavonoid Content

The total phenolic content and flavonoid content of the extracts were estimated by standard procedures [38,39]. The flowering top extract (HMF) possessed maximum total phenol and flavonol content with 38.6 and 33.48 mg/g of extract, respectively, followed by leaves, aerial parts, stem and root (Table 1).

Table 1. Total flavonol and phenol content of different extracts of *Hypericum mysorense* (HM).

Part of Plant	Total Flavonol Content * (mg/g of Extract)	Total Phenol Content * (mg/g of Extract)
HMF	33.48 ± 2.1	38.6 ± 3.66
HML	28.76 ± 1.44	37.07 ± 2.90
HMA	27.52 ± 1.67	32.7 ± 1.23
HMS	26.54 ± 3.56	30.7 ± 3.14
HMR	15.84 ± 0.84	20.7 ± 1.11

* The average of three determinations; values are the mean ± S.E.M. HMF, flowering tops; HML, leaves; HMA, aerial parts; HMS, stem; HMR, root.

3.3. In Vitro Antioxidant Activity

Results of the *in vitro* studies carried out for determining the antioxidant capacity of the methanolic extracts of different parts of HM in scavenging DPPH$^{\bullet}$, ABTS$^{\bullet-}$, NO$^{\bullet}$, $O_2^{\bullet-}$ and $^{\bullet}$OH radicals, model lipid and H_2O_2 are shown in Table 2. Positive correlations were observed between the results from total phenolic and total flavonoid contents (Table 1) with that of *in vitro* antioxidant activity using different assays (Table 2). HMF had the highest IC_{50} values, followed by HML, HMA, HMS and HMR, respectively. A comparison of the *in vitro* antioxidant efficiencies of the extracts with the standards, especially in the case of $DPPH^•$, $^•OH$ (*p*-NDA), $O_2^{•-}$, lipid peroxidation and total antioxidant capacity, showed that the HMF had better scavenging efficiency than the corresponding standards.

The ability of extracts to inhibit lipid peroxidation by inactivating free radicals was determined by preventing the oxidation of egg lecithin, using the TBA colorimetric method. The good efficiency of extracts rich in total phenols/flavonoids to inhibit lipid peroxidation may be due to the scavenging of free radicals and partly due to their ability to form stronger chelates with iron/copper ions, thus rendering them inactive towards undergoing the Fenton reaction in contrast to butylated hydroxyanisole and the α-tocopherol used as standards.

Many oxidase enzymes are known to generate H_2O_2 endogenously. Though by itself a weak oxidant, it can undergo a Fenton-type reaction to form potent $^•OH$ radical; hence, it was of interest to study the scavenging of H_2O_2. The present studies showed that the extracts were relatively less efficient (by 1.5- to three-times) in scavenging H_2O_2 in comparison to rutin, used as a standard. The very high IC_{50} values in the $^•OH$ radical scavenging by the well-known deoxyribose method, as well as by *p*-NDA methods showed that extracts, as well as the standards do not scavenge the radicals well. The reason for this phenomenon is rather obscure. The hydroxyl radical reacts with phenolic compounds present in the extracts by different mechanisms: firstly, by direct abstraction of hydrogen atom present in the $^•OH$ group of the phenol, a typical example being the scavenging of $DPPH^•$ radical; secondly, by the electron transfer process from the phenol to the free radical, followed by rapid proton transfer.

The *in vitro* $ABTS^{•-}$, $DPPH^•$, $O_2^{•-}$ radical scavenging methods allow one to determine, exclusively, the intrinsic ability of an antioxidant compound or of similar compounds present in extracts, to donate hydrogen atoms/electrons to these radicals in a homogenous system. The results obtained from these methods, though useful, however, cannot be directly extrapolated to biological systems, where the species are distributed in micro-heterogeneous systems according to their lipophilicities.

3.4. In Vivo Antioxidant and Hepatoprotective Studies

Among the five extracts tested, the HMF and HML showed potent *in vitro* antioxidant activity and total phenol and flavonol content. Hence, these two extracts were selected for *in vivo* antioxidant studies using the CCl_4-intoxicated model using male albino rats of the Wister strain.

A significant increase in the levels of ASAT, ALAT, ALP and total bilirubin and a significant decrease in the levels of total proteins in liver and serum were observed in CCl_4-intoxicated rats when compared to the normal control group. The HMF at 100 and 200 mg/kg, and HML at 200 mg/kg significantly ($p < 0.001$) restored the biochemical parameters towards normal. The HML at 100 mg/kg restored ASAT, ALAT and ALP levels significantly, but did not show significant restoration of total protein and bilirubin levels. HMF at 200 mg/kg and silymarin at 100 mg/kg showed potent restoration of all biochemical parameters towards a normal level (Table 3).

Table 2. *In vitro* antioxidant activity of methanol extracts of different parts of *Hypericum mysorense*. ABTS, diammonium salt; DPPH, 1,1-diphenyl-2-picrylhydrazyl; *p*-NDA, *p*-nitroso dimethyl aniline.

Extracts/Standards	IC_{50} Values ± S.E.M. (μg/mL) * by Methods							Total Antioxidant Capacity
	ABTS	DPPH	p-NDA	Hydrogen Peroxide	Lipid per Oxidation	Nitric Oxide	Alkaline DMSO	
HMF	$1.53 \pm 0.04^{a,b}$	$3.65 \pm 0.02^{a,b}$	$690.15 \pm 11.16^{b,c}$	$57.56 \pm 2.34^{a,b}$	$13.68 \pm 1.62^{c,d}$	208.35 ± 9.36	$822.56 \pm 18.93^{a,b,c}$	0.30 ± 0.01^{d}
HML	$2.05 \pm 0.04^{a,b}$	$4.05 \pm 0.03^{a,b}$	>1000	$68.34 \pm 3.26^{a,b}$	$18.47 \pm 1.32^{c,d}$	250.53 ± 12.38	$923.84 \pm 22.45^{a,b,c}$	0.43 ± 0.01^{d}
HMA	2.97 ± 0.04^{a}	$5.23 \pm 0.04^{a,b}$	>1000	74.44 ± 3.32^{a}	$28.26 \pm 1.76^{c,d}$	301.38 ± 12.57	>1000	0.66 ± 0.02^{d}
HMS	3.63 ± 0.02^{a}	5.95 ± 0.03	>1000	80.50 ± 4.02^{a}	$33.32 \pm 1.34^{c,d}$	365.64 ± 15.64	>1000	0.96 ± 0.03^{d}
HMR	4.60 ± 0.04^{a}	8.32 ± 0.06	>1000	97.53 ± 2.98^{a}	$40.22 \pm 2.13^{c,d}$	408.24 ± 14.75	>1000	1.43 ± 0.06^{d}
STANDARDS								
Ascorbic acid	11.25 ± 0.49	2.69 ± 0.05	-	187.33 ± 3.93	-	-	>1000	-
Rutin	0.51± 0.01	3.91 ± 0.10	>1000	36.66 ± 0.22	-	65.44 ± 2.56	>1000	-
Butylated hydroxyl anisole	-	-	>1000	24.88 ± 0.16	112.66 ± 1.32		>1000	
α-Tocopherol	-	-	-	-	91.66 ± 4.92	-	-	3.41 ± 0.47

* The average of three determinations; values are the mean ± S.E.M. For the deoxyribose method, the IC_{50} values of all the extracts were >1000 μg/mL. For total antioxidant capacity, the values are expressed as the equivalent of ascorbic acid per gram of extract. ^{a} $p < 0.05$, ^{b} $p < 0.05$, ^{c} $p < 0.05$, ^{d} $p < 0.05$ between extracts and standards of ascorbic acid, rutin, butylated hydroxyl anisole and α-tocopherol, respectively.

CCl_4-intoxicated rats, showed a significant decrease in the levels of CAT and SOD and a significant increase in the TBARS levels when compared to the normal control rats. The HMF and HML at 200 mg/kg showed a significant ($p < 0.001$) reduction in the TBARS levels with an increase in SOD and CAT levels. The HMF and HML at 100 mg/kg showed moderate restoration of SOD, CAT and TBARS levels towards normal. HMF at 200 mg/kg showed potent restoration of enzymes and lipid peroxidation, comparable to that of standard silymarin ($p < 0.001$) (Figures 1 and 2, Table 4).

Figure 1. The effect of HMF and HML on CAT enzyme levels in liver and serum.

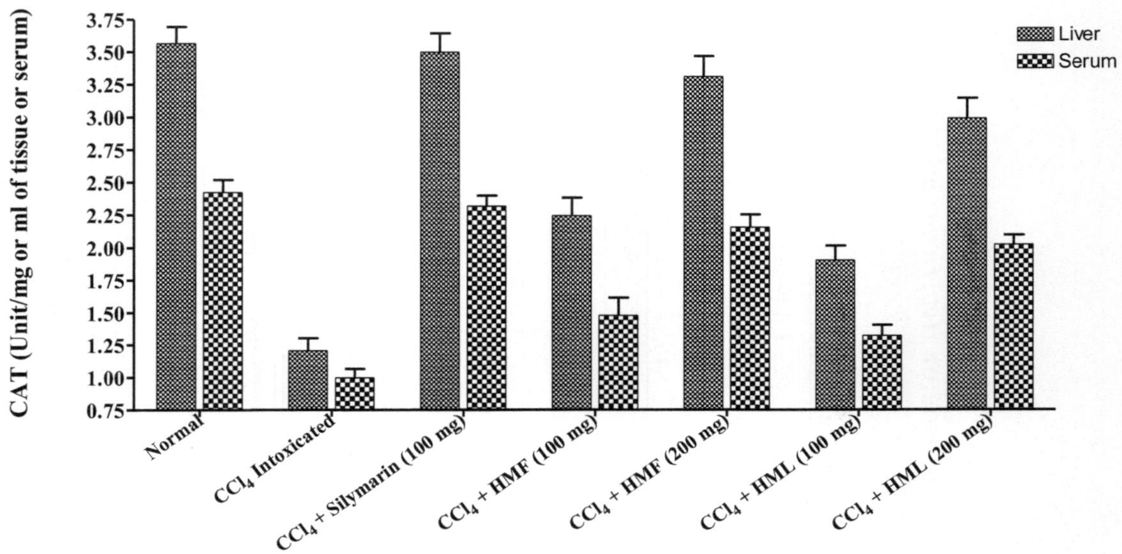

Figure 2. The effect of HMF and HML on SOD enzyme levels in liver and serum.

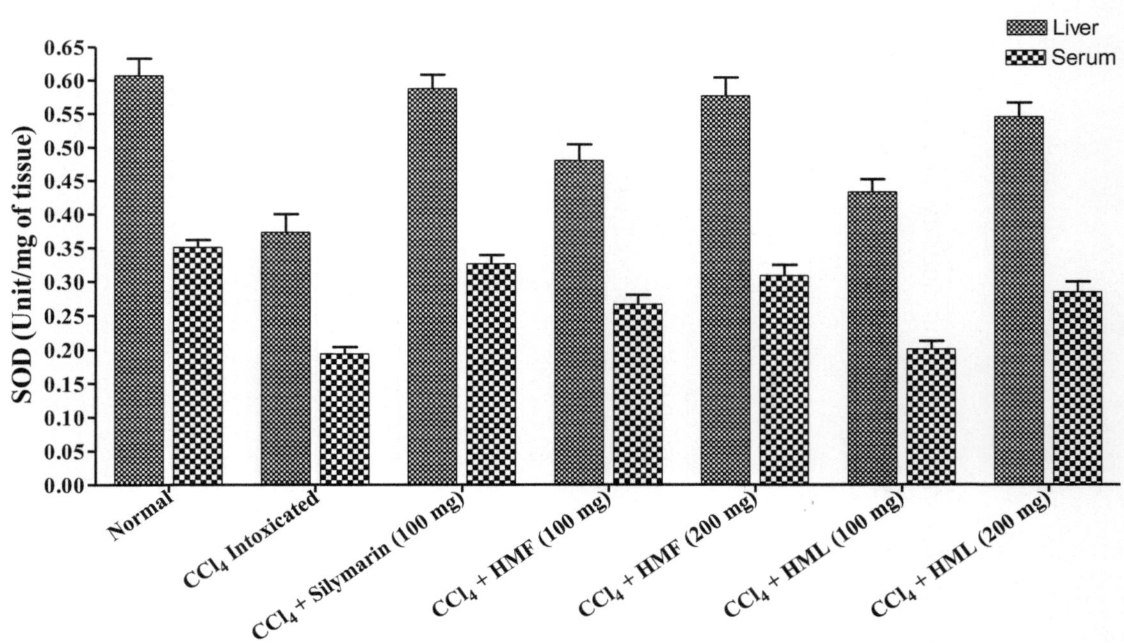

Table 3. The effects of treatment with HMF and HML on the biochemical hepatoprotective parameters of CCl_4-intoxicated rats. ASAT, aspartate amino transferase; ALAT, alanine amino transferase; ALP, alkaline phosphatase.

Treatment	Dose (mg or mL/Kg b.w.)	ASAT (U/L)		ALAT (U/L)		ALP (U/L)		Total Protein (G/dL)		Total Bilirubin (mg/dL)	
		Liver	Serum	Liver	Serum	Liver	Serum	Liver	Serum	Liver	Serum
Normal	-	101.52 ± 1.078	123.39 ± 1.244	51.02 ± 0.926	69.49 ± 1.435	197.83 ± 4.321	260.31 ± 6.622	6.917 ± 0.175	6.283 ± 0.207	0.516 ± 0.031	0.702 ± 0.036
CCl_4 intoxicated	1 mL	390.74 ± 1.254 [a]	450.23 ± 1.630 [a]	198.57 ± 1.708 [a]	237.58 ± 1.931 [a]	515.23 ± 11.746 [a]	691.05 ± 15.282 [a]	4.867 ± 0.088 [a]	4.692 ± 0.129 [a]	1.783 ± 0.047 [a]	2.017 ± 0.127 [a]
CCl_4 + Silymarin	1 mL + 100 mg	143.07 ± 1.633 [b]	188.82 ± 1.493 [b]	64.16 ± 1.071 [b]	94.02 ± 1.317 [b]	256.28 ± 9.387 [b]	289.54 ± 7.784 [b]	6.283 ± 0.105 [b]	5.983 ± 0.194 [b]	0.708 ± 0.063 [b]	0.966 ± 0.042 [b]
CCl_4 + HMF	1 mL + 100 mg	292.75 ± 1.414 [b]	304.62 ± 2.139 [b]	160.34 ± 1.838 [b]	180.47 ± 2.072 [b]	428.52 ± 11.455 [b]	547.53 ± 11.846 [b]	5.556 ± 0.131 [c]	4.933 ± 0.185	1.310 ± 0.068 [b]	1.517 ± 0.047 [b]
	1 mL + 200 mg	152.73 ± 1.062 [b]	219.79 ± 1.282 [b]	66.19 ± 1.052 [b]	107.73 ± 1.606 [b]	282.37 ± 10.147 [b]	328.59 ± 9.316 [b]	6.023 ± 0.116 [b]	5.758 ± 0.180 [c]	0.753 ± 0.062 [b]	0.903 ± 0.036 [b]
CCl_4 + HML	1 mL + 100 mg	315.24 ± 1.695 [b]	331.32 ± 2.274 [b]	171.93 ± 1.517 [b]	194.76 ± 1.942 [b]	469.83 ± 14.269	584.38 ± 16.682 [b]	5.032 ± 0.066	4.796 ± 0.169	1.483 ± 0.054 [c]	1.717 ± 0.063 [d]
	1 mL + 200 mg	187.03 ± 1.732 [b]	254.42 ± 1.904 [b]	76.69 ± 1.217 [b]	121.59 ± 1.585 [b]	307.27 ± 9.665 [b]	361.31 ± 11.926 [b]	5.767 ± 0.168 [b]	5.413 ± 0.171	0.883 ± 0.043 [b]	1.220 ± 0.066 [b]

The results are the mean ± S.E.M. (n = 6), [a] $p < 0.001$, between the normal and CCl_4-intoxicated groups. [b] $p < 0.001$, [c] $p < 0.01$, [d] $p < 0.05$, between the CCl_4-intoxicated and treated groups.

Table 4. The effect of HMF, HML and silymarin on antioxidant enzymes and lipid peroxidation in CCl_4-induced rats. TBARS, 2-thiobarbituric acid reactive substance; MDA, malondialdehyde.

Treatment	Dose (mg/kg Body Weight)	CAT (Unit/mg of Tissue)		SOD (Unit/mg of Tissue)		TBARS (n mole of MDA/mg of Protein)	
		Liver	Serum	Liver	Serum	Liver	Serum
Normal	0.5 mL Sodium CMC	3.564 ± 0.128	2.425 ± 0.094	0. 607 ± 0.026	0.351 ± 0.011	4.872 ± 0.178	3.845 ± 0.065
Control (CCl_4)	1 mL	1.207 ± 0.096 [a]	0.997 ± 0.069 [a]	0.373 ± 0.027 [c]	0.194 ± 0.010 [a]	8.425 ± 0.149 [a]	6.583 ± 0.176 [a]
Silymarin + CCl_4	100	3.495 ± 0.145 [b]	2.318 ± 0.082 [b]	0.587 ± 0.021 [b]	0.326 ± 0.013 [b]	5.102 ± 0.170 [b]	4.207 ± 0.123 [b]
HMF + CCl_4	100	2.245 ± 0.137 [d]	1.481 ± 0.133 [b]	0.480 ± 0.024 [c]	0.267 ± 0.014 [d]	7.214 ± 0.243 [b]	5.512 ± 0.114 [b]
	200	3.310 ± 0.154 [b]	2.156 ± 0.098 [b]	0.576 ± 0.028 [b]	0.309 ± 0.016 [b]	5.456 ± 0.162 [b]	4.417 ± 0.107 [b]
HML + CCl_4	100	1.906 ± 0.109	1.323 ± 0.084 [d]	0.433 ± 0.019	0.201 ± 0.012	7.676 ± 0.196	5.878 ± 0.134 [c]
	200	2.987 ± 0.156 [b]	2.023 ± 0.075 [b]	0.545 ± 0.021 [d]	0.285 ± 0.015 [b]	5.873 ± 0.112 [b]	4.765 ± 0.124 [b]

The results are the mean ± S.E.M. (n = 6), [a] $p < 0.001$, between the normal and CCl_4-intoxicated groups. [b] $p < 0.001$, [c] $p < 0.01$, [d] $p < 0.05$, between the CCl_4-intoxicated and treated groups.

Antioxidant action has been reported to play a crucial role in the hepatoprotective capacity of many plants, such as *Curcuma longa*, *Ganoderma formosanum*, *Solanum nigrum*, *Boehmeria nivea* and *Spirulina maxima* [47–51]. Thus, the search for drugs of plant origin with antioxidant activity has become a central focus of study of hepatoprotection. This may prove effective in alleviating tissue damage prevalent in organisms as a consequence of exposure to toxins of extrinsic or intrinsic origin. Natural antioxidants strengthen the endogenous antioxidant defenses, by ROS scavenging and restoring the optimal balance by neutralizing the reactive species. They are gaining immense importance by virtue of their critical role in disease prevention.

The preventive action against liver damage by CCl_4 has been widely used as an indicator of the liver protective activity of drugs in general [52]. Since the changes associated with CCl_4-induced liver damage are similar to that of acute viral hepatitis [53], CCl_4-mediated hepatotoxicity was chosen as the experimental model. It has been established that CCl_4 is accumulated in hepatic parenchyma cells and metabolically activated by cytochrome P450-dependent monooxygenases to form a trichloromethyl radical (CCl_3). The CCl_3 radical alkylates cellular proteins and other macromolecules with a simultaneous attack on polyunsaturated fatty acids, in the presence of oxygen, to produce lipid peroxides, leading to liver damage [54]. Thus, antioxidant or free radical generation inhibition is important in protection against CCl_4-induced liver lesions [41]. ASAT, ALAT, ALP, TB and TP are the most sensitive tests for the diagnosis of liver diseases [55]. Hepatotoxic compounds, such as CCl_4, are known to cause marked elevation in serum enzymes and bilirubin levels. It causes a marked decrease in TP levels. The present study revealed a significant increase in the activities of ASAT, ALAT, ALP and TB and a significant decrease in TP within 24 h of exposure to CCl_4, in toxicant control animals, indicating considerable hepatocellular injury. Silymarin is used as a standard hepatoprotective compound, since it is reported to have a protective effect on the plasma membrane of hepatocytes [56]. Administration of HM extracts, especially HMF, attenuated the increased levels of the serum enzymes, produced by CCl_4, and caused a subsequent recovery towards normalization, almost like that of the silymarin treatment, as reported [57].

Thus, the antioxidant activity or the inhibition of the generation of free radicals is important for the protection against CCl_4-induced hepatopathy [41]. The body has an effective defense mechanism to prevent and neutralize the free radical-induced damage. This is accomplished by a set of endogenous antioxidant enzymes, such as SOD and CAT. These enzymes constitute a mutually-supportive team of defense against ROS [58]. In CCl_4-induced hepatotoxicity, the balance between ROS production and these antioxidant defenses may be lost, and "oxidative stress" results, which, through a series of events, deregulates the cellular functions, leading to hepatic necrosis. The reduced activities observed for SOD and catalase point to the hepatic damage in the rats administered with CCl_4 [59]. However, the extract-treated groups showed a significant increase in the level of these enzymes, which indicates the antioxidant potential of the HMF and HML.

The level of lipid peroxide is a measure of membrane damage and alterations in the structure and function of cellular membranes. In the present study, the elevation of lipid peroxidation in the liver of rats treated with CCl_4 was observed. The increase in malondialdehyde (MDA) levels in liver suggests enhanced lipid peroxidation, leading to tissue damage and the failure of antioxidant defense mechanisms to prevent the formation of excessive free radicals [60]. Treatment with HMF and HML significantly reversed these changes. From the results, it is clear that the drugs show dose-dependent activity, among which, the HMF and HML at a dose level of 200 mg/kg p.o. showed greater activity, which is comparable with the standard drug, silymarin.

It is already been discussed that HMF and HML successfully restored the level of MDA after CCl_4 intoxication towards normal. Both of the extracts prevented the lipid peroxidation in a dose-dependent manner, thereby preventing the hepatotoxicity, indicating the anti-lipid peroxidative effect. This suggested the possibility that HM extracts are able to condition the hepatocytes, so as to cause accelerated regeneration of parenchyma cells, thus protecting against membrane fragility and decreasing the leakage of the marker enzymes into circulation.

3.5. Histopathology

Histological examination of the liver tissues under light microscope was done to observe the effects of HMF and HML on the structural integrity of the cells. The liver of normal animals showed a normal histological appearance (Figure 3a). The CCl_4-intoxicated animal liver showed fat changes, liver necrosis and hepatic degeneration (Figure 3b). The animals treated with standard silymarin at the 100 mg/kg body weight dose and HMF at 200 and 100 mg/kg body weight doses exhibited an almost normal histological appearance of liver cells, except a few lymphocytic collections in the portal area (Figure 3c–e). The animals treated with HML at the 200 mg/kg body weight dose also showed normal histology with intact hepatocytes with slight inflammation (Figure 3f,g), whereas, 100 mg/kg body weight showed slightly more inflammatory changes compared to normal.

Figure 3. Histology of liver stained with hematoxylin-eosin (×100) of the groups of mice. (**a**) Normal; (**b**) CCl_4-intoxicated; (**c**) CCl_4 + silymarin treated; (**d**) CCl_4 + HMF (200 mg/kg b.w.); (**e**) CCl_4 + HMF (100 mg/kg b.w.); (**f**) CCl_4 + HML (200 mg/kg b.w.); (**g**) CCl_4 + HML (100 mg/kg b.w.).

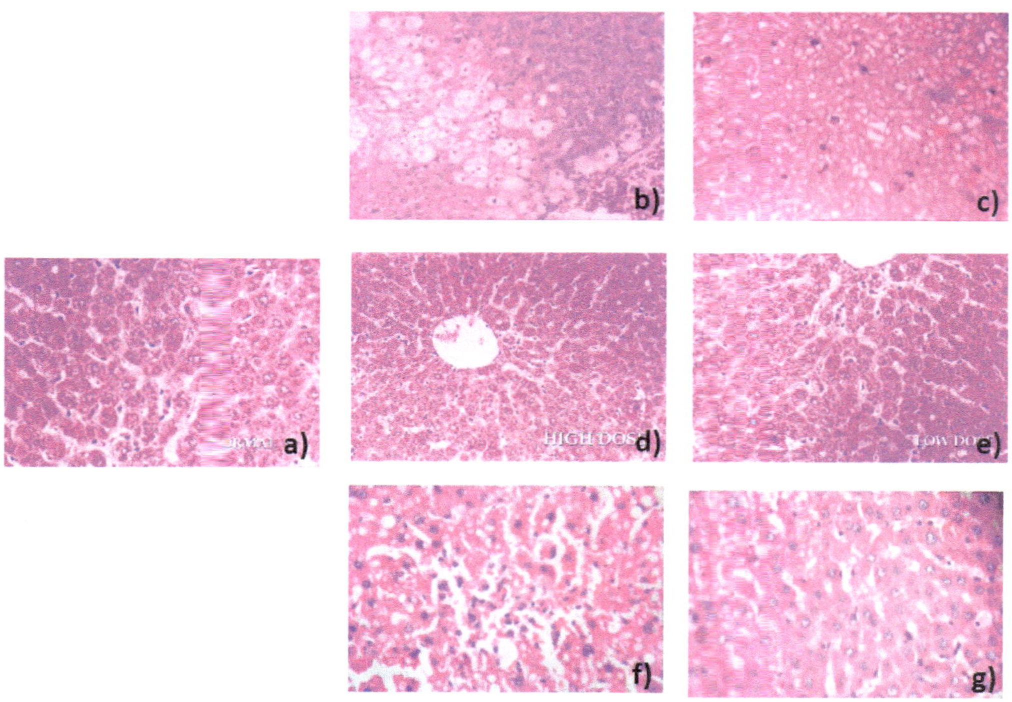

3.6. HPLC Quantitation

Typical chromatograms of hyperoside and rutin and of HMF and HML are shown in Figures 4–6, respectively. The amount of hyperoside present in the HMF and HML was 1.981% ± 0.12% and 1.165% ± 0.09% w/w, respectively. The amount of rutin present in HMF and HML was 1.527% ± 0.1% and 1.238% ± 0.09% w/w, respectively.

Figure 4. HPLC chromatographs of hyperoside and rutin.

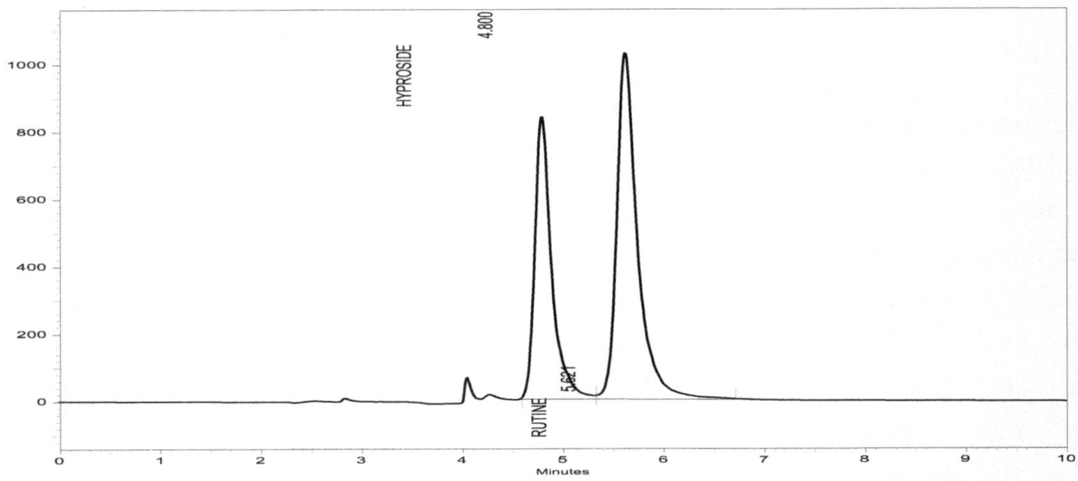

Figure 5. HPLC chromatographs of HMF.

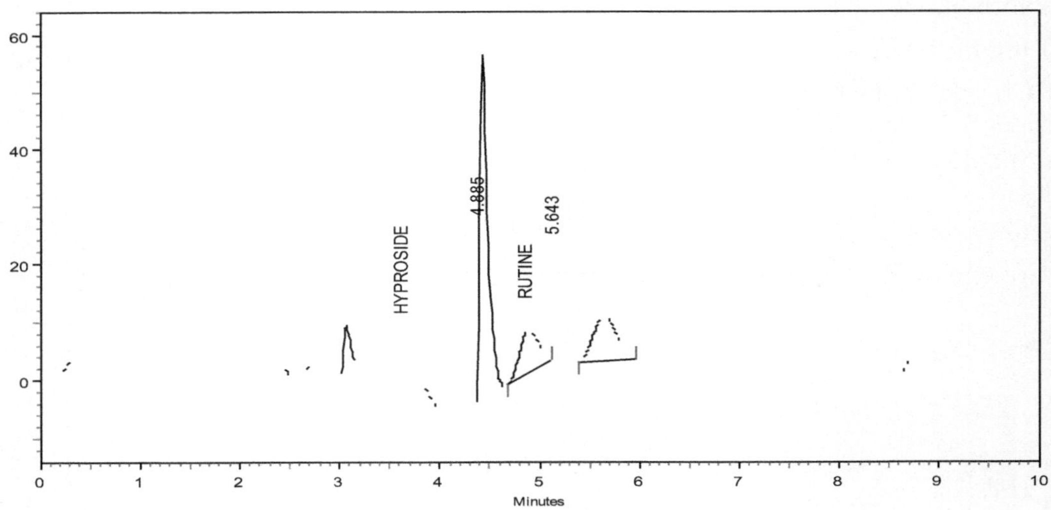

Figure 6. HPLC chromatographs of HML.

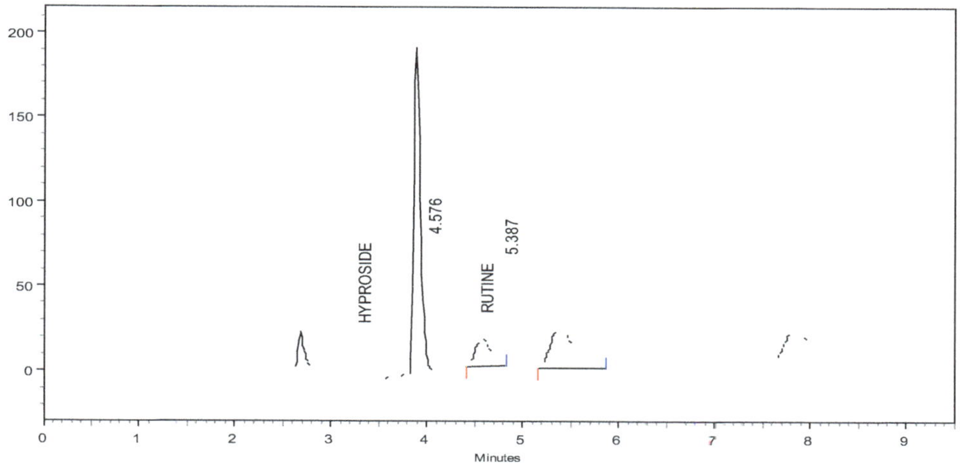

4. Conclusions

The protective effect exhibited by HMF and HML against free radical-induced toxicity could be due to the protection of hepatic drug metabolizing enzymes and their antioxidant activities. The hepatic injury caused by CCl_4 is associated with damage to the endoplasmic reticulum, and any compound capable of preventing the toxicity of CCl_4 must have some direct or indirect effect on the liver. Both HMF and HML extracts have a maximum quantity of phenols and flavonols in them. The antioxidant activity of phenolics and flavonoids is well known and widely accepted. HMF and HML showed potent *in vitro* and *in vivo* antioxidant and hepatoprotective activity among the various extracts of HM. The antioxidant and hepatoprotective activity of HM may be due to its rich flavonoid content. Two compounds were isolated from the HMF and HML, namely, hyperoside and rutin.

Acknowledgements

The authors would like to acknowledge the authorities of JSS College of Pharmacy, Ooty and Manipal College of Pharmacy, Manipal for providing necessary research facilities.

Author Contributions

Raghu C. Hariharapura has designed and executed the experimental work. Ramamurthy Srinivasan, Godavarthi Ashok and Santoshkumar H. Dongre have helped in analysis and interpretation of the data. Raghu C. Hariharapura and Hitesh V. Jagani have prepared and edited the manuscript. Pottekkad Vijayan was the main supervisor and has designed the experiments for this project. All the authors have read and approved the final manuscript.

Conflicts of Interest

The authors declare no conflict of interest.

References

1. Ben-Yoseph, O.; Boxer, P.A.; Ross, B.D. Assessment of the role of the glutathione and pentose phosphate pathways in the protection of primary cerebrocortical cultures from oxidative stress. *J. Neurochem.* **1996**, *66*, 2329–2337.
2. Harman, D. Free radical theory of aging: Origin of life, evolution, and aging. *Age* **1980**, *3*, 100–102.
3. Moskovitz, J.; Yim, K.A.; Choke, P.B. Free radicals and disease. *Arch. Biochem. Biophys.* **2002**, *397*, 354–359.
4. Hollman, P.C.H.; Katan, M.B. Absorption, metabolism, and bioavailability of flavonoids. In *Flavonoids in Health and Disease*; Rice-Evans, C.A., Packer, L., Eds.; Marcel Dekker: New York, NY, York, 1996; pp. 483–522.
5. Rice-Evans, C.A.; Miller, N.J.; Paganga, G. Structure antioxidant activities of flavonoids as bioactive components of food. *Free Radic. Biol. Med.* **1996**, *20*, 933–956.
6. Rice-Evans, C.A.; Miller, N.J.; Paganga, G. Antioxidant properties of phenolic compounds. *Trends Plant Sci.* **1997**, *2*, 152–159.
7. Bors, W.; Michel, C. Antioxidant capacity of flavonols and gallate esters: Pulse radiolysis studies. *Free Radic. Biol. Med.* **1999**, *27*, 1413–1426.
8. Torrel, J.; Cillard, J.; Cillard, P. Antioxidant activity of flavonoids and reactivity with peroxyl radical. *Phytochemistry* **1986**, *25*, 383–385.
9. Van Acker, S.A.B.E.; van den Berg, D.J.; Tromp, M.N.J.L.; Griffioen, D.H.; van Bennekom, W.P.; van der Vijgh, W.J.F.; Bast, A. Structural aspect of antioxidant activity of flavonoids. *Free Radic. Biol. Med.* **1996**, *20*, 331–342.
10. Yazaki, K.; Okada, T. Hypericum erectum Thunb (St. John's wort): *In vitro* culture and the production of procynadins. *Biotechnol. Agric. For.* **1994**, *26*, 167–178.
11. Hu, L.H.; Sim, K.Y.; Sampsoniones, A.-M. A unique family of caged pilyprenylated benzoylphloroglucinol derivatives, from Hypericum sampsonii. *Tetrahedron* **2000**, *56*, 1379–1386.
12. Decosterd, L.; Hoffmann, E.; Kyburz, R.; Bray, D.; Jostettmann, K. A new phloroglucinol derivative from Hypericum calycinum with antifungal and *in vitro* antimalarial activity. *Planta Med.* **1991**, *57*, 548–551.
13. Ishiguro, K.; Yamaki, M.; Kashihara, M.; Takagi, S.; Isoi, K. Srothraling: A new antimicrobial compound from *Hypericum japonicum*. *Planta Med.* **1990**, *56*, 274–276.
14. Hudson, J.B.; Lopez-Bazzocchi, I.; Towers, G.H.N. Antiviral activities of hypericin. *Antivir. Res.* **1991**, *15*, 101–112.
15. Agostinins, P.; Vantieghem, A.; Merlevede, W.; de Witte, P.A.M. Hypericin in cancer treatment: More light on the way. *Int. J. Biochem. Cell Biol.* **2002**, *34*, 221–241.
16. Veronika, B.; Guido, J.; Adolf, N.; Hilke, W. Flavonoids from Hypericum perforaturm show antidepressant activity in the forced swimming test. *Planta Med.* **2000**, *66*, 3–6.

17. Luo, L.; Sun, Q.; Mao, Y.Y.; Lu, Y.H.; Tan, R.X. Inhibitory effects of flavonoids from *Hypericum perforatum* on nitric oxide synthesis. *J. Ethnopharmacol.* **2004**, *93*, 221–225.
18. Sara, C.; Franco, O.R.; Aleessandro, R.; Nicola, M.; Antonella, C.; Piero, M.; Grancesca, B.A.; Mauro, P. Interaction with Type II estrogen binding sites and antiproloferateve activity of tamoxifen and quercetin in human non-small-cell lung cancer. *Am. J. Respir. Cell. Mol. Biol.* **1997**, *17*, 51–59.
19. Cakir, A.; Mavi, A.; Yildirim, A.; Duru, M.E.; Harmandar, M.; Kazaz, C. Isolation and characterization of antioxidant phenolic compounds from the aerial part of Hypericum *hyssopifolium* L. by activity-guided fractionation. *J. Ethnopharmacol.* **2003**, *87*, 73–83.
20. Gamble, J.S. *Flora of the Presidency of Madras*; Bishen Singh & Mahendra Pal Singh: Dehradun, India, 1984; Volume 1, pp. 69–71.
21. Asolkar, L.V.; Kakkar, K.K.; Chakre, O.J. *Second Supplement of Glossary of Indian Medicinal Plants with Active Principles*; Publication and Information Directorate, CSIR: New Delhi, India, 1992; Volume 1, pp. 138–139.
22. Vijayan, P.; Raghu, C. Ashok, G.; Dhanaraj, S.A.; Suresh, B. Antiviral activity of medicinal plants of Nilgiris. *Indian J. Med. Res.* **2004**, *120*, 24–29.
23. Vijayan, P.; Vinod Kumar, S.; Dhanaraj, S.A.; Mukherjee, P.K.; Suresh, B. *In vitro* cytotoxicity and antitumour properties of *Hypericum mysorense* and *Hypericum patulum*. *Phytother. Res.* **2003**, *17*, 952–956.
24. Raghu Chandrashekhar, H.; Venkatesh, P.; Arumugam, M.; Vijayan, P. Estimation of total phenols with special emphasis to antioxidant potentials of few hypericum species. *Pharmacologyonline 1* **2009**, *1*, 680–687.
25. Re, R.; Pellegrini, N.; Proteggente, A.; Pannala, A.; Yang, M.; Rice-Evans, C. Antioxidant activity applying an improved ABTS radical cation decolorization assay. *Free Radic. Biol. Med.* **1999**, *26*, 1231–1237.
26. Hwang, B.Y.; Kim, H.S.; Lee, J.H.; Hong, Y.S.; Lee, K.S.; Lee, J.J. Antioxidant benzoylated flavan-3-ol glycoside from Celastrus orbiculatus. *J. Nat. Prod.* **2001**, *64*, 82–84.
27. Halliwell, B.; Gutteridge, J.M.C.; Aruoma, O.I. The deoxyribose method: A simple "test-tube" assay for determination de-oxyribose of rate constants for reactions of hydroxyl radicals. *Anal. Biochem.* **1987**, *165*, 215–219.
28. Bors, W.; Michel, C.; Saran, M. On the nature of biochemically generated hydroxyl radicals studies using the bleaching of p-nitrosodimethylaniline as a direct assay method. *Eur. J. Biochem.* **1979**, *95*, 621–627.
29. Jayaprakasha, G.K.; Jaganmohan Rao, L.; Sakariah, K.K. Antioxidant activity of flavidin in different *in vitro* model systems. *Bioorg. Med. Chem.* **2004**, *12*, 5141–5147.
30. Duh, P.D.; Yen, G.C.; Yen, W.J.; Chang, L.W. Antioxidant effects of water extracts from barley (*Hordeum vulgare*) prepared under different roasting temperatures. *J. Agric. Food Chem.* **2001**, *49*, 1455–1463.
31. Fukuzawa, K.; Tokumura, A.; Ouchi, S.; Tsukatani, H. Antioxidant activities of tocopherols on Fe^{2+}-ascorbate-induced lipid peroxidation in lecithin liposomes. *Lipids* **1982**, *17*, 511–513.
32. Marcocci, L.; Packer, L.; Droy-Lefaix, M.T.; Sekaki, A.; Gardes-Albert, M. Antioxidant action of Ginko biloba extracts EGB 761. *Methods Enzymol.* **1994**, *234*, 462–475.

33. Garrat, D.C. The Quantitative Analysis of Drugs. *Quant. Anal. Drugs* **1964**, doi:10.1007/978-1-4613-3380-7_1.
34. Elizabeth, K.; Rao, M.N.A. Oxygen radical scavenging activity of curcumin. *Int. J. Pharm.* **1990**, *58*, 237–240.
35. Prieto, P.; Pineda, M.; Aquilar, M. Spectrophotometric quantitation of antioxidant capacity through the formation of a phosphomolybdenum complex: Specific application to the determination of vitamin E. *Anal. Biochem.* **1999**, *269*, 337–341.
36. Sadasivam, S.; Manikam, A. *Biochemical Methods for Agricultural Sciences*; Wiley Eastern Limited: New Delhi, India, 1992.
37. Zhishen, J.; Mengcheng, T.; Jianming, W. The determination of flavonoid contents in mulberry and their scavenging effects on superoxide radicals. *Food Chem.* **1999**, *64*, 555–559.
38. Evans, W.C. *Trease and Evans' Pharmacognosy*; Elsevier Health Sciences: Philadelphia, PA, USA, 2009.
39. Trease, G.E.; Evans, W.C. *A Textbook of Pharmacognosy*; Bailliere Tindall: London, UK, 1989; p 388.
40. Bacon, B.R.; Tavill, A.S.; Brittenham, G.M.; Park, C.H.R.; Recknagel, O. Hepatic lipid peroxidation *in vivo* in rats with chronic iron overload. *J. Clin. Investig.* **1983**, *71*, 429–439.
41. Castro, J.A.; DeFerreyra, E.C.; DeCastro, C.R.; Fenoes, O.M.; Sasame, H.; Gillette, J.R. Prevention of carbon tetrachloride induced necrosis by inhibitors of drug metabolism—Further studies on their mechanism of action. *Biochem. Pharmacol.* **1974**, *23*, 295–302.
42. Lin, C.C.; Yen, M.H.; Lo, T.S.; Lin, J.M. Evaluation of the hepatoprotective and antioxidant activity of *Boehmeria nivea* Var. *nivea* and *B. nivea* Var, *tenacissma*. *J. Ethnopharmacol.* **1998**, *60*, 9–17.
43. Ohkawa, H.; Ohishi, N.; Yagi, K. Assay for lipid peroxides in animal tissues by thiobarbituric acid reaction. *Anal. Biochem.* **1979**, *95*, 351–358.
44. Fujii, T. Toxicological correlation between changes in blood biochemical parameters and liver histopathological findings. *J. Toxicol. Sci.* **1997**, *22*, 161–183.
45. Vijayan, P.; Vinod Kumar, S.; Shrishailappa, B.; Mukherjee, P.K.; Dhanaraj, S.A.; Suresh, B. Selective *in vitro* cytotoxicity of *Hypericum hookerianum* towards cancer cell lines. *Orient. Pharm. Exp. Med.* **2003**, *3*, 141–146.
46. Mukherjee, P.K.; Suresh, B. Studies on *in vivo* wound healing activity of leaf extract of *Hypericum mysorense* with different wound model in rats. *Nat. Prod. Sci.* **2000**, *6*, 73–78.
47. Mukherjee, P.K.; Saritha, G.S.; Suresh, B. Antimicrobial potential of two different *Hypericum* species available in India. *Phytother. Res.* **2002**, *16*, 692–695.
48. Selvam, R.; Subramonian, L.; Gayathri, R.; Angayarkanni, N. The Antioxidant activity of turmeric (*Curcuma longa*). *J. Ethnopharmacol.* **1995**, *47*, 59–67.
49. Lin, J.M.; Lin, C.C.; Chen, M.F.; Ujiie, T.; Takada, T. Radical scavenger and antihepatotoxic activity of *Ganoderma formosanum*, *Ganoderma lucidum* and *Ganodermaneo japonicum*. *J. Ethnopharmacol.* **1995**, *47*, 33–41.
50. Sultana, S.; Pervaiz, S.; Iqbal, M.; Athar, M. Crude extracts of hepatoprotective plants, *Solanum nigrum* and *Cichorum intybus* inhibits free radical-mediated DNA Damage. *J. Ethnopharmacol.* **1995**, *45*, 189–192.

51. Torres-Duran, P.V.; Miranda Zamora, R.; Paredes-Carbajal, M.C. Studies on the preventive effect of *Spirulina maxima* on fatty liver development induced by carbon tetrachloride, in the rat. *J. Ethnopharmacol.* **1999**, *64*, 141–147.
52. Clauson, G.A. Mechanism of carbon tetrachloride hepatotoxicity. *Pathol. Immunopathol. Res.* **1989**, *8*, 104–112.
53. Rubinstein, D. Epinephrine release and liver glycogen levels after carbon tetrachloride administration. *Am. J. Physiol.* **1962**, *203*, 1033–1037.
54. Bishayee, A.; Sarkar, A.; Chatterjee, M. The hepatoprotective activity of carrot (*Daucas carota* L.) against carbon tetrachloride intoxication in mouse liver. *J. Ethnopharmacol.* **1995**, *47*, 69–74.
55. Mahendale, H.M.; Gupta, P.K.; Shalunkhe, D.K. *Hepatic Toxicity*; Metropolitan Books: New Delhi, India, 1985; Volume 1, p. 225.
56. Ramellini, G.; Meldolesi, J. Liver protection by silymarin. *In vitro* effect on dissociated rat hepatocytes. *Arzneim. Forsch.* **1976**, *26*, 69–73.
57. Morazzoni, P.; Bombardelli, E. *Silybum marianum* (*Carduus marianus*). *Fitoterapia* **1995**, *66*, 3–42.
58. Venukumar, M.R.; Latha, M.S. Antioxidant activity of *Curculigo orchioides* in carbon tetrachloride induced hepatopathy in rats. *Indian J. Clin. Biochem.* **2002**, *17*, 80–87.
59. Bandyopadhyay, U.; Das, D.; Ranajit Banerjee, K. Reactive oxygen species: Oxidative damage and pathogenesis. *Curr. Sci.* **1999**, *77*, 658–665.
60. Shenoy, K.A.; Somayaji, S.N.; Bairy, K.L. Evaluation of hepatoprotective activity of *Gingo biloba* in rats. *Indian J. Pharmacol.* **2002**, *46*, 167–174.

4

Evaluation of Antioxidant and Hepatoprotective Activities of *Moringa oleifera* Lam. Leaves in Carbon Tetrachloride-Intoxicated Rats

Dharmendra Singh [1,2], Priya Vrat Arya [2], Ved Prakash Aggarwal [2] and Radhey Shyam Gupta[1,*]

[1] Centre for Advanced Studies, Department of Zoology, University of Rajasthan, Jaipur 302 055, India; E-Mail: d.singh2009@gmail.com

[2] Department of Zoology, Dyal Singh College, University of Delhi, Lodhi Road, New Delhi 110 003, India; E-Mails: zoology.dsc@gmail.com (P.V.A.); vpa541@gmail.com (V.P.A.)

* Author to whom correspondence should be addressed; E-Mail: gupta_rs@hotmail.com

---

Abstract: The antioxidant and hepatoprotective activities of the extract of *Moringa oleifera* leaves were investigated against CCl_4-induced hepatotoxicity in rats. Hepatotoxic rats were treated with ethanol extract of *Moringa oleifera* for a period of 60 days at the following three dose levels; 100, 200 and 400 mg/kg body weight/day, orally. The activities were studied by assaying the serum marker enzymes like SGOT, SGPT, GGT, LDH, ALP, ACP, as well as total bilirubin, total protein and albumin in serum concomitantly with the activities of LPO, SOD, CAT, GSH, GR and GPx in liver. The activities of all parameters registered a significant ($p \leq 0.001$) alteration in CCl_4 treated rats, which were significantly recovered towards an almost normal level in rats co-administered with *M. oleifera* extract in a dose-dependent manner. All the biochemical investigations were confirmed by the histopathological observations and compared with the standard drug. silymarin. Results suggest that the antioxidant and hepatoprotective activities of *M. oleifera* leaves are possibly related to the free radical scavenging activity which might be due to the presence of total phenolics and flavonoids in the extract and/or the purified compounds β-sitosterol, quercetin and kaempferol, which were isolated from the ethanol extract of *M. oleifera* leaves.

Keywords: antioxidants; free radicals; hepatoprotection; *Moringa oleifera*

---

1. Introduction

Moringa oleifera Lam. is a drumstick tree of the Moringaceae family, known as sahinjan in Hindi. It is a native of India and now grown extensively in many southeastern Asian countries particularly in Thailand, Philippines and Pakistan *etc.* [1]. Traditionally, *Moringa oleifera* is considered to be one of the most useful trees in the world, as almost every part of the tree has some nutritional, medicinal and other valuable properties [2]. The leaves, especially young shoots, are eaten as salads, in vegetable curries, and as pickles. Additionally, the shade dried leaves of *Moringa oleifera* are widely utilized in developing countries as a good source of protein, calcium, vitamin A, C and E, β-carotene, amino acids, various polyphenolics and some natural anti-oxidizing agents [3]. Therefore, it is used as an alternative source of nutritional supplements and growth promoters in various countries [4].

Apart from nutritional benefits, *Moringa oleifera* has been extensively used as an antioxidant, and for the following applications; wound healing, anti-tumor, anti-fertility, hypotensive, antipyretic, antihepatotoxic, antiepileptic, anti-inflammatory, antiulcer, diuretic, hypocholesterolaemic, antifungal, antibacterial and anti-cardiovascular agent, *etc.* [5,6]. The extract of *Moringa oleifera* leaves is also capable of reducing hyperglycemia, dyslipidemia [7], and diabetes mellitus [8]. Hence, the present study was carried out in an attempt to evaluate the antioxidant and hepatoprotective activities of *M. oleifera* leaves extract in carbon tetrachloride CCl_4-intoxicated rats which might be due to the presence of total phenolics and flavonoids in the extract and/or isolated active constituents β-sitosterol, quercetin and kaempferol.

2. Material and Methods

2.1. Plant Material

Fresh leaves of *Moringa oleifera* Lam. were collected from the University Campus, University of Rajasthan, Jaipur and authenticated by the Department of Botany, University of Rajasthan, Jaipur (Herbarium Sheet No. RUBL-20287).

2.2. Extraction and Isolation

The leaves were shade-dried and pulverized. The powder was treated with petroleum ether for defatting as well as to remove chlorophyll. The powder was packed into a soxhlet apparatus and subjected to hot continuous percolation using alcohol (95% v/v) as solvent for 48 h at 58–60 °C. The extract was concentrated under vacuum, dried in a vacuum desiccator, and yielded 7.4% w/w of a dark greenish-brown solid mass. The solid mass was then powdered, and washed with chloroform to remove the remaining chlorophyll content present in the extract. Half of the extract was suspended in an appropriate volume of olive oil to prepare the desired concentration for oral administration to rats during experimentation.

The rest of the extract (30 g) was subjected to traditional column chromatography by fractionation with different solvents. For this purpose, a column (1.4 m × 5 cm) filled with 900 g Si-gel (60–120 mesh) was used. The purity of fractions was checked by qualitative thin layer chromatography using different solvent systems. After ascertaining the purity of compounds, it was subjected to detailed spectral analysis (IR, ^{1}H NMR, ^{13}C NMR and MS) to establish the structure. As a result, the compounds (A, B & C) were isolated, purified and characterized.

2.2.1. Isolation and Characterization of Compound A

Compound A was obtained when the column was eluted with chloroform and benzene in the ratio 1:1. After removal of solvent, A was obtained as yellowish crystalline solid. Further purification by re-column chromatography yielded β-sitosterol, colorless needles, 1.8 g/30 g (6% w/w), R_f 0.56($CHCl_3$)$_3$ m.p. 136–137 °C and responded positively to the Liebermann-Burchard test for sterols. It was identified by a mixed melting point and Co-TLC with an authentic sample. IR (ν_{max}) cm^{-1} (KBr): 3450, 2940, 2880, 1600, 1040; ^{1}HNMR (δ ppm, $CDCl_3$): 0.65 (3H, s), 0.85 (3H, s), 0.90 (3H, s), 0.95 (3H, s), 0.98 (3H, s), 1.25 (3H, s), 1.45 to 1.85 (for 26H, 10CH_2 and 6CH), 1.85 (H, d), 2.05 (1H, d), 2.25 (1H, d), 3.50 (1H, m), 5.30 (1H, d); ^{13}CNMR (δ ppm, $CDCl_3$): 31.3(C-1), 31.7(C-2), 71.8(C-3), 42.3(C-4), 141.0(C-5), 121.7(C-6), 31.9(C-7), 45.9(C-8), 50.1(C-9), 36.1(C-10), 21.1(C-11), 28.2(C-12), 42.3(C-13), 56.8(C-14), 24.3(C-15), 39.8(C-16), 56.1(C-17), 11.8(C-18), 19.3(C-19), 36.1(C-20), 19.0(C-21), 36.1(C-22), 24.3(C-23), 39.8(C-24), 28.2(C-25), 23.1(C-26), 23.1(C-27), 31.9(C-28), 29.2(C-29); MS *m*/*z*: 414(M$^+$), 399, 383, 369, 256, 215, 174, 159, 145, 134, 120, 107, *etc.*

On the basis of ^{1}HNMR, ^{13}CNMR and mass spectral studies of compound A, it was characterized as β-sitosterol (Figure 1) with molecular formula $C_{29}H_{50}O$ and comparable with the literature of β-Sitosterol [9,10].

Figure 1. Compound A.

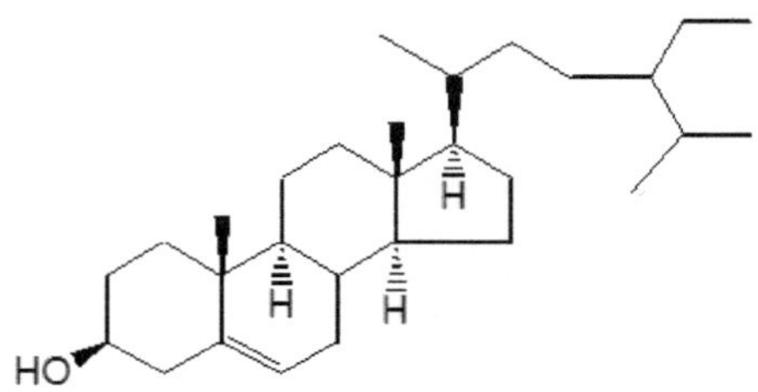

2.2.2. Isolation and Characterization of Compound B

A light brown solid was obtained after removal of the solvent of acetone and methanol (1:1) as light yellow needles, 2.85 g/30 g (9.5% w/w), m.p. 301–302 °C. The compound was insoluble in pet ether, sparingly soluble in benzene, ethyl acetate and acetone, soluble in methanol and NaOH solution. It gave a blue-green color with alcoholic $FeCl_3$, a reddish brown colour in Shinoda's test and a yellow color showing light green fluorescence with conc. H_2SO_4 indicating its flavonoid nature. It gave a dark bright yellow spot on the TLC plate when viewed in UV light. IR (ν_{max}) cm^{-1} (KBr): 3450–3100 (broad), 3040, 3010, 1660, 1590, 1520, 1230, 1200, 1180, 910, 830, 820 and 790; ^{1}HNMR (δ ppm, $CDCl_3$ + DMSO-d_6): 12.31 (OH, s), 10.25 (OH, s), 8.87 (OH, s), 8.68 (OH, s), 8.31 (OH, s), 7.81–7.62 (2H, m), 7.00 (1H, d), 6.50 (1H, d) and 6.32 (1H, d); MS *m*/*z*: 302(M$^+$), 301,235, 284, 152, 137, 135, 132, 105, 95, 89, 77, *etc.*

On the basis of ^{1}HNMR and mass spectral studies of compound B, it was characterized as quercetin (Figure 2) with molecular formula $C_{15}H_{10}O_7$ and comparable with the literature of quercetin [9,11].

Figure 2. Compound B.

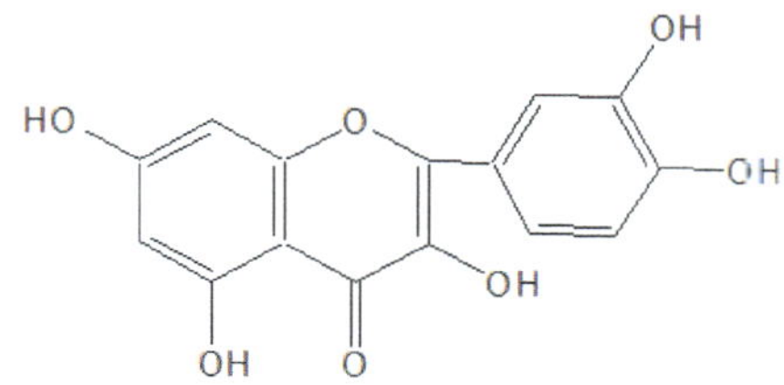

2.2.3. Isolation and Characterization of Compound C

The methanol fraction afforded a greenish-yellow solid after removal of solvent, which was recrystallized with aqueous ethanol as light yellow needles, 4.95 g/30 g (16.5% w/w), m.p. 274–276 °C. It dissolved in alkali, to give a green colour with alcoholic $FeCl_3$ and a fluorescent blue colour with conc. H_2SO_4. It gave the positive Shinoda's test characteristic for flavonoids (to a pinch of substance in 1 mL alcohol, magnesium and a few drops of conc. HCl were added) where it gave a dark red color. In UV light on TLC plates it displayed a yellow color spot with an R_f value 0.95 in the following system; ethyl acetate: formic acid: glacial acetic acid: water (51:11:11:27). IR (ν_{max}) cm^{-1} (KBr): 3380, 3050, 3020, 1680, 1590, 1490, 1410, 1220, 1150, 910, 830, and 780; ^{1}HNMR (δ ppm, $CDCl_3$ + DMSO-d_6): 12.25 (1H, s), 10.18 (1H, s), 9.56 (1H, s), 8.12 (2H, d), 7.62 (1H, s), 6.93 (2H, d), 6.43 (1H, d) and 6.25 (1H, d); MS *m*/*z*: 286(M^+), 285, 269, 268, 152, 121, 105, 95, 89, 77, *etc.*

On the basis of ^{1}HNMR and mass spectral studies of compound C, it was characterized as kaempferol (Figure 3) with molecular formula $C_{15}H_{10}O_6$ and comparable with the literature of kaempferol [11,12].

Figure 3. Compound C.

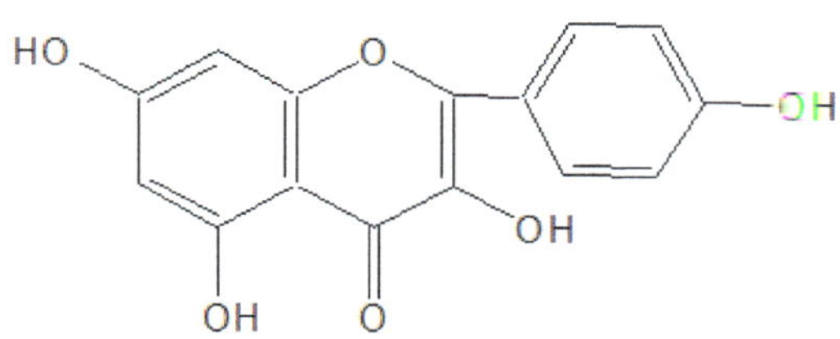

2.3. Silymarin

Silymarin was purchased from MP Biomedicals, France and it was dissolved in olive oil for oral administration to rats during experimentation at the dose level-25 mg/kg body weight/day [13].

2.4. Chemicals

All chemicals were analytical grade and chemicals required for all biochemical assays were obtained from Sigma Chemicals Co., St. Louis, MO, USA.

2.5. Animal Model

Colony bred healthy, adult male albino rats (wistar strain) (*Rattus norvegicus*) weighing 175–200 g were used in the present study. The rats were housed in polypropylene cages under controlled conditions of temperature (23–26 °C), humidity (60%–70%) and light (12 h light/dark cycle). They were provided with a nutritionally adequate standard laboratory diet (Lipton, India Ltd., Bangalore, India) and tap water *ad libitum*.

2.6. Ethical Aspects

The study was approved by the ethical committee (Protocol No. 1678/Go/a/12/CPCSEA/73) of the University Department of Zoology, Jaipur, India. Indian National Science Academy, New Delhi, (INSA, 2000) guidelines were followed for maintenance and use of the experimental animals.

2.7. Chronic Toxicity

The extract of plant material was administered to all the test groups in graded doses ranging up to 3 g/kg body weight and the rats were observed for signs of toxicity and mortality for 60 days afterward. The extract was found to be practically non-toxic when given orally to rats and its LD_{50} value was found to be higher than 3 g/kg body weight [data not shown]. The minimum dose levels viz. 100, 200 and 400 mg/kg body weight were used for oral administration to rats during experimentation [14].

2.8. Treatment Design

After acclimatization of 15 days, the animals were divided into the following groups containing 06 animals in each group:

- Group I: Vehicle treated rats were kept on normal diet and served as control for 60 days.
- Group II: Rats were intoxicated with carbon tetrachloride (CCl_4) at the dose level of 0.3 mL/kg body weight/twice a week, intra-peritoneally for 60 days.
- Group III: Rats orally received *M. oleifera* extract at 100 mg/kg body weight/day, and CCl_4 as Group II for 60 days, simultaneously.
- Group IV: Rats orally received *M. oleifera* extract at 200 mg/kg body weight/day, and CCl_4 as Group II for 60 days, simultaneously.
- Group V: Rats orally received *M. oleifera* extract at 400 mg/kg body weight/day, and CCl_4 as Group II for 60 days, simultaneously.
- Group VI: Rats orally received silymarin (as a reference standard drug) at 25 mg/kg body weight/day and CCl_4 as Group II for 60 days, simultaneously.

2.9. Autopsy Schedule

After the last dose-delivery, rats of each group were kept on starvation for 24 h and after that anaesthetized under mild ether anesthesia. Blood samples were collected by cardiac puncture. The blood samples of each animal were taken and allowed to clot at 37 °C and the serum was separated by centrifugation then stored at 4 °C until assayed.

After the collection of blood, the liver was immediately excised, washed with cold normal saline, blotted, and weighed on an electrical balance. Half of the liver was fixed in Bouin's fixative for histological studies and the remaining half was immediately frozen (at −20°/−70 °C) for biochemical analysis.

2.10. Analysis and Processing of the Samples

The biochemical analysis of enzymes in serum samples *viz.* serum glutamic oxaloacetic transaminase (SGOT), serum glutamic pyruvic transaminase (SGPT), gamma glutamyl transpeptidase (GGT), lactate dehydrogenase (LDH), alkaline phosphatase (ALP), acid phosphatase ACP) and total bilirubin, total protein and albumin were performed using kit methods. SGOT (Batch No. 61105), SGPT (Batch No. 60865) and GGT (Batch No. 34004) kits were purchased from Accurex Biomedical Pvt. Ltd.; Mumbai, India. LDH (LOT. No. 6854), ALP (LOT. No.7093), ACP (LOT. No.6666), total bilirubin (LOT. No. 6801), total protein (LOT. No. 6808) and albumin (LOT. No. 6988) kits were purchased from Span Diagnostics Ltd., Surat, India, respectively.

In tissue samples, a part of liver tissue was minced and homogenized in ice-cold 1.15% w/v KCl in a Potter Elvehjem Teflon glass homogenizer for 1 min to make a 10% w/v liver homogenate. Lipid peroxidation (LPO) [15] was measured in the liver homogenate. The quantitative estimation of hepatic antioxidant enzymes such as superoxide dismutase (SOD) [16], catalase (CAT) [17], reduced glutathione (GSH) [18], glutathione reductase (GR) [19], and glutathione peroxidase (GPx) [20] were performed in liver homogenate also, respectively.

2.11. Histopathology

Liver was fixed in Bouin's fixative for 24 h and after that dehydrated in ethanol series (50%–100%), cleared in xylene, and embedded in paraffin using the standard microtechnique. Sections of the liver (5 μm) were stained with alum haematoxylin and eosin (H-E) for histopathological changes.

2.12. Statistical Analysis

Statistical analysis was performed using one-way analysis of variance (ANOVA) followed by student "*t*" test. The values are mean ± S.E. for six rats in each group. p values ≤0.05 were considered as significant.

3. Results

CCl_4-intoxication to rats for the period of 60 days resulted in a significant ($p \leq 0.001$) rise in the levels of SGOT, SGPT, GGT, LDH, ALP, ACP and total bilirubin along with notable reduction ($p \leq 0.01$) in the levels of total protein and albumin in serum when compared with normal controls (Figures 4–7).

The effect of *M. oleifera* leaves extract on serum—SGOT, SGPT, GGT, LDH, ALP, ACP and total bilirubin in CCl_4-induced rats—was found to be reduced significantly ($p \leq 0.001$) along with remarkable elevation in the total protein and albumin at all three dose levels (Group III–V) as compared to CCl_4-treated Group II. The dose level of 400 mg/kg of *M. oleifera* was most effective but the attenuation of altered serum parameters was not as high as in silymarin treated rats of Group VI (Figures 4–7).

Figure 4. Changes in the activity of serum glutamic oxaloacetic transaminase (SGOT), serum glutamic pyruvic transaminase (SGPT), gamma glutamyl transpeptidase (GGT), lactate dehydrogenase (LDH) in serum after various treatments of *M. oleifera* leaves extract and silymarin in rats. Data points with different symbol and letter notations are significantly different at *** $p \leq 0.001$: Group II compared to Group I, [a] $p \leq 0.001$: Group III–VI compared to Group II, [d] $p \leq 0.001$: Group IV–VI compared to Group III, [g] $p \leq 0.001$: Group V & VI compared to Group IV, [j] $p \leq 0.001$; [k] $p \leq 0.01$: Group VI compared to Group V.

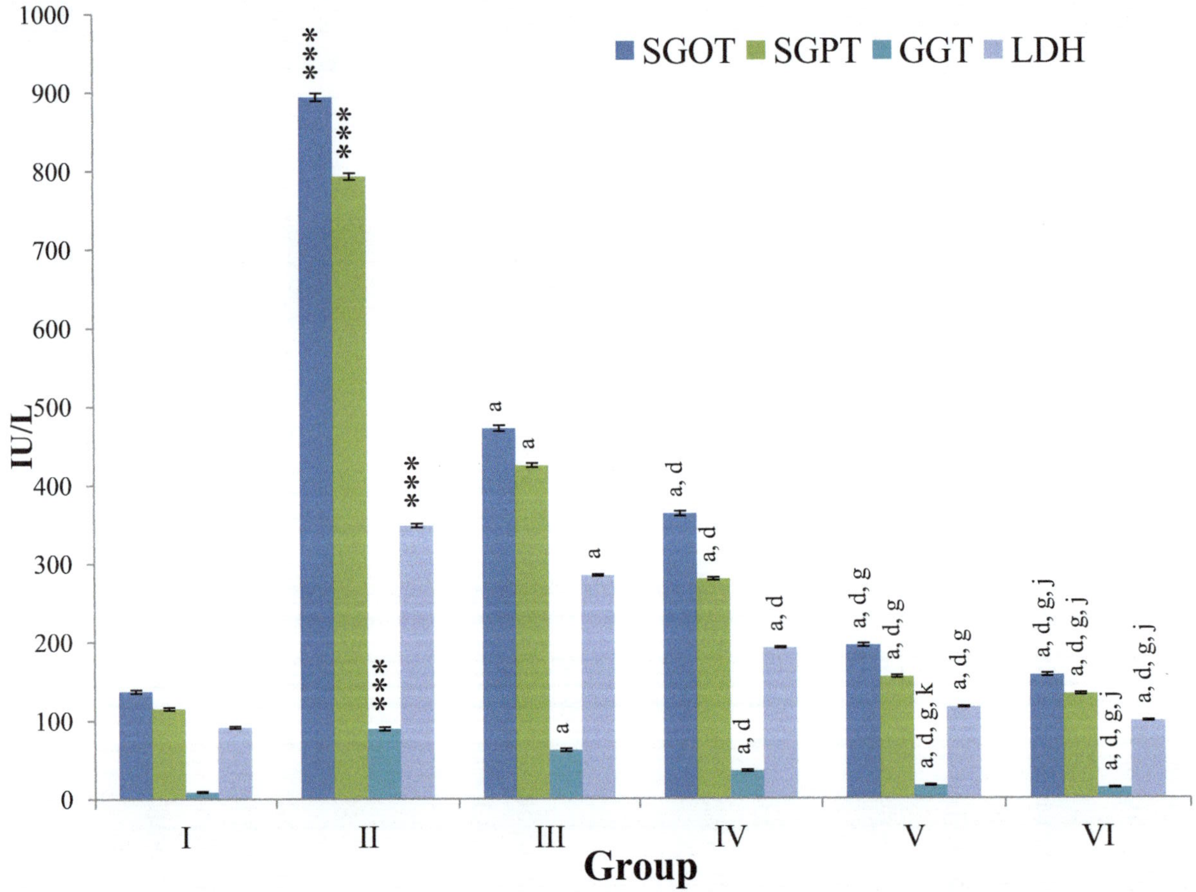

Figure 5. Changes in the activity of alkaline phosphatase (ALP), and acid phosphatase (ACP) in serum after various treatments of *M. oleifera* leaves extract and silymarin in rats. Data points with different symbol and letter notations are significantly different at $^{***}p \leq 0.001$ Group II compared to Group I, $^{a}p \leq 0.001$: Group III–VI compared to Group II, $^{d}p \leq 0.001$: Group IV–VI compared to Group III, $^{g}p \leq 0.001$: Group V & VI compared to Group IV, $^{k}p \leq 0.01$; $^{l}p \leq 0.05$: Group VI compared to Group V.

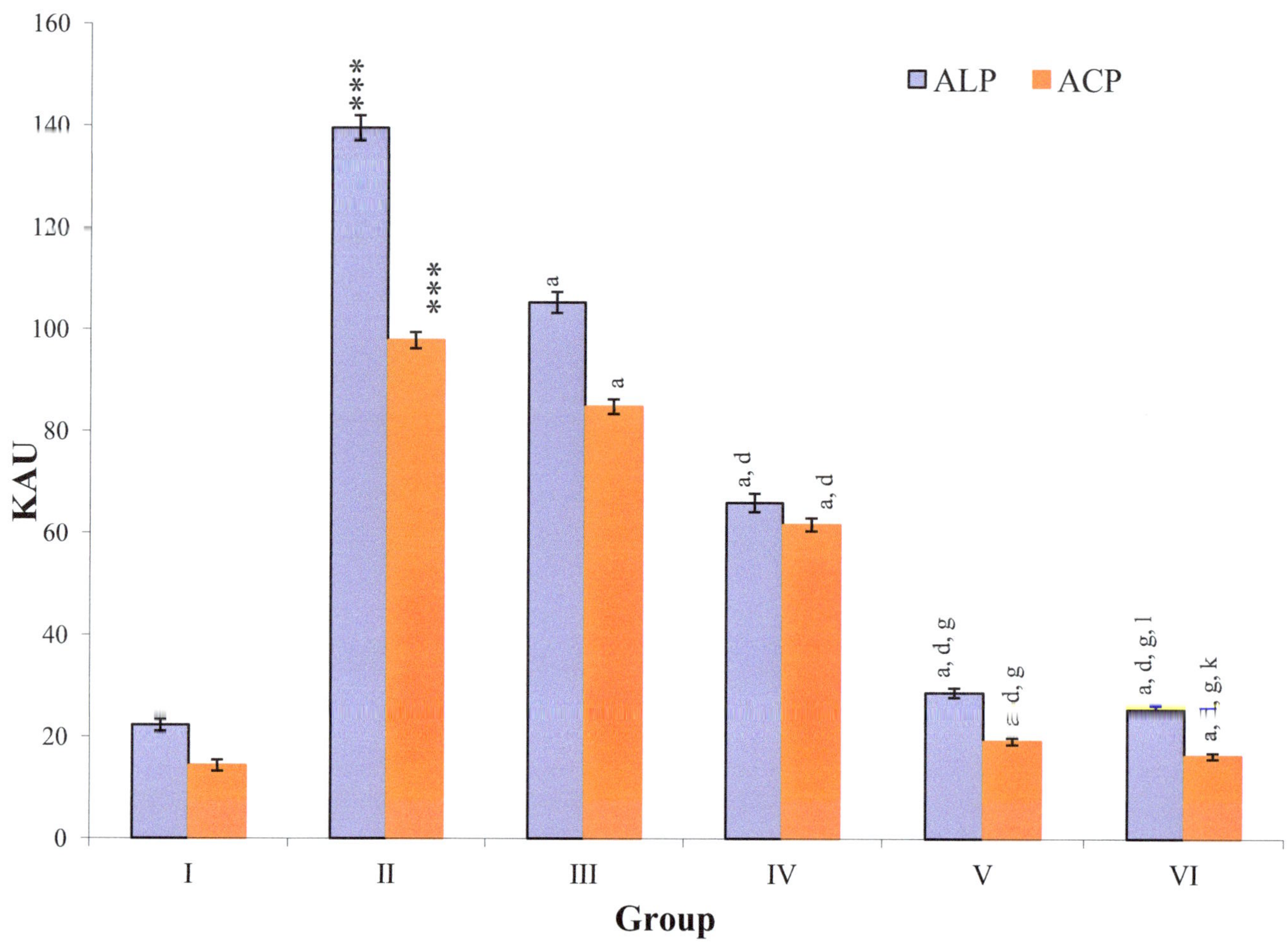

Figure 6. Changes in the total bilirubin concentration in serum after various treatments of *M. oleifera* leaves extract and silymarin in rats. Data points with different symbol and letter notations are significantly different at $^{***}p \leq 0.001$ Group II compared to Group I, $^{a}p \leq 0.001$; $^{b}p \leq 0.01$; ^{ns} non significant: Group III–VI compared to Group II, $^{d}p \leq 0.001$: Group IV–VI compared to Group III, $^{g}p \leq 0.001$: Group V & VI compared to Group IV, ^{ns} non significant: Group VI compared to Group V.

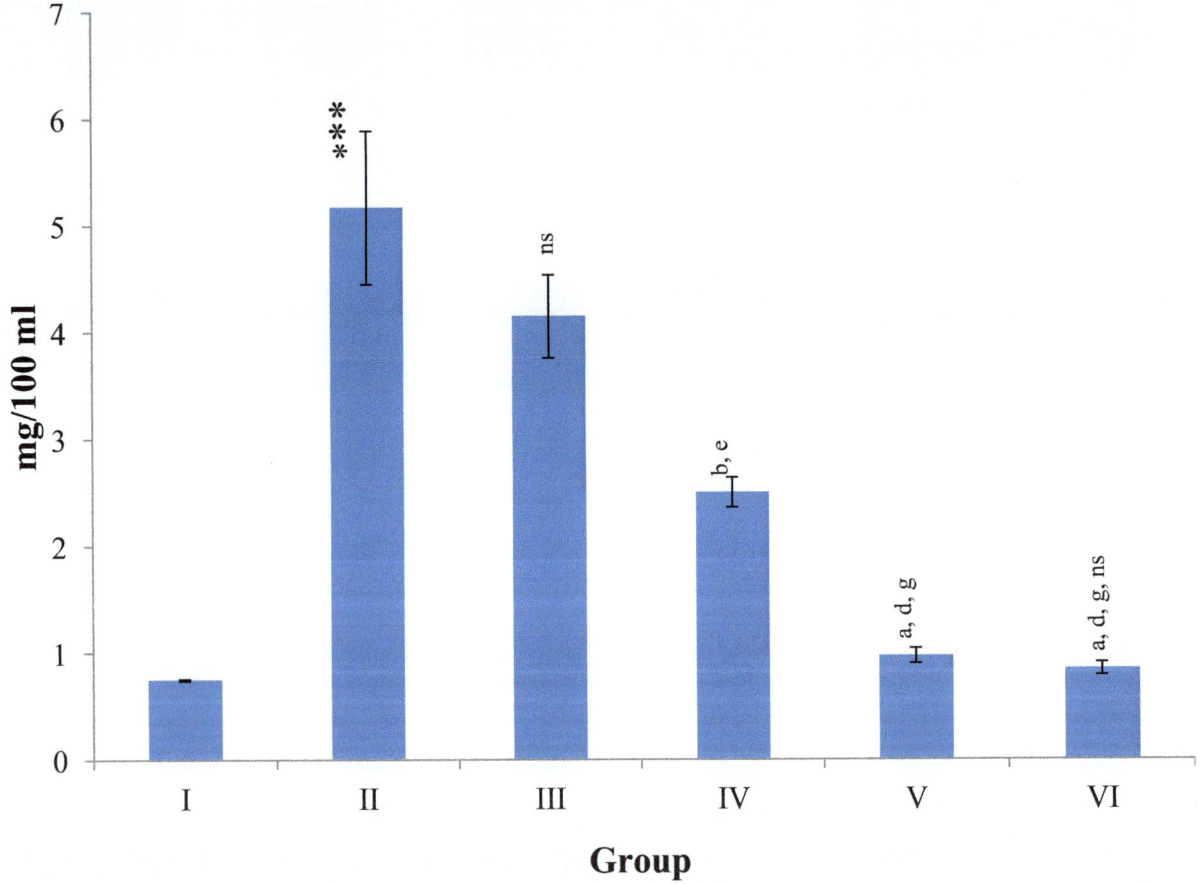

Figure 7. Changes in the total protein and albumin in serum after various treatments of *M. oleifera* leaves extract and silymarin in rats. Data points with different symbol and letter notations are significantly different at $^{**}p \leq 0.01$ Group II compared to Group I, $^{a}p \leq 0.001$; $^{b}p \leq 0.01$; $^{c}p \leq 0.05$; ^{ns} non significant: Group III–VI compared to Group II, $^{d}p \leq 0.001$; $^{f}p \leq 0.05$; ^{ns} non significant: Group IV–VI compared to Group III, $^{g}p \leq 0.001$; $^{h}p \leq 0.01$; ^{ns} non significant: Group V & VI compared to Group IV, ^{ns} non significant: Group VI compared to Group V.

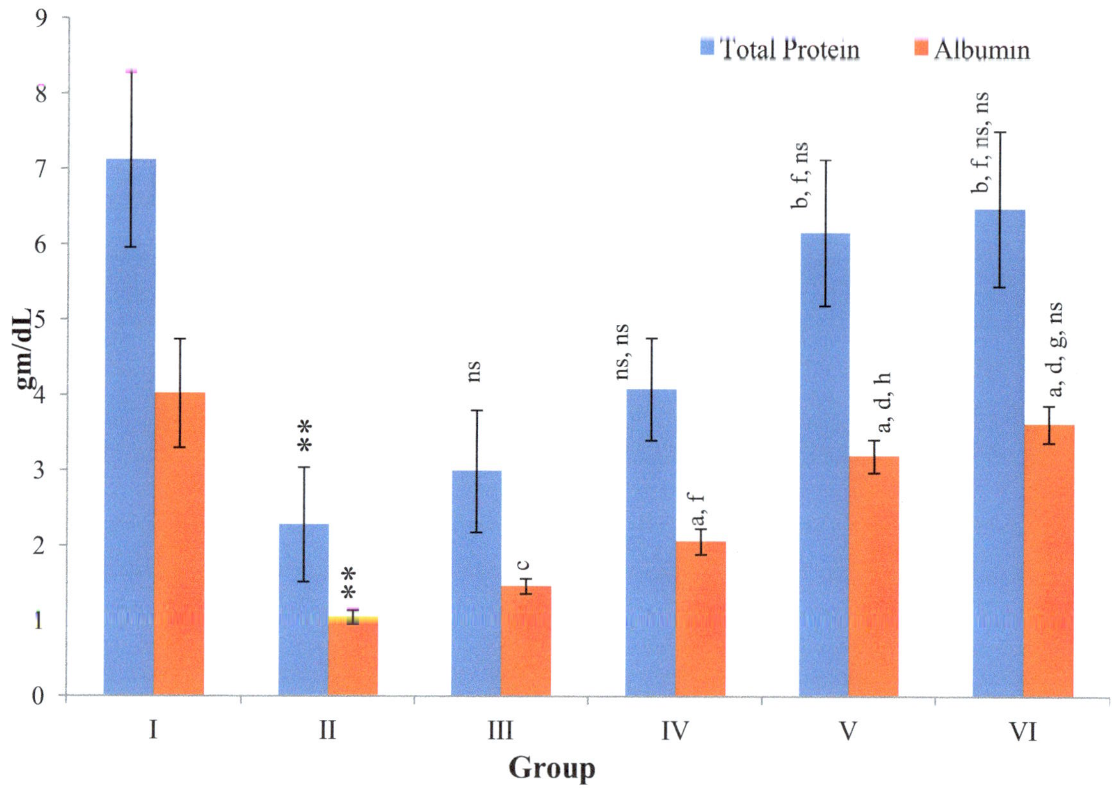

Figure 8 illustrates a significant ($p \leq 0.001$) increase in the level of hepatic LPO in CCl_4 intoxicated rats as compared to normal controls. Treatment with *M. oleifera* leaves extract significantly ($p \leq 0.05$; $p \leq 0.001$) prevented this rise in LPO level at all three dose levels (Group III–V). The silymarin treated group VI showed non-significant decline in the level of hepatic LPO as compared to higher dose level (400 mg/kg) of *M. oleifera* extract treated rats (Group V).

Figure 8. Changes in the lipid peroxidation in liver after various treatments of *M. oleifera* leaves extract and silymarin in rats. Data points with different symbol and letter notations are significantly different at *** $p \leq 0.001$: Group II compared to Group I, ^{a} $p \leq 0.001$; ^{c} $p \leq 0.05$: Group III–VI compared to Group II, ^{d} $p \leq 0.001$; ^{e} $p \leq 0.01$: Group IV–VI compared to Group III, ^{g} $p \leq 0.001$: Group V & VI compared to Group IV, ^{ns} non significant: Group VI compared to Group V.

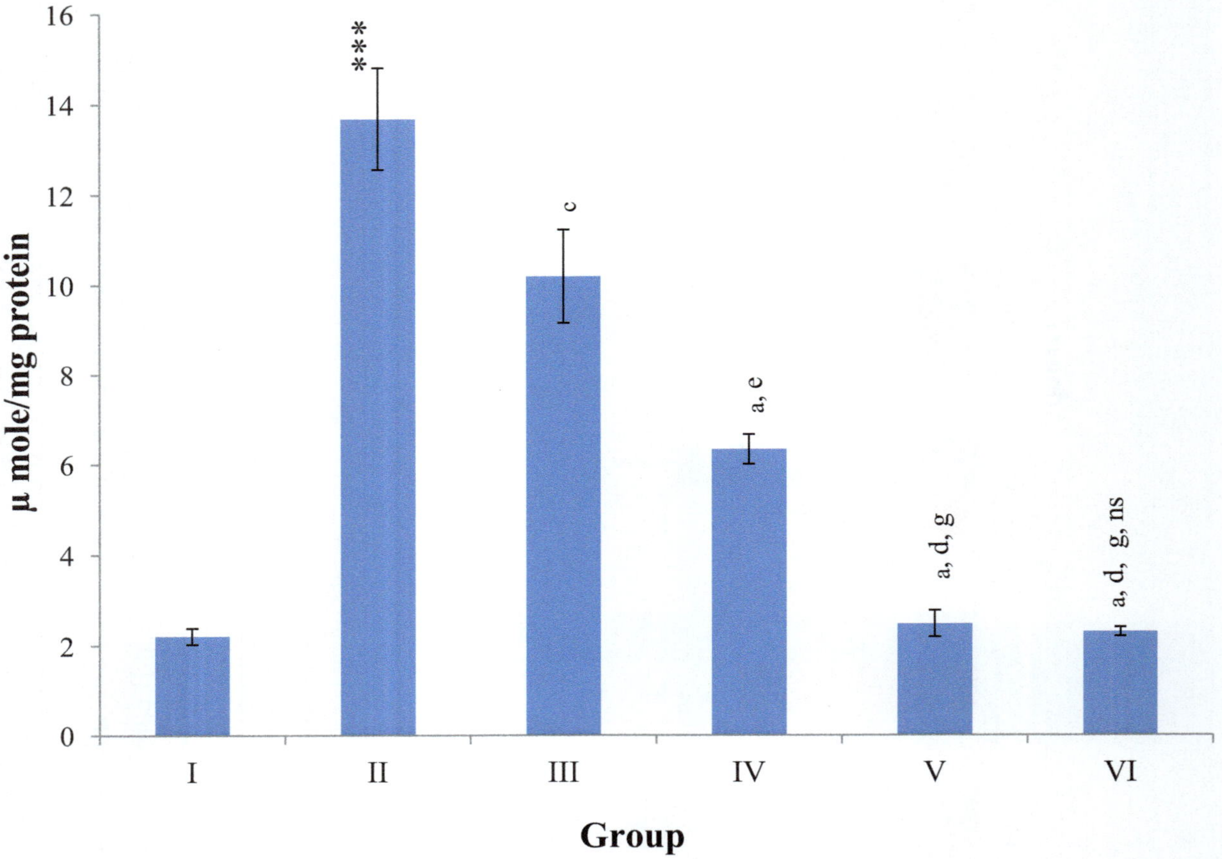

Hepatic SOD, CAT, GSH, GR and GPx contents were elevated significantly ($p \leq 0.001$) in extract treated animals at 400 mg/kg dose level (Group V) but also showed non-significant to significant ($p \leq 0.05$; $p \leq 0.01$; $p \leq 0.001$ respectively) elevation in the levels of all the above antioxidant parameters at 100 and 200 mg/kg dose levels (Group III and VI) whereas CCl_4-intoxicated Group II was shown to have a highly significant ($p \leq 0.001$) decrease in the all above antioxidant contents as compared to normal controls. Therefore, the dose levels of 400 mg/kg of *M. oleifera* extract also exhibited again as a most effective dose but showed a non-significant elevation compared to silymarin treated rats of Group VI (Figures 9–12).

Figure 9. Changes in the superoxide dismutage (SOD) in liver after various treatments of *M. oleifera* leaves extract and silymarin in rats. Data points with different symbol and letter notations are significantly different at *** $p \leq 0.001$: Group II compared to Group I, ^{a} $p \leq 0.001$; ^{c} $p \leq 0.05$: Group III–VI compared to Group II, ^{d} $p \leq 0.001$; ^{f} $p \leq 0.05$: Group IV–VI compared to Group III, ^{h} $p \leq 0.01$: Group V & VI compared to Group IV, ^{ns} non significant: Group VI compared to Group V.

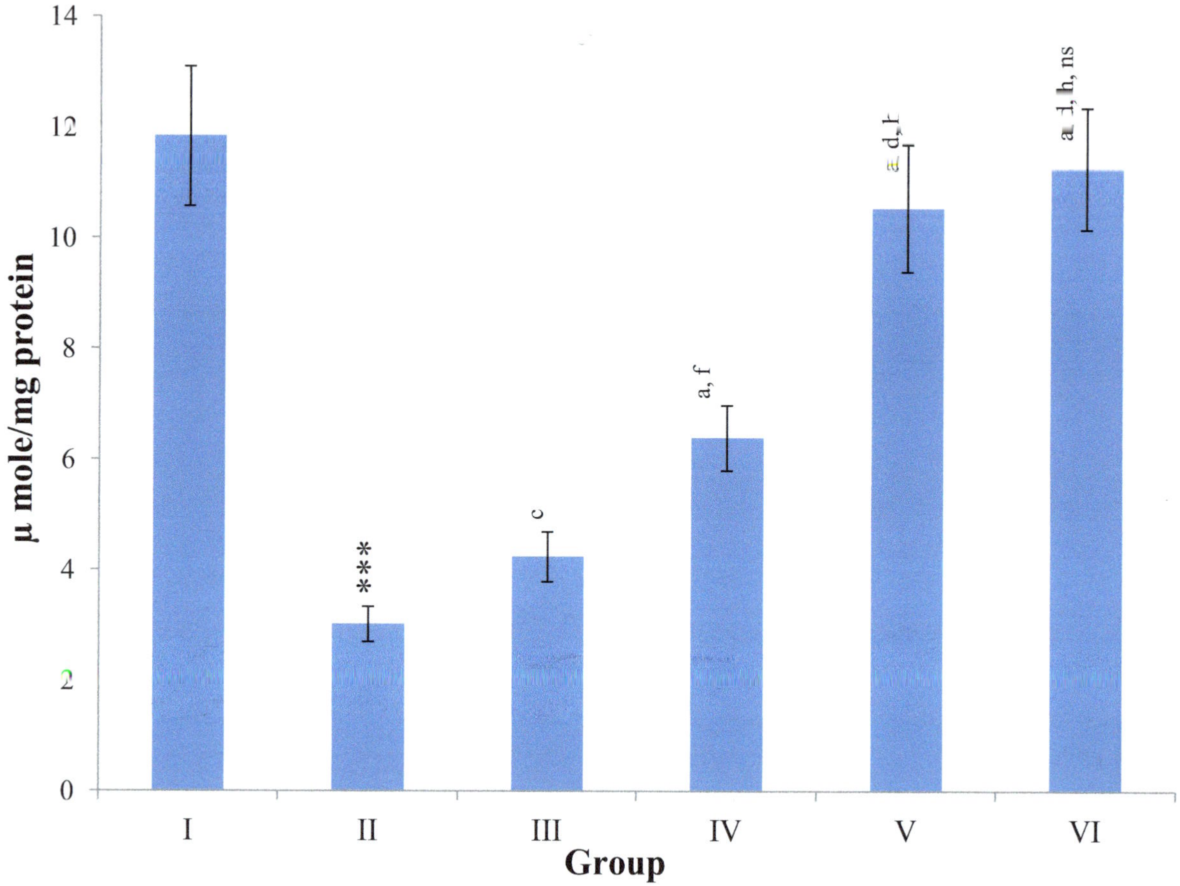

Figure 10. Changes in the catalase in liver after various treatments of *M. oleifera* leaves extract and silymarin in rats. Data points with different symbol and letter notations are significantly different at *** $p \leq 0.001$: Group II compared to Group I, ^{a} $p \leq 0.001$: Group III–VI compared to Group II, ^{d} $p \leq 0.001$: Group IV–VI compared to Group III, ^{g} $p \leq 0.001$: Group V & VI compared to Group IV, ^{ns} non significant: Group VI compared to Group V.

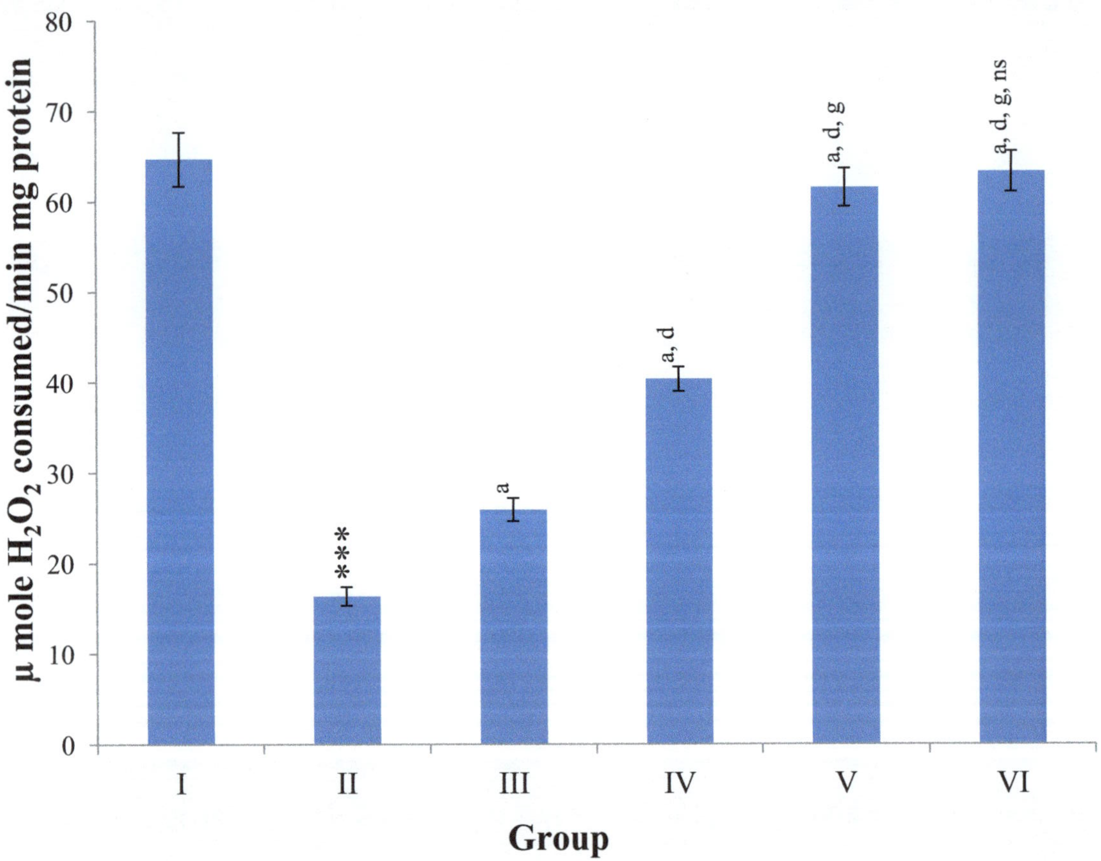

Figure 11. Changes in the glutathione (reduced) in liver after various treatments of *M. oleifera* leaves extract and silymarin in rats. Data points with different symbol and letter notations are significantly different at *** $p \leq 0.001$: Group II compared to Group I, ^{a} $p \leq 0.001$; ^{b} $p \leq 0.01$: Group III–VI compared to Group II, ^{d} $p \leq 0.001$; ^{f} $p \leq 0.05$: Group IV–VI compared to Group III, ^{g} $p \leq 0.001$: Group V & VI compared to Group IV, ^{ns} non significant: Group VI compared to Group V.

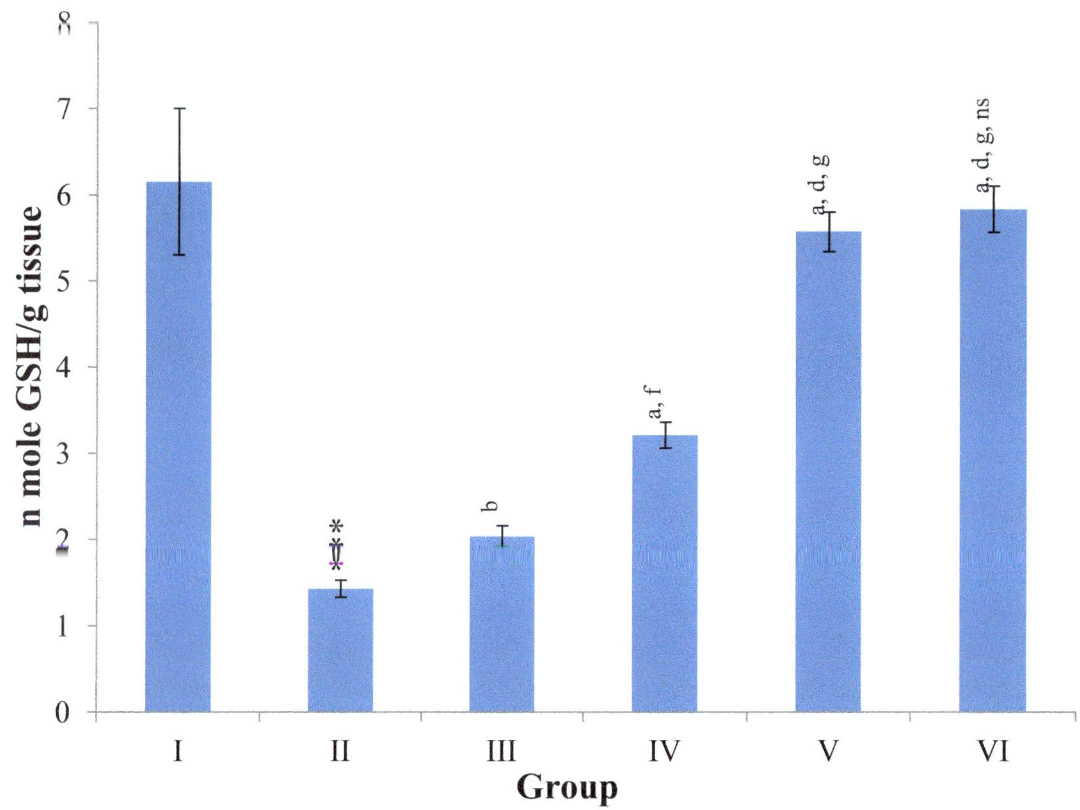

Figure 12. Changes in the glutathione reductase (GR) and glutathione peroxidase (GPx) in liver after various treatments of *M. oleifera* leaves extract and silymarin in rats. Data points with different symbol and letter notations are significantly different at *** $p \leq 0.001$: Group II compared to Group I, $^{a}p \leq 0.001$; $^{c}p \leq 0.05$; ^{ns} non significant: Group III–VI compared to Group II, $^{d}p \leq 0.001$; $^{e}p \leq 0.01$; ^{ns} non significant: Group IV–VI compared to Group III, $^{h}p \leq 0.01$; $^{i}p \leq 0.05$: Group V & VI compared to Group IV, ^{ns} non significant: Group VI compared to Group V.

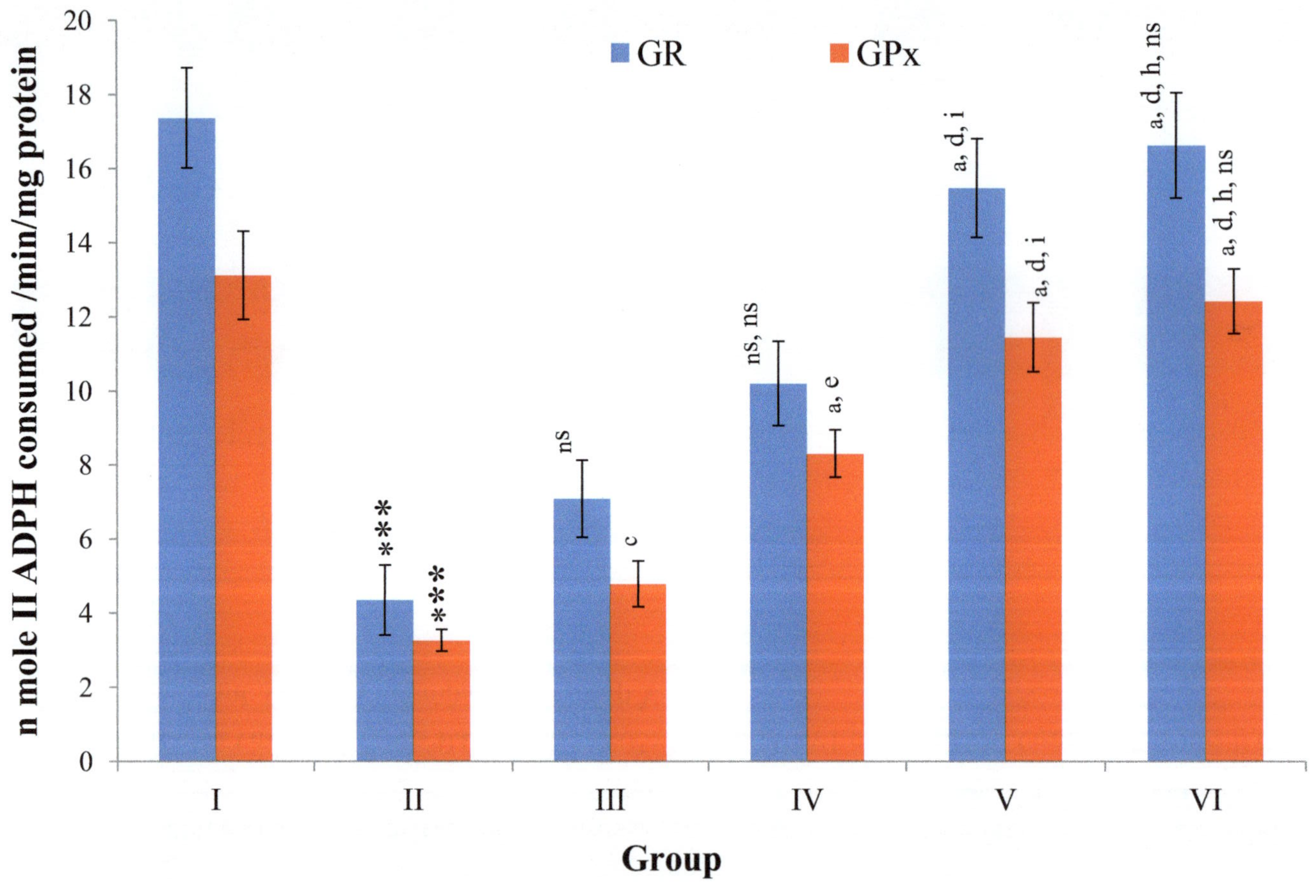

The histopathology of CCl_4-intoxicated rats when compared with normal hepatic architecture (Figure 13) showed massive fatty changes, necrosis, ballooning degeneration and the loss of cellular boundaries (Figure 14). The liver sections of *M. oleifera* extract at 100 mg/kg dose level plus CCl_4-treated rats (Group III) showed mild prevention of CCl_4-induced degenerative changes with the few pyknotic nuclei and fatty vacuolization in cytoplasm (Figure 15). The liver sections of extract treated rats at the dose level of 200 mg/kg along with CCl_4 (Group VI) indicated partial amelioration of degenerative effects in hepatocytes but still showed cloudy swelling and mild fatty changes (Figure 16). Histomorphological picture of liver sections of *M. oleifera* extract at the dose level of 400 mg/kg along with CCl_4-induction to rats (Group V) showed more or less normal lobular pattern with the devoid of degenerative changes and preserved cytoplasm with prominent nucleus without intracellular lipid accumulation (Figure 17) almost comparable to the normal control and silymarin treated Group VI (Figure 18).

Figure 13. Photomicrograph of control rat liver section (60 days) showing well brought central vein, hepatic cells with preserved cytoplasm and prominent nucleus at H & E × 100.

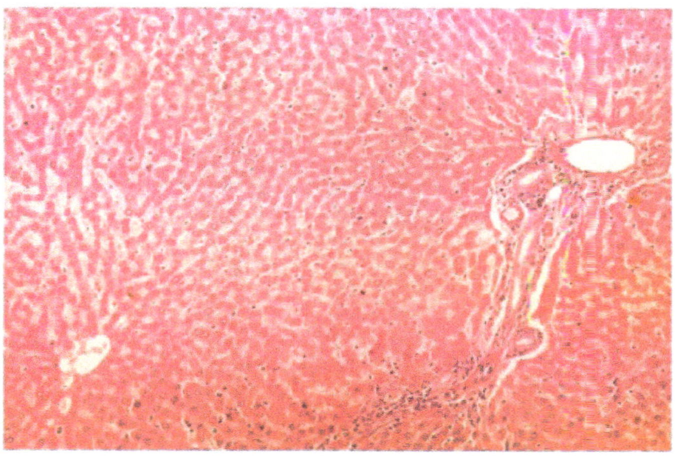

Figure 14. Photomicrograph of rat liver section with CCl_4 treatment (60 days) showing marked steatosis of the hepatocytes with ballooning degeneration and distended portal veins and necrosis at H & E × 100.

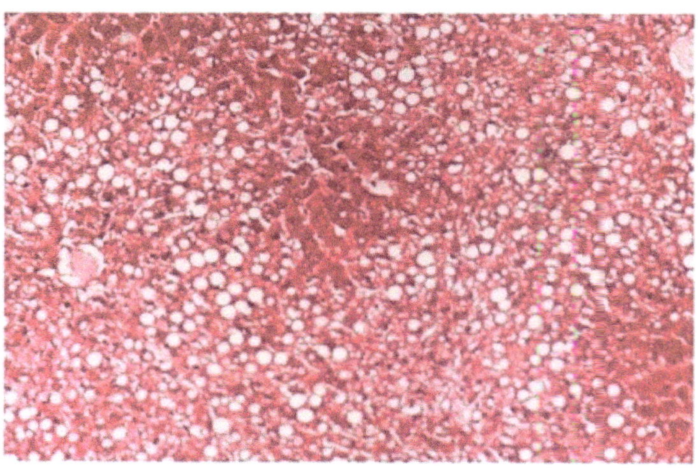

Figure 15. Photomicrograph of rat liver section of CCl_4 + *M. oleifera* extract at 100 mg/kg (60 days) showing slight reduction in fatty degenerative changes with congestion of sinusoids, necrosis and infiltration of polymorphonucleocytes at H & E × 100.

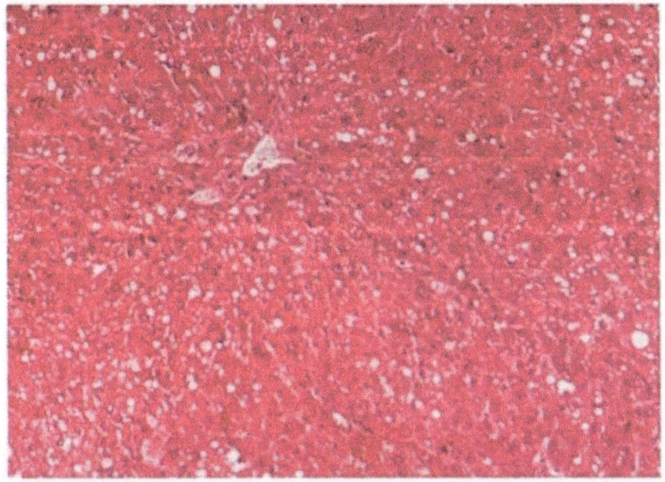

Figure 16. Photomicrograph of rat liver section of CCl_4 + *M. oleifera* extract at 200 mg/kg (60 days) showing considerable reduction in necrosis and fatty changes with pyknotic nuclei and cytoplasmic clearing at H & E × 100.

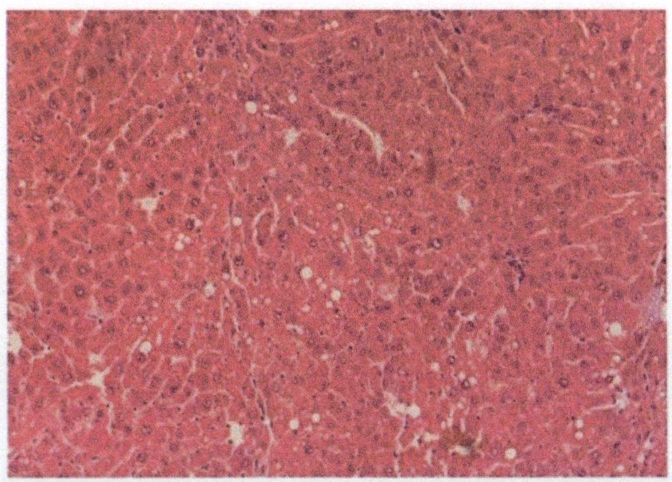

Figure 17. Photomicrograph of rat liver section of CCl_4 + *M. oleifera* extract at 400 mg/kg (60 days) showing moderately brought central vein, hepatic cells with preserved cytoplasm and prominent nucleus at H & E × 100.

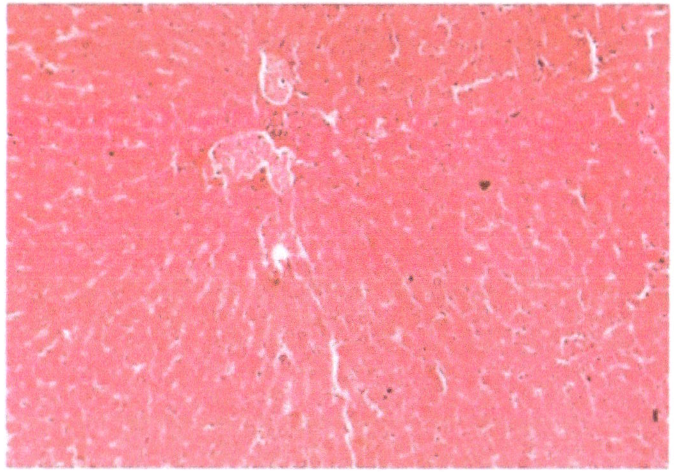

Figure 18. Photomicrograph of rat liver section of CCl_4 + silymarin at 25 mg/kg (60 days) depicting histological pattern almost similar to liver of normal rats with preserved cytoplasm and prominent nucleus at H & E × 100.

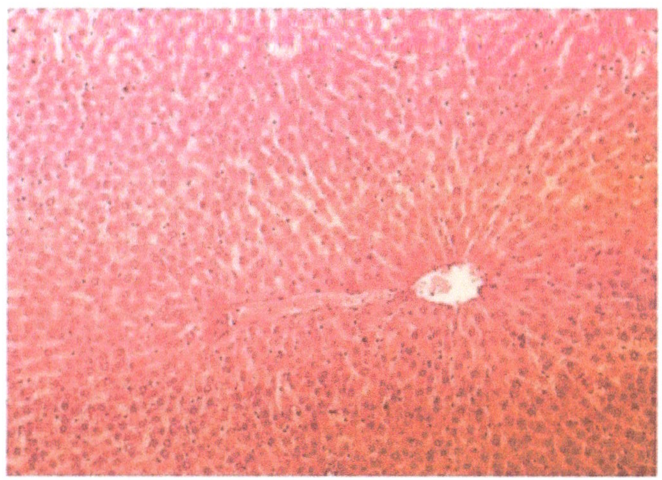

4. Discussion

It is generally accepted in the scientific world that the hepatotoxicity induced by CCl_4 is due to the formation of the active metabolite, trichloromethyl free radical ($CCl_3^{\bullet}$). This then readily interacts with molecular oxygen to form the trichloromethyl peroxy radical ($CCl_3OO^{\bullet}$). Both radicals are capable of binding to proteins and other macromolecules with simultaneous attack on poly-unsaturated fatty acids to produce lipid peroxidation leading to hepatotoxicity [21].

Lipid peroxidation of hepatic cell membrane is one of the principle causes of hepatic injury induced by CCl_4 or other hepatotoxicants. This is because lipid peroxidation is viewed as a complicated biochemical reaction involving free radicals, metal ions, oxygen and a host of many different factors in the biological system. Also in recent years, lipids and their derivatives have been recognized as important molecules in signal transduction [22].

The efficacy of any liver curative drug depends on its capacity of either reducing the harmful effect or restoring the normal hepatic physiology that has been made anxious by CCl_4 and/or other hepatotoxicants [23]. In our present study, the measurement of LPO in the liver tissue is a convenient method to monitor oxidative cell damage. Inhibition of elevated LPO has been observed in *M. oleifera* extract and silymarin treated groups due to its antioxidant and free radical scavenging activities through re-establishment of biomembranes of hepatic parenchymal cells [24].

In agreement with results obtained in previous investigations [25,26], our present study elicited a significant increase in the activities of SGOT, SGPT, GGT, LDH, ALP, and ACP with the exposure to CCl_4 which is indicated by cellular leakage and loss of functional integrity of the hepatic cell membrane [27,28]. Oral treatment with *M. oleifera* extract and silymarin attenuated these increased enzyme activities produced by CCl_4 and a subsequent recovery towards normalization of these enzymes strongly suggests the possibility of *M. oleifera* extract being able to affect the hepatocytes so as to cause accelerated regeneration of parenchymal cells and lysosomes, thus protecting against lysosomal integrity and cell membrane fragility, and therefore decreasing the leakage of marker enzymes into the circulation [25]. Stabilization of serum total bilirubin level by the administration of *M. oleifera* extract is further a clear signal of the improvement of the functional status of the hepatic cells [29].

The significant reduction in the total protein and albumin levels in serum with exposure to CCl_4 causes considerable liver damage through induction of peroxidation of lipids and finally inhibits the protein synthesis due to trichloromethyl free radical covalent bindings [30]. The treatment with *M. oleifera* extract and silymarin stabilized the serum total protein and albumin levels. The stabilization of proteins might be considered as an indication of enhanced protein synthesis in the hepatic cells due to inhibition of peroxidation of lipids and scavenge of the free radicals [31].

The antioxidant defense mechanisms include enzymatic and non-enzymatic antioxidants playing a significant role in the sustaining of physiological levels of O_2 and H_2O_2 and eradicating the peroxides generated from inadvertent exposure to toxic drugs. Any natural medications with antioxidant profiles may help to maintain health when continuously taken as components of dietary food, spices or remedies. Among the antioxidant enzymes, SOD and catalase are the first line of defense against CCl_4 induced hepatic oxidative damage. SOD is the primary step of the defense mechanism in the antioxidant system against oxidative stress by catalyzing the dismutation of superoxide radicals (O^{2-})

into molecular oxygen (O_2) and hydrogen peroxide (H_2O_2). H_2O_2 is neutralized by the action of catalase [32]. A significant depletion in the activities of hepatic SOD and catalase during CCl_4 intoxication to rats might be due to the enhanced superoxide radical formation leading to oxidative stress in the tissue. Administration of *M. oleifera* extract to CCl_4 treated rats enhanced the SOD and catalase profiles, dose-dependently, by acting as a strong free radical quencher and protecting the hepatic cells. Therefore SOD and catalase are essential for the endogenous antioxidative defense system to scavenge reactive oxygen species and maintain the cellular redox balance [33,34].

GSH is one of the most abundant tripeptide, non-enzymatic biological antioxidants present in the hepatocytes, which is a key component of the overall antioxidant defense system that protects the membrane protein thiols of hepatocytes from deleterious effects of reactive oxygen metabolites such as hydrogen peroxide and superoxide radicals [35]. The decline of GSH level in the CCl_4 treated group might be due to its utilization by the excessively generated quantity of free radicals in the hepatocytes leading to hepatic injury. However, the subsequent recovery in rats treated with *M. oleifera* extract might be due to *de-novo* GSH synthesis or GSH regeneration (GSSG to GSH), dose-dependently.

After the CCl_4 induced oxidative liver damage, GPx along with catalase metabolize H_2O_2 to water and other non-toxic substances. This antioxidant system also consists of GSH and a range of functionally interrelated enzymes, of which GR and GPx are responsible for the regeneration of GSH or from GSSG to GSH, where both enzymes work together with GSH in the decomposition of hydrogen peroxide and also other biological hydroperoxides [36]. The dose-dependent reversal of GR and GPx activity to near normal level with the *M. oleifera* extract treatment showed the antioxidant activity of plant extract by scavenging the endogenous metabolic peroxides generated after CCl_4 induced damage in the liver tissue.

Histopathological observations suggested that the reactive oxygen species and lipid peroxidation may play an important role in pathogenesis of hepatocytes as hepatic fibrosis and necrosis with the loss of normal liver architecture. Because of CCl_4 toxicity, a toxic reactive metabolite trichloromethyl free radical was produced which binds covalently to macromolecules of the lipid membranes of adipose tissue and causes peroxidative degradation. As a result, fats from the adipose tissue are translocated and accumulated in the hepatocytes [24,36,37]. The degenerative changes were shown to be minimal or absent with the plant extract treatment, dose-dependently. This might be due to lower fat accumulation and re-establishment of the antioxidant defense system in the liver tissue through the antioxidant and hepatoprotective nature of *M. oleifera* leaves.

5. Conclusions

The antioxidant and hepatoprotective potential of *M. oleifera* leaves extract may be attributed to the presence of total phenolics and flavonoids in the extract and/or isolated active constituents—β-sitosterol, quercetin and kaempferol—which have hydroxyl group(s). The hydroxyl group(s), because of its resonance property, easily donates e^- to free radicals and effectively neutralizes them. Also, the presence of a hydroxyl group(s) increases its antioxidant potential through intermolecular hydrogen bonding involving the -SH group of non-protein thiols and enzymes resulting in the restoration of the antioxidant system against oxidative damage in mammalian liver tissue.

Acknowledgments

The authors are thankful to the Coordinator, Centre for Advanced Studies, and Head, Department of Zoology, University of Rajasthan, Jaipur, India and the Principal, Dyal Singh College, University of Delhi, New Delhi, India and also gratified to M. P. Dobhal, Department of Chemistry, University of Rajasthan, Jaipur, India, for providing the necessary amenities.

Author Contributions

Dharmendra Singh and Radhey Shyam Gupta contributed in experimental design and data analysis. Dharmendra Singh, Priya Vrat Arya, Ved Prakash Aggarwal and Radhey Shyam Gupta have done manuscript preparation and data interpretation. All authors read and approved the final manuscript.

Conflicts of interest

The authors declare no conflict of interest.

References

1. Charoensin, S. Antioxidant and anticancer activities of *Moringa oleifera* leaves. *J. Med. Plants Res.* **2014**, *8*, 318–325.
2. Florence, I.F.; Adeboye, A.O.; Stephen, I.O. Comparative evaluation of *in vitro* antioxidant properties of *Cajanus cajan* seed and *Moringa oleifera* leaf extracts. *Int. J. Biochem. Res. Rev.* **2014**, *4*, 163–172.
3. Luqman, S.; Srivastava, S.; Kumar, R.; Maurya, A.K.; Chanda, D. Experimental assessment of *Moringa oleifera* leaf and fruit for its antistress, antioxidant, and scavenging potential using *in vitro* and *in vivo* assays. *Evid. Based Complement. Alternat. Med. eCAM* **2012**, *519084*, 1–12.
4. Anwar, F.; Latif, S.; Ashraf, M.; Gilani, A.H. *Moringa oleifera*: A food plant with multiple medicinal uses. *Phytother. Res.* **2007**, *21*, 17–25.
5. Hussain, S.; Malik, F.; Mahmood, S. Review: An exposition of medicinal preponderance of *Moringa oleifera* (Lank.). *Pak. J. Pharm. Sci.* **2014**, *27*, 397–403.
6. Jung, I.L. Soluble Extract from *Moringa oleifera* leaves with a new anticancer activity. *PLoS One* **2014**, *9*, e95492.
7. Mbikay, M. Therapeutic potential of *Moringa oleifera* leaves in chronic hyperglycemia and dyslipidemia: A review. *Front. Pharmacol.* **2012**, *3*, 1–12.
8. Yassa, H.D.; Tohamy, A.F. Extract of *Moringa oleifera* leaves ameliorates streptozotocin-induced diabetes mellitus in adult rats. *Acta Histochem.* **2014**, in press.
9. Faizi, S.B.; Siddiqui, R.; Saleem, S.; Siddiqui, K.A.; Gillani, A. Isolation and structure elucidation of new nitrite and mustard oil glycosides from *Moringa oleifera* and their effect on blood pressure. *J. Nat. Prod.* **1994**, *57*, 1256–1261.
10. Guevara, A.P.; Vargas, C.; Sakurai, H.; Fujiwara, Y.; Hashimoto, K.; Maoka, T.; Kozuka, M.; Ito, Y.; Tokuda, H.; Nishino, H. An antitumor promoter from *Moringa oleifera* Lam. *Mutat. Res.* **1999**, *440*, 181–188.

11. Singh, B.N.; Singh, B.R.; Singh, R.L.; Prakash, D.; Dhakarey, R.G.; Upadhyay, G.; Singh, H.B. Oxidative DNA damage protective activity, antioxidant and anti-quorum sensing potentials of *Moringa oleifera*. *Food Chem. Toxicol.* **2009**, *47*, 1109–1116.
12. Manquro, L.O.; Lemmen, P. Phenolics of *Moringa oleifera* leaves. *Nat. Prod. Res.* **2007**, *21*, 56–68.
13. Raja, S.; Nazeer Ahmed, K.F.H.; Kumar, V.; Mukherjee, K.; Bandyopadhyay, A.; Mukherjee, P.K. Antioxidant effect of *Cytisus scoparius* against carbon tetrachloride treated liver injury in rats. *J. Ethnopharmacol.* **2007**, *109*, 41–47.
14. Porchezhian, E.; Ansari, S.H. Hepatoprotective activity of *Abutilon indicum* on experimental liver damage in rats. *Phytomedicine* **2005**, *12*, 62–64.
15. Ohkawa, H.; Ohishi, N.; Yagi, K. Assay for lipid peroxidation in animal tissue by thiobarbituric acid reaction. *Anal. Biochem.* **1979**, *95*, 351–358.
16. Marklund, S.; Marklund, G. Involvement of superoxide anion radical in auto-oxidation of pyrogallol and a convenient assay for superoxide dismutase. *Eur. J. Biochem.* **1974**, *47*, 469–474.
17. Aebi, H. Catalase *in vitro*. In *Methods in Enzymology*; Calowick, S.P., Kaplan, N.O., Eds.; Academic Press: New York, NY, USA, 1984; Volume 105, pp. 121–126.
18. Moron, M.S.; Depierre, J.W.; Mannervick, B. Levels of glutathione, glutathione reductase and glutathione-*s*-transferase activities in rat lung and liver. *Biochem. Biophys. Acta* **1979**, *582*, 67–78.
19. Carlberg, I.; Mennervick, B. Glutathione reductase. In *Methods in Enzymology*; Academic Press: New York, NY, USA, 1985; Volume 113, pp. 484–490.
20. Paglia, D.E.; Velentine, W.M. Studies on the quantitative and qualitative characterization of erythrocyte glutathione peroxidase. *J. Lab. Clin. Med.* **1967**, *70*, 158–169.
21. Zeashan, H.; Amresh, G.; Singh, S.; Rao, C.V. Hepatoprotective activity of *Amaranthus spinosus* in experimental animals. *J. Food Chem. Toxicol.* **2008**, *46*, 3417–3421.
22. Manubolu, M.; Goodla, L.; Ravilla, S.; Thanasekaran, J.; Dutta, P.; Malmlöf, K.; Obulum, V.R. Protective effect of *Actiniopteris radiata* (Sw.) Link. against CCl_4 induced oxidative stress in albino rats. *J. Ethnopharmacol.* **2014**, *153*, 744–752.
23. Mani Senthilkumar, K.T.; Rajkapoor, B.; Kavimani, S. Protective effect of *Enicostemma littorale* against CCl_4-induced hepatic damage in rats. *Pharmaceuti. Biol.* **2005**, *43*, 485–487.
24. Singh, D.; Singh, R.; Singh, P.; Gupta, R.S. Effects of embelin on lipid peroxidation and free radical scavenging activity against liver damage in rats. *Basic Clin. Pharmacol. Toxicol.* **2009**, *105*, 243–248.
25. Bishayee, A.; Sarkar, A.; Chatterjee, M. Hepatoprotective activity of carrot (*Daucus carota* L.) against carbon tetrachloride intoxication in mouse liver. *J. Ethnopharmacol.* **1995**, *47*, 69–74.
26. Shaaban, A.A.; Shaker, M.E.; Zalata, K.R.; El-kashef, H.A.; Ibrahim, T.M. Modulation of carbon tetrachloride-induced hepatic oxidative stress, injury and fibrosis by olmesartan and omega-3. *Chemi. Biol. Interact.* **2014**, *207*, 81–91.
27. Gupta, R.S.; Singh, D. Hepatomodulatory role of *Enicostemma littorale* Blume against oxidative stress induced liver injury in rats. *Afr. J. Agric. Res.* **2007**, *2*, 131–138.

28. Kalegari, M.; Gemin, C.A.; Araújo-Silva, G.; Brito, N.J.; López, J.A.; Oliveira Tozetto, S.D.; das Graças Almeida, M.; Miguel, M.D.; Stien, D.; Miguel, O.G. Chemical composition, antioxidant activity and hepatoprotective potential of *Rourea induta* Planch. (Connaraceae) against CCl_4-induced liver injury in female rats. *Nutrition* **2014**, *6*, 713–718.
29. Shah, N.A.; Khan, M.R.; Ahmad, B.; Noureen, F.; Rashid, U.; Khan, R.A. Investigation on flavonoid composition and anti-free radical potential of *Sida cordata*. *BMC Comp. Altern. Med.* **2013**, *13*, 276–288.
30. Lee, K.J.; Woo, E.; Choi, C.Y.; Shin, D.W.; Lee, D.G.; You, H.J.; Jeong, H.G. Protective effect of acteoside on carbon tetrachloride-induced hepatotoxicity. *Life Sci.* **2004**, *74*, 1051–1064.
31. Mandal, P.K.; Bishayee, A.; Chatterjee, M. Stimulation of tissue repair by *Mikania cordata* root extract in carbon tetrachloride-induced liver injury in mice. *Phytother. Res.* **1993**, *7*, 103–105.
32. Salvi, M.; Battaglia, V.; Brunati, A.M.; LaRocca, N.; Tibaldi, E.; Pietrangeli, P.; Marcocci, L.; Mondovi, B.; Rossi, C.A.; Toninello, A. Catalase takes part in rat liver mitochondria oxidative stress defense. *J. Biol. Chem.* **2007**, *282*, 24407–24415.
33. Molina, M.F.; Sanchez-Reus, I.; Iglesias, I.; Benedi, J. Quercetin, a flavonoid antioxidant, prevents and protects against ethanol induced oxidative stress in mouse liver. *Biol. Pharm. Bull.* **2003**, *26*, 1398–1402.
34. Parimoo, H.A.; Sharma, R.; Patil, R.D.; Sharma, O.P.; Kumar, P.; Kumar, N. Hepatoprotective effect of *Ginkgo biloba* leaf extract on lantadenes-induced hepatotoxicity in guinea pigs. *Toxicon* **2014**, *81*, 1–12.
35. Meister, A. Glutathione. In *The Liver, Biology and Pathobiology*; Arias, I.M., Boyer, J.L., Jakoby, W.B., Fausto, D., Schacter, D., Shafritz, D.A., Eds.; Ravan Press: New York, 1994; pp. 401–417.
36. Huo, H.Z.; Wang, B.; Liang, Y.K.; Bao, Y.Y.; Gu, Y. Hepatoprotective and Antioxidant Effects of Licorice Extract against CCl_4-Induced Oxidative Damage in Rats. *Int. J. Mol. Sci.* **2011**, *12*, 6529–6543.
37. Okuno, H.; Hazama, H.; Mutazo, T.; Shiozaki, Y.; Somoshima, Y.T. Drug metabolizing activity in rats with chronic liver injury, induced by carbon tetrachloride relationship with the hydroxyproline content in liver. *Jpn. J. Pharmacol.* **1998**, *41*, 363–369.

5

Friedreich's Ataxia: A Neuronal Point of View on the Oxidative Stress Hypothesis

Barbara Carletti * and Fiorella Piemonte *

Unit of Neuromuscular and Neurodegenerative diseases, Children's Hospital and Research Institute "Bambino Gesù", 00165 Rome, Italy

* Authors to whom correspondence should be addressed; E-Mails: carletti.barbara@tiscali.it (B.C.); fiorella.piemonte@opbg.net (F.P.)

Abstract: A prominent feature of Friedreich's ataxia (FRDA) is the neurodegeneration of the central and peripheral nervous systems, but little information is available about the mechanisms leading to neuronal damage in this pathology. Currently, no treatments delay, prevent, or reverse the inexorable decline that occurs in this condition. Evidence of oxidative damage has been demonstrated in Friedreich's ataxia, and this damage has been proposed as the origin of the disease. Nevertheless, the role of oxidative stress in FRDA remains debatable. The lack of direct evidence of reactive oxygen species overproduction in FRDA cells and tissues and the failure of exogenous antioxidants to rescue FRDA phenotypes questions the role of oxidative stress in this pathology. For example, the antioxidant "idebenone" ameliorates cardiomyopathy in FRDA patients, but this therapy does not improve neurodegeneration. To date, no known pharmacological treatment with antioxidant properties cures or delays FRDA neuropathology. This review reports and discusses the evidence of oxidative stress in FRDA and focuses on the existing knowledge of the apparent ineffectiveness of antioxidants for the treatment of neuronal damage.

Keyword: Friedreich's ataxia; oxidative stress; neurodegeneration; antioxidants

---

1. Introduction

Friedreich's ataxia (FRDA) is an inherited autosomal recessive disorder caused by severely reduced levels of the mitochondrial iron chaperone protein, frataxin, as a result of a large GAA triplet-repeat expansion within the first intron of the frataxin gene. The GAA expansion interferes with gene transcription and determine a reduction in the amount of frataxin protein. The residual amount of frataxin protein in FRDA patients varies between 5% and 35% of normal levels. The prominent feature of FRDA pathology is neurodegeneration in the central and peripheral nervous systems. A distal length-related axonal degeneration affects the upper motor neurons of the corticospinal tract, the posterior columns of the spinal cord, the spinocerebellar tract and the large sensory fibers of the peripheral nerves [1]. Clinical symptoms appear during childhood or adolescence, and they are characterized by a progressive relentless ataxia associated with dysarthria, loss of reflexes and decrease of deep sensation [2]. Patients typically require wheelchairs within 10 to 20 years after symptoms begin. A hypertrophic cardiomyopathy is the second important clinical trait that presents in two-thirds of the patients, and it is the most frequent cause of early death. Additional non-neurological features are skeletal deformities and diabetes mellitus. The similarities of FRDA with vitamin E deficiency suggested from the beginning a role of oxidative damage in the pathogenesis of this disorder [3]. However, a prolonged debate began to emerge as the importance of oxidative stress in FRDA became increasingly evident. Is oxidative stress a secondary event of disease progression, or does it represent the primary cause of cell damage in the target tissues? If oxidative damage contributes to the pathogenesis of neurodegeneration in FRDA, why are antioxidant therapies unsuccessful in ameliorating nervous system clinical symptoms? This review provides an overview of the oxidative stress findings in FRDA and analyzes the possible role of redox markers in FRDA neuronal damage to delineate the cause of the selective vulnerability of specific neurons to frataxin deficiency and their apparent unresponsiveness to antioxidants.

2. Frataxin Function

Oxidative stress is caused by an imbalance between the production of reactive oxygen species (ROS) and the cellular antioxidant defense, which usually detoxifies reactive intermediates and repairs the resulting damage. ROS production occurs during normal cellular aerobic metabolism, primarily during mitochondrial respiration during the incomplete reduction of oxygen to water. ROS includes both free radicals that contain a highly reactive unpaired electron, such as superoxide anion (O_2^-) and hydroxyl radical (OH), and other molecular species, such as hydrogen peroxide (H_2O_2). All of these species react with cellular components that oxidize proteins, lipids and DNA [4]. The cell controls the flux of ROS under normal physiological conditions by neutralizing and preventing ROS production to maintain the redox equilibrium. Oxidative stress occurs when ROS levels overwhelm the antioxidant systems. A vicious circle was hypothesized very early on that considered oxidative stress as primarily responsible for the cellular consequences of frataxin loss of function [5,6].

Frataxin is a ubiquitous mitochondrial protein involved in intracellular iron homeostasis that participates in heme biogenesis [7], iron binding storage and detoxification [8,9], iron chaperone activity [10], and the biosynthesis of iron-sulfur complexes (ISCs) [11–18]. The proposed interpretation for FRDA pathogenesis focuses on ISC biosynthesis. ISCs act as prosthetic groups for several proteins that participate in energy metabolism, respiration, iron metabolism, purine synthesis and DNA repair. Frataxin likely contributes to ISC assembly by making ferrous iron available [10]. Several studies suggest that a frataxin deficiency underlies an inefficient use of iron during ISC synthesis with a consequent accumulation of the metal and defects in ISC-containing enzymes [19,20]. Frataxin involvement in Fe/S formation was confirmed by ISC enzyme impairment in FRDA patients' tissues and yeasts and animal models [5,21–23]. These studies showed particular dysfunction in Fe/S containing enzymes such as aconitase and complexes I, II and III of the mitochondrial respiratory chain with consequent defects in mitochondrial respiration, lower ATP production and iron accumulation.

The observations of mitochondrial enzyme deficiencies and iron accumulation in animal models and affected tissues suggested that the loss of frataxin determined the presence of unbound reactive free iron, which generates ROS within the mitochondrion via the Fenton reaction [23,24]. This process would lead to oxidative damage which might inactivate mitochondrial enzymes and determine a further generation of free radicals. In fact, Fe/S enzymes of the mitochondrial respiratory chain comprise the major ROS generators and are thus more exposed to the oxidative damage. ROS production during mitochondrial respiration consists of prematurely leaking electrons, mostly at complexes I and III. Electrons react with molecular oxygen to generate the superoxide anion (O_2^-). Frataxin deficiency in FRDA underlies the dysfunctional biogenesis of the ISC-containing complexes with reduced activity of the mitochondrial respiratory chain enzymes. This process presumably enhances superoxide generation, which can be converted to H_2O_2 by the dismutation catalyzed by superoxide dismutase (SOD) or Fe^{3+}. The excess of Fe^{2+} and Fe^{3+} derived from the frataxin defect may generate more toxic OH from the hydrogen peroxide via the Fenton reaction ($Fe^{2+} + H_2O_2 \rightarrow Fe^{3+} + OH + OH^-$ or $Fe^{3+} + H_2O_2 \rightarrow Fe^{2+} + OOH + H^+$), which causes further respiratory chain damage and ROS production. Several aspects of frataxin function remain controversial, but it is now commonly accepted that frataxin prevents the highly redox-reactive iron from oxidative stress generation, thus frataxin deficiency might render the cell more vulnerable to oxidative stress [16].

3. Evidence for Oxidative Stress in FRDA

Unequivocal findings for increased ROS production in frataxin-deficient cells are lacking. However, several markers of oxidative stress have been revealed in FRDA cells and patient tissues. Increased plasma level of malondialdehyde (a lipid peroxidation product) [25] and increased urinary 8-hydroxy-2′-deoxiguanosine (a marker of oxidative DNA damage) were found in FRDA patients [26]. Additional confirmations also came from the dysregulation of glutathione homeostasis. Glutathione is a critical component of antioxidant cellular defense, and one key aspect of the redox status is the equilibrium between the reduced and oxidized forms of this tri-peptide (GSH/GSSG). The increase in the oxidized form of GSSG during oxidative stress conditions induces a process termed glutathionylation, which forms mixed disulfides between glutathione and protein cysteine residues. Our studies using blood or cells from FRDA patients suggest that frataxin deficiency leads to an impairment of glutathione equilibrium [27,28]. A considerable reduction in free glutathione levels and a significant increase in glutathione bound to hemoglobin were observed in the blood of FRDA patients, and GSSG concentrations increase in cultured fibroblasts and lymphoblasts from FRDA patients. We also associated the loss of cytoskeletal organization to the constitutive glutathionylation of cytoskeletal proteins and its increase in FRDA fibroblasts and spinal cord compared to healthy controls [29–31]. The altered glutathione status was further confirmed by analyses of yeast and human frataxin-deficient cells showing a low GSH/GSSG ratio, thiol modification of key mitochondrial proteins and changes in GSH-dependent enzymes [32,33].

A direct demonstration of increased ROS production in FRDA is limited to two studies that showed an overproduction of peroxide in patients' lymphoblasts and frataxin-deficient P19 cells [34,35]. Although we have scarce information on ROS production in FRDA, a wide variety of frataxin-deficient cells and FRDA tissues show an oversensitivity to oxidants, which indicates that they are under oxidative stress conditions [36–39]. Anderson and collaborators [40] reported that the administration of H_2O_2, but not superoxide, scavenging enzymes rescue the pathological phenotype in a drosophila FRDA model, which suggests hydrogen peroxide as the reactive species involved in FRDA damage.

In addition to the possibility of ROS overproduction, several reports also highlighted a disabled recruitment of antioxidant defenses. An impaired induction of SOD under oxidative stimuli has been reported in FRDA fibroblasts [37,41], and a significant increase in the activity ratio between SOD and glutathione peroxidase (GPX) has been detected by our group in the blood of FRDA patients [42]. SOD plays a fundamental role in modulating ROS toxicity as catalyzes the dismutation of superoxide into oxygen and hydrogen peroxide, subsequently reduced to water by GPX. Thus, a disequilibrium in SOD activity might alter the redox status of the cell towards oxidative stress. A further demonstration of impaired antioxidant defense in FRDA cells was provided also by Paupe and colleagues (2009) which reported that FRDA fibroblasts showed disorganization and impairment of the Nrf2 signaling pathway [43]. Nrf2 is a key transcription factor that responds to oxidants by binding to the antioxidant responsive element (ARE) and activating the transcription of Phase II antioxidant genes. These genes encode for several enzymes, such as SOD, catalase and the enzymes responsible for glutathione synthesis. Nrf2 does not translocate to the nucleus in FRDA fibroblasts or induce the transcription of antioxidant enzymes under oxidative stress conditions, which increases their vulnerability. Similarly, Marmolino *et al.* (2010) showed that frataxin-deficient cells presented reduced levels of PGC-1α, a transcription factor that emerged as a key player in the induction of several antioxidant pathways [44]. PGC-1α is a transcriptional regulator of mitochondrial biogenesis and metabolism that ensures a global positive impact on oxidative metabolism by increasing mitochondrial functions and minimizing the buildup of its oxidant by-products [45]. This specific pathway represents a physiological response activated by ROS that might be impaired in FRDA, where a decrease in PGC-1α expression is suggested to result in oxidative sufferance for diminished ROS-detoxifying capacity. These observations support the possibility of a further ROS overload due to an inadequate contribution of the antioxidant defense system. Therefore, whether oxidative status in FRDA arises from a ROS overproduction or a disabled antioxidant defense or both, an increasing body of evidence indicates that this overload may underlie the cell damage and play a key role in the pathogenesis of this disorder.

4. Neuronal Damage

Antioxidant therapy received increasing attention in clinical neurology, and many trials have been performed in common neurologic disorders as well as rare conditions supposed to be associated to oxidative stress [46]. However the lack of a proper understanding of the complex free radical biochemistry in neuron diseases determined conflicting and unsuccessful results. Unfortunately, this condition is also common to Friedreich's ataxia.

The successful results of the treatment of FRDA patients with the antioxidant idebenone were initially very encouraging. An early trial demonstrated that low doses of idebenone reduced cardiac hypertrophy in the majority of patients [26,45,47–49], but no influence was detected on the neurological progression. A comprehensive review of all randomized clinical trials using antioxidant drugs confirmed that none of the tested pharmacological treatments had significant neurological benefits in FRDA patients [50]. This disappointing translation of the oxidative stress hypothesis into useful antioxidant therapy to ameliorate the neurological symptoms suggests more complex cellular interactions than initially thought.

FRDA neuropathology includes atrophy of the dorsal root ganglia (DRG) with a progressive destruction of the larger neurons and thicker myelinated axons, which accounts for the thinning of the dorsal root and sensory nerve neuropathy [51,52]. The impact of DRG degeneration on the downstream structures of the spinal cord and brainstem underlies secondary damage, with atrophy of the Clarke and dorsal column, gracile and cuneate nucleus and spinocerebellar tract. Atrophy of Betz cells and the corticospinal tract is the second purely intrinsic CNS lesion of FRDA. How does a global event, such as oxidative stress, result in the selective loss of specific neurons? In addition, FRDA is a genetic disorder, and frataxin expression in different tissues does not explain this selective vulnerability. We might speculate that DRG neurons and upper motor neurons are among the longest in the body, and therefore, present a high-energy demand for axonal transport. A high ATP requirement combined with mitochondrial dysfunction may render these neurons more vulnerable to oxidative stress and degeneration than other neuronal groups. This hypothesis is consistent with the neurodegenerative phenotype associated with a selective defect of the retrograde axonal transport reported in a drosophila model of FRDA [53]. These authors tracked individual organelles along the axon using mito-GFP and showed that retrogradely moving mitochondria were profoundly affected with an excess accumulation at the neuromuscular junctions. Shidara and colleagues [53] suggested that the transport deficiency is an effect of a deficient mitochondrial metabolism and an inadequate production of ATP. In fact, mitochondria accumulation in the distal axons and synapses are profoundly depolarized and denies an adequate energy support.

Nevertheless, scarce data are available on the mechanisms of neuronal damage in FRDA pathology, and clear indications of oxidative damage in neurons, which paralleled existing data on other FRDA cell types, were obtained with difficulties. In 2000, Bradley and collaborators [54] performed a comprehensive analysis of mitochondrial respiratory chain and aconitase activities from FRDA frozen tissues, including cerebellum and DRG, but surprisingly, they detected normal activity values in DRG samples. These results were most likely justifiable by the loss of the larger ganglion cells at the time of sample collection. To date, dysfunctional mitochondrial respiratory chain activities have not been detected in FRDA target neurons, and the analysis of iron overload did not evidence a clear accumulation of this metal in neurons. However, an altered distribution of Fe-handling proteins has been found, which suggests a metal transfer from degenerating DRG neurons to activated satellite cells [55]. Nonetheless, an accurate analysis performed on DRG cells from the YG8R mouse model evidenced oxidative stress caused by impaired glutathione redox status and antioxidant protection [56]. Microarray analysis of DRG tissue identified decreased transcripts encoding several antioxidant enzymes and a significant reduction in Nrf2 expression. Consistent with these data, we also found a defective Nrf2 expression in frataxin-deficient NSC34 neuronal cells after treatment with oxidized glutathione and a reduced basal expression of this transcription factor compared to control cells [57]. In addition, by analyzing the patterns of glutathionylation in the spinal cords of FRDA patients, Sparaco *et al.* (2009) found that cytoskeletal abnormalities co-localized with an increase in protein glutathionylation, which suggested a role for glutathione in FRDA pathogenesis [30].These results confirm the presence of oxidative stress in FRDA neurons and encourage the investigation of the source of ROS generation in the target cells of nervous tissue. These results also highlight that oxidative stress is a global event that is likely to produce many different downstream effects collectively and depict a complex neurodegenerative scenario.

The consequences of oxidative stress may be different and numerous, but several studies evidenced a common final outcome of the neurodegenerative cascade in the apoptotic pathways that most likely occurs in FRDA neuropathy. An increased susceptibility to apoptosis has been detected in fibroblasts and lymphoblasts from FRDA patients and frataxin-deficient cell lines [35,36,58–60], but a more stringent result came from two recent works on neuronal cells. Palomo *et al.* (2011) knocked down frataxin expression in the human neuroblastoma cell line SH-SY5Y using lentiviral vectors [61]. The SH-SY5Y cell line retain the ability to stop proliferating under specific condition, and to differentiate into postmitotic cells with the characteristic features of mature neurons. These authors demonstrated that differentiated neuron-like cells were very susceptible to oxidative stress and underwent a characteristic apoptotic cell death accompanied by p53 induction and caspase 3 activation. The authors argue that oxidative stress may play a causative role in p53 activation, which triggers the apoptotic cascade through the expression of the downstream genes PUMA and Bax. This work extended a previous finding of an enhanced apoptosis in frataxin-deficient embryonic P19 stem-like cells induced to differentiate into neurons [35]. More recently, Mincheva-Tasheva and collaborators explored the neurodegenerative process occurring in primary rat DRG neurons after frataxin depletion and observed an apoptotic cell death associated with a marked increase in intracellular Ca^{2+} levels (2013) [62]. The authors did not investigate the possible involvement of oxidative stress, but it has long been known that ROS can alter Ca^{2+} homeostasis and cause an increase in the intracellular ion concentration, which may disrupt normal metabolism and lead to cell death.

The notion that ROS may act on redox-sensitive transcription factors to alter the pattern of gene expression and determine the decision between cell survival and death increases the complexity of the dangerous mechanisms potentially activated by oxidative stress and introduces several further considerations for successful antioxidant therapies. The apoptotic pathway represents the last stage of the FRDA neuronal response to a chronic oxidative stress condition and a downstream target in the neurodegenerative cascade. The neurodegenerative process is the result of a progressive attrition of dysfunctional neurons that, although triggered from an oxidative insult, may then progress and evolve over time in an oxidative-independent manner. This pathway implies that the search for early events in oxidative stress-mediated pathogenesis is the real focus for the development of beneficial antioxidant therapies. Antioxidants should directly block the origin of the oxidative damage and be administered at an early stage before the neurodegenerative process begins. A clear understanding of the mechanisms generating oxidative stress in FRDA target neurons is essential for an efficacious antioxidant therapy.

Oxidative stress is most likely differentially generated in diverse tissues and directly or indirectly initiates several dangerous cell type-specific metabolic pathways, which may frustrate the general use of antioxidants not specifically targeting the cause of the damage. One possible explanation for the unsuccessful treatment of the neurological symptoms with idebenone may reside in a similar phenomenon. Idebenone is a short-chain coenzyme Q that acts as a substrate for complexes II and III and ameliorates the function of these respiratory chain proteins. In 1997, Rustin *et al.* demonstrated that idebenone protected complex II, lipids and aconitase from iron injury in heart homogenates [5] and, encouraged by these findings, the authors observed a significant reduction of hypertrophic cardiomyopathy in three treated patients [47]. Complexes II, III and aconitase activities were impaired in FRDA heart tissue, and the beneficial effects of idebenone prove the success of a treatment directly targeting one of the possible causes of damage in cardiac cells. Nevertheless, the pathogenesis may be not the same in the nervous tissue. For example, idebenone marginally inhibits complex I and strongly favors succinate oxidation [63]. We recently found that mitochondrial complex I is severely affected in frataxin deficient NSC34 motoneuronal cells [64]. In our model the NSC34 cell line has been silenced for frataxin gene by means of specific shRNA lentiviral vectors and reproduced some major biochemical and morphological features of FRDA. Whether this model recapitulate the mitochondrial damage in FRDA target neurons, idebenone treatment by inhibiting complex I may worsen the condition of the nervous tissue at the target sites. Therefore, a systematic analysis of potential sites and mechanisms of increased ROS production and impaired cellular antioxidant defense systems in FRDA damaged neurons is demanded. A limit to the effectiveness of antioxidants may be for example that they randomly diffuse through the cell, with only a small proportion of them reaching the site of damage. Accordingly, Jauslin and colleagues (2003) demonstrated that targeting antioxidants to mitochondria improve their effectiveness [65]. Thus, a subcellular compartmentalization of oxidative sites is critical to direct effective therapeutic treatments, and an analysis of *in vivo* imaging of redox-sensitive proteins targeted to the cytosol, mitochondrial matrix and the intermembrane space should be performed. These investigations may enable the dissection of the pathogenetic mechanisms and the role of oxidative stress in FRDA neuron damage and enable the identification of possible neuron-specific antioxidant molecules.

5. Conclusions

Despite the mounting evidence that oxidative stress is involved in the FRDA neuron damage that contributes to the pathogenesis of this disorder, clear research documenting sites and mechanisms of oxidative stress generation is lacking. Recent reports highlighted significant reductions in antioxidant protection and impairments in the glutathione redox status in frataxin-deficient neurons, but a causative mechanism documenting the role of oxidative stress in determining the FRDA neurodegenerative cascade is far from being discovered. The new findings on the apoptotic pathways as the final result of FRDA neuron damage definitely opens a complex scenario and suggests that oxidative stress most likely triggers many different downstream effects ending in a common outcome. Therefore, the early events in the oxidative process could prove decisive for an efficacious therapy targeting oxidative stress, whereas the final stages of neurodegeneration may not be responsive to an antioxidant treatment. For this reason, we remark that major efforts should be performed to elucidate the mechanisms of ROS production in FRDA. An efficacious antioxidant therapy should act upstream of the neurodegenerative process at the origin of oxidative stress generation to interrupt the dangerous cellular interactions of ROS and prevent the breakdown of target enzymes that trigger the neurodegenerative pathways. A general use of antioxidants that act as scavengers rather than blockers of the source of ROS generation may be ineffective. A more complete knowledge of the pathogenetic mechanisms induced by oxidative stress and the causes underlying these processes are needed to enable the development of useful antioxidant treatments. Only then we can identify molecules with suitable pharmacological antioxidant properties.

Acknowledgment

This article is dedicated to the memory of Ferdinando Rossi.

Conflicts of Interest

The authors declare no conflict of interest.

References

1. Koeppen, A.H.; Mazurkiewicz, J.E. Friedreich ataxia: Neuropathology revised. *J. Neuropathol. Exp. Neurol.* **2013**, *72*, 78–90.
2. Pandolfo, M. Friedreich ataxia: The clinical picture. *J. Neurol.* **2009**, *256*, 3–8.
3. Koenig, M.; Mandel, J.L. Deciphering the cause of Friedreich ataxia. *Curr. Opin. Neurobiol.* **1997**, *7*, 689–694.
4. Sies, H. *Oxidative Stress*; Academic Press: London, UK, 1985.
5. Rötig, A.; de Lonlay, P.; Chretien, D.; Foury, F.; Koenig, M.; Sidi, D.; Munnich, A.; Rustin, P. Aconitase and mitochondrial iron-sulphur protein deficiency in Friedreich ataxia. *Nat. Genet.* **1997**, *17*, 215–217.
6. Bayot, A.; Santos, R.; Camadro, J.M.; Rustin, P. Friedreich's ataxia: The vicious circle hypothesis revisited. *BMC Med.* **2011**, *9*, 112.
7. Yoon, T.; Cowan, J.A. Frataxin-mediated iron delivery to ferrochelatase in the final step of heme biosynthesis. *J. Biol. Chem.* **2004**, *279*, 25943–25946.
8. Cavadini, P.; O'Neill, H.A.; Benada, O.; Isaya, G. Assembly and iron-binding properties of human frataxin, the protein deficient in Friedreich ataxia. *Hum Mol. Genet.* **2002**, *11*, 217–227.
9. Gakh, O.; Park, S.; Liu, G.; Macomber, L.; Imlay, J.A.; Ferreira, G.C.; Isaya, G. Mitochondrial iron detoxification is a primary function of frataxin that limits oxidative damage and preserves cell longevity. *Hum. Mol. Genet.* **2006**, *15*, 467–479.

10. Yoon, T.; Cowan, J.A. Iron-sulfur cluster biosynthesis. Characterization of frataxin as an iron donor for assembly of [2Fe-2S] clusters in ISU-type proteins. *J. Am. Chem. Soc.* **2003**, *125*, 6078–6084.
11. Martelli, A.; Wattenhofer-Donzé, M.; Schmucker, S.; Bouvet, S.; Reutenauer, L.; Puccio, H. Frataxin is essential for extramitochondrial Fe-S cluster proteins in mammalian tissues. *Hum. Mol. Genet.* **2007**, *16*, 2651–2658.
12. Richardson, D.R.; Huang, M.L.; Whitnall, M.; Becker, E.M.; Ponka, P.; Suryo Rahmanto, Y. The ins and outs of mitochondrial iron-loading: The metabolic defect in Friedreich's ataxia. *J. Mol. Med.* **2010**, *88*, 323–329.
13. Santos, R.; Lefevre, S.; Sliwa, D.; Seguin, A.; Camadro, J.M.; Lesuisse, E. Friedreich ataxia: Molecular mechanisms, redox considerations, and therapeutic opportunities. *Antioxid. Redox Signal.* **2010**, *13*, 651–690.
14. Schmucker, S.; Martelli, A.; Colin, F.; Page, A.; Wattenhofer-Donzé, M.; Reutenauer, L.; Puccio, H. Mammalian frataxin: An essential function for cellular viability through an interaction with a preformed ISCU/NFS1/ISD11 iron-sulfur assembly complex. *PLoS* One **2011**, *6*, e16199.
15. Shan, Y.; Cortopassi, G. HSC20 interacts with frataxin and is involved in iron-sulfur cluster biogenesis and iron homeostasis. *Hum. Mol. Genet.* **2012**, *21*, 1457–1469.
16. Pastore, A.; Puccio, H. Frataxin: A protein in search for a function. *J. Neurochem.* **2013**, *126* (Suppl. 1), 43–52.
17. Prischi, F.; Konarev, P.V.; Iannuzzi, C.; Pastore, C.; Adinolfi, S.; Martin, S.R.; Svergun, D.I.; Pastore, A. Structural bases for the interaction of frataxin with the central components of iron-sulphur cluster assembly. *Nat. Commun.* **2010**, *1*, 95.
18. Pandolfo, M.; Pastore, A. The pathogenesis of Friedreich ataxia and the structure and function of frataxin. *J. Neurol.* **2009**, *256* (Suppl. 1), 9–17.
19. Radisky, D.C.; Babcock, M.C.; Kaplan, J. The yeast frataxin homologue mediates mitochondrial iron efflux. Evidence for a mitochondrial iron cycle. *J. Biol. Chem.* **1999**, *274*, 4497–4499.
20. Chen, O.S.; Crisp, R.J.; Valachovic, M.; Bard, M.; Winge, D.R. Kaplan, J. Transcription of the yeast iron regulon does not respond directly to iron but rather to iron-sulfur cluster biosynthesis. *J. Biol. Chem.* **2004**, *279*, 29513–29518.
21. Babcock, M.; de Silva, D.; Oaks, R.; Davis-Kaplan, S.; Jiralerspong, S.; Montermini, L.; Pandolfo, M.; Kaplan, J. Regulation of mitochondrial iron accumulation by Yfh1p, a putative homolog of frataxin. *Science* **1997**, *276*, 1709–1712.
22. Foury, F.; Cazzalini, O. Deletion of the yeast homologue of the human gene associated with Friedreich's ataxia elicits iron accumulation in mitochondria. *FEBS Lett.* **1997**, *411*, 373–377.
23. Puccio, H.; Simon, D.; Cossée, M.; Criqui-Filipe, P.; Tiziano, F.; Melki, J.; Hindelang, C.; Matyas, R.; Rustin, P.; Koenig, M. Mouse models for Friedreich ataxia exhibit cardiomyopathy, sensory nerve defect and Fe-S enzyme deficiency followed by intramitochondrial iron deposits. *Nat. Genet.* **2001**, *27*, 181–186.
24. Lodi, R.; Cooper, J.M.; Bradley, J.L.; Manners, D.; Styles, P.; Taylor, D.J.; Schapira, A.H. Deficit of *in vivo* mitochondrial ATP production in patients with Friedreich ataxia. *Proc. Natl. Acad. Sci. USA* **1999**, *96*, 11492–11495.

25. Emond, M.; Lepage, G.; Vanasse, M.; Pandolfo, M. Increased levels of plasma malondialdehyde in Friedreich ataxia. *Neurology* **2000**, 55, 1752–1753.
26. Schulz, B.; Dehmer, T.; Schöls, L.; Mende, H.; Hardt, C.; Vorgerd, M.; Bürk, K.; Matson, W.; Dichgans, J.; Beal, M.F.; *et al.* Oxidative stress in patients with Friedreich ataxia. *Neurology* **2000**, *55*, 1719–1721.
27. Piemonte, F.; Pastore, A.; Tozzi, G.; Tagliacozzi, D.; Santorelli, F.M.; Carrozzo, R.; Casali, C.; Damiano, M.; Federici, G.; Bestini, E. Glutathione in blood of patients with Friedreich's ataxia. *Eur. J. Clin. Investig.* **2001**, *31*, 1007–1011.
28. Pastore, A.; Piemonte, F.; Locatelli, M.; Lo Russo, A.; Gaeta, L.M.; Tozzi, G.; Federici, G. Determination of blood total, reduced, and oxidized glutathione in pediatric subjects. *Clin. Chem.* **2001**, *47*, 1467–1469.
29. Sparaco, M.; Gaeta, L.M.; Tozzi, G.; Bertini, E.; Pastore, A.; Simonati, A.; Santorelli, F.M.; Piemonte, F. Protein glutathionylation in human central nervous system: Potential role in redox regulation of neuronal defense against free radicals. *J. Neurosci. Res.* **2006**, *83*, 256–263.
30. Pastore, A.; Tozzi, G.; Gaeta, L.M.; Bertini, E.; Serafini, V.; di Cesare, S.; Bonetto, V.; Casoni, F.; Carrozzo, R.; Federici, G.; *et al.* Actin glutathionylation increases in fibroblasts of patients with Friedreich's ataxia: A potential role in the pathogenesis of the disease. *J. Biol. Chem.* **2003**, *278*, 42588–42595.
31. Sparaco, M.; Gaeta, L.M.; Santorelli, F.M.; Passarelli, C.; Tozzi, G.; Bertini, E.; Simonati, A.; Scaravilli, F.; Taroni, F.; Duyckaerts, C.; *et al.* Friedreich's ataxia: Oxidative stress and cytoskeletal abnormalities. *J. Neurol. Sci.* **2009**, *287*, 111–118.
32. Auchère, F.; Santos, R.; Planamente, S.; Lesuisse, E.; Camadro, J.M. Glutathione-dependent redox status of frataxin-deficient cells in a yeast model of Friedreich's ataxia. *Hum. Mol. Genet.* **2008**, *17*, 2790–2802.
33. Bulteau, A.L.; Planamente, S.; Jornea, L.; Dur, A.; Lesuisse, E.; Camadro, J.M.; Auchère, F. Changes in mitochondrial glutathione levels and protein thiol oxidation in Δyfh1 yeast cells and the lymphoblasts of patients with Friedreich's ataxia. *Biochim. Biophys. Acta* **2012**, *1822*, 212–225.
34. Tan, G.; Napoli, E.; Taroni, F.; Cortopassi, G. Decreased expression of genes involved in sulfur amino acid metabolism in frataxin-deficient cells. *Hum. Mol. Genet.* **2003**, *12*, 1699–1711.
35. Santos, M.M.; Ohshima, K.; Pandolfo, M. Frataxin deficiency enhances apoptosis in cells differentiating into neuroectoderm. *Hum. Mol. Genet.* **2001**,*10*, 1935–1944.
36. Wong, A.; Yang, J.; Cavadini, P.; Gellera, C.; Lonnerdal, B.; Taroni, F.; Cortopassi, G. The Friedreich's ataxia mutation confers cellular sensitivity to oxidant stress which is rescued by chelators of iron and calcium and inhibitors of apoptosis. *Hum. Mol. Genet.* **1999**, *8*, 425–430.
37. Chantrel-Groussard, K.; Geromel, V.; Puccio, H.; Koenig, M.; Munnich, A.; Rötig, A.; Rustin, P. Disabled early recruitment of antioxidant defenses in Friedreich's ataxia. *Hum. Mol. Genet.* **2001**, *10*, 2061–2067.
38. Vázquez-Manrique, R.P.; González-Cabo, P.; Ros, S.; Aziz, H.; Baylis, H.A.; Palau, F. Reduction of Caenorhabditis elegans frataxin increases sensitivity to oxidative stress, reduces lifespan, and causes lethality in a mitochondrial complex II mutant. *FASEB J.* **2006**, *20*, 172–174.

39. Llorens, J.V.; Navarro, J.A.; Martínez-Sebastián, M.J.; Baylies, M.K.; Schneuwly, S.; Botella, J.A.; Moltó, M.D. Causative role of oxidative stress in a Drosophila model of Friedreich ataxia. *FASEB J.* **2007**, *21*, 333–344.
40. Anderson, P.R.; Kirby, K.; Orr, W.C.; Hilliker, A.J.; Phillips, J.P. Hydrogen peroxide scavenging rescues frataxin deficiency in a Drosophila model of Friedreich's ataxia. *Proc. Natl. Acad. Sci.USA* **2008**, *105*, 611–616.
41. Jiralerspong, S.; Ge, B.; Hudson, T.J.; Pandolfo, M. Manganese superoxide dismutase induction by iron is impaired in Friedreich ataxia cells. *FEBS Lett.* **2001**, *509*, 101–105.
42. Tozzi, G.; Nuccetelli, M.; Lo Bello, M.; Bernardini, S.; Bellincampi, L.; Ballerini, S.; Gaeta, L.M.; Casali, C.; Pastore, A.; Federici, G.; *et al.* Antioxidant enzymes in blood of patients with Friedreich's ataxia. *Arch. Dis. Child.* **2002**, *86*, 376–379.
43. Paupe, V.; Dassa, E.P.; Goncalves, S.; Auchère, F.; Lönn, M.; Holmgren, A.; Rustin, P. Impaired nuclear Nrf2 translocation undermines the oxidative stress response in Friedreich ataxia. *PLoS One* **2009**, *4*, e4253.
44. Marmolino, D.; Manto, M.; Acquaviva, F.; Vergara, P.; Ravella, A.; Monticelli, A.; Pandolfo, M. PGC-1alpha down-regulation affects the antioxidant response in Friedreich's ataxia. *PLoS One* **2010**, *5*, e10025.
45. St-Pierre, J.; Drori, S.; Uldry, M.; Silvaggi, J.M.; Rhee, J.; Jäger, S.; Handschin, C.; Zheng, K.; Lin, J.; Yang, W.; *et al.* Suppression of reactive oxygen species and neurodegeneration by the PGC-1 transcriptional coactivators. *Cell* **2006**, *127*, 397–408.
46. Delanty, N.; Dichter, M.A. Antioxidant therapy in neurologic disease. *Arch. Neurol.* **2000**, *57*, 1265–1270.
47. Rustin, P.; von Kleist-Retzow, J.C.; Chantrel-Groussard, K.; Sidi, D.; Munnich, A.; Rötig, A. Effect of idebenone on cardiomyopathy in Friedreich's ataxia: A preliminary study. *Lancet* **1999**, *354*, 477–479.
48. Rustin, P.; Rötig, A.; Munnich, A.; Sidi, D. Heart hypertrophy and function are improved by idebenone in Friedreich's ataxia. *Free Radic. Res.* **2002**, *36*, 467–469.
49. Hausse, A.O.; Aggoun, Y.; Bonnet, D.; Sidi, D.; Munnich, A.; Rötig, A.; Rustin, P. Idebenone and reduced cardiac hypertrophy in Friedreich's ataxia. *Heart* **2002**, *87*, 346–349.
50. Kearney, M.; Orrell, R.W.; Fahey, M.; Pandolfo, M. Antioxidants and other pharmacological treatments for Friedreich ataxia. *Cochrane Database Syst. Rev.* **2009**, *4*, CD007791.
51. Koeppen, A.H. Nikolaus Friedreich and degenerative atrophy of the dorsal columns of the spinal cord. *J. Neurochem.***2013**, *126*, 4–10.
52. Koeppen, A.H.; Morral, J.A.; Davis, A.N.; Qian, J.; Petrocine, S.V.; Knutson, M.D.; Gibson, W.M.; Cusack, M.J.; Li, D. The dorsal root ganglion in Friedreich's ataxia. *Acta Neuropathol.* **2009**, *118*, 763–776.
53. Shidara, Y.; Hollenbeck, P.J. Defects in mitochondrial axonal transport and membrane potential without increased reactive oxygen species production in a Drosophila model of Friedreich ataxia. *J. Neurosci.* **2010**, *30*, 11369–11378.
54. Bradley, J.L.; Blake, J.C.; Chamberlain, S.; Thomas, P.K.; Cooper, J.M.; Schapira, A.H. Clinical, biochemical and molecular genetic correlations in Friedreich's ataxia. *Hum. Mol. Genet.* **2000**, *9*, 275–282.

55. Koeppen, A.H.; Kuntzsch, E.C.; Bjork, S.T.; Ramirez, R.L.; Mazurkiewicz, J.E.; Feustel, P.J. Friedreich ataxia: Metal dysmetabolism in dorsal root ganglia. *Acta Neuropathol. Commun.* **2013**, *1*, 26.
56. Shan, Y.; Schoenfeld, R.A.; Hayashi, G.; Napoli, E.; Akiyama, T.; Iodi Carstens, M.; Carstens, E.E.; Pook, M.A.; Cortopassi, G.A. Frataxin deficiency leads to defects in expression of antioxidants and Nrf2 expression in dorsal root ganglia of the friedreich's ataxia YG8R mouse model. *Antioxid. Redox Signal.* **2013**, *19*, 1481–1493.
57. D'Oria, V.; Petrini, S.; Travaglini, L.; Priori, C.; Piermarini, E.; Petrillo, S.; Carletti, B.; Bertini, E.; Piemonte, F. Frataxin deficiency leads to reduced expression and impaired translocation of NF-E2-Related Factor (Nrf2) in cultured motor neurons. *Int. J. Mol. Sci.* **2013**, *14*, 7853–7865.
58. Condò, I.; Ventura, N.; Malisan, F.; Tomassini, B.; Testi, R. A pool of extramitochondrial frataxin that promotes cell survival. *J. Biol. Chem.* **2006**, *281*, 16750–16756.
59. Kakhlon, O.; Manning, H.; Breuer, W.; Melamed-Book, N.; Lu, C.; Cortopassi, G.; Munnich, A.; Cabantchik, Z.I. Cell functions impaired by frataxin deficiency are restored by drug-mediated iron relocation. *Blood* **2008**, *112*, 5219–5227.
60. Pianese, L.; Busino, L.; de Biase, I.; de Cristofaro, T.; Lo Casale, M.S.; Giuliano, P.; Monticelli, A.; Turano, M.; Criscuolo, C.; Filla, A.; *et al.* Up-regulation of c-Jun *N*-terminal kinase pathway in Friedreich's ataxia cells. *Hum. Mol. Genet.* **2002**, *11*, 2989–2996.
61. Palomo, G.M.; Cerrato, T.; Gargini, R.; Diaz-Nido, J. Silencing of frataxin gene expression triggers p53-dependent apoptosis in human neuron-like cells. *Hum. Mol. Genet.* **2011**, *20*, 2807–2822.
62. Mincheva-Tasheva, S.; Obis, E.; Tamarit, J.; Ros, J. Apoptotic cell death and altered calcium homeostasis caused by frataxin depletion in dorsal root ganglia neurons can be prevented by BH4 domain of Bcl-xL protein. *Hum. Mol. Genet.* **2013**, *23*, 1829–1841.
63. Brière, J.J.; Schlemmer, D.; Chretien, D.; Rustin, P. Quinone analogues regulate mitochondrial substrate competitive oxidation. *Biochem. Biophys. Res. Commun.* **2004**, *316*, 1138–1142.
64. Carletti, B.; Piermarini, E.; Tozzi, G.; Travaglini, L.; Torraco, A.; Pastore, A.; Sparaco, M.; Petrillo, S.; Carrozzo, R.; Bertini, E.; *et al.* Frataxin silencing inactivates mitochondrial complex I in NSC34 motoneuronal cells and alters glutathione homeostasis. *Int. J. Mol. Sci.* **2014**, *15*, 5789–5806.
65. Jauslin, M.L.; Meier, T.; Smith, R.A.; Murphy, M.P. Mitochondria-targeted antioxidants protect Friedreich Ataxia fibroblasts from endogenous oxidative stress more effectively than untargeted antioxidants. *FASEB J.* **2003**, *17*, 1972–1974.

Optimisation of Ultrasound-Assisted Extraction Conditions for Phenolic Content and Antioxidant Capacity from *Euphorbia tirucalli* Using Response Surface Methodology

Quan V. Vuong [1,*], Chloe D. Goldsmith [1], Trung Thanh Dang [1,2], Van Tang Nguyen [1,2], Deep Jyoti Bhuyan [1], Elham Sadeqzadeh [1], Christopher J. Scarlett [1] and Michael C. Bowyer [1]

1 Pancreatic Cancer Research, Nutrition Food & Health Research Group, School of Environmental and Life Sciences, University of Newcastle, NSW 2258, Australia;
E-Mails: chloe.d.goldsmith@uon.edu.au (C.D.G.); trung.dang@uon.edu.au (T.T.D.); vantang.nguyen@uon.edu.au (V.T.N.); deepjyoti.bhuyan@uon.edu.au (D.J.B.); elham.sadeqzadeh@newcastle.edu.au (E.S.); c.scarlett@newcastle.edu.au (C.J.S.); michael.bowyer@newcastle.edu.au (M.C.B.)

2 Faculty of Food Technology, Nha Trang University, No. 2 Nguyen Dinh Chieu, Nha Trang, Khanh Hoa 8458, Vietnam

* Author to whom correspondence should be addressed; E-Mail: van.vuong@uon.edu.au

---

Abstract: *Euphorbia tirucalli* (*E. tirucalli*) is now widely distributed around the world and is well known as a source of traditional medicine in many countries. This study aimed to utilise response surface methodology (RSM) to optimise ultrasonic-assisted extraction (UAE) conditions for total phenolic compounds (TPC) and antioxidant capacity from *E. tirucalli* leaf. The results showed that ultrasonic temperature, time and power effected TPC and antioxidant capacity; however, the effects varied. Ultrasonic power had the strongest influence on TPC; whereas ultrasonic temperature had the greatest impact on antioxidant capacity. Ultrasonic time had the least impact on both TPC and antioxidant capacity. The optimum UAE conditions were determined to be 60 °C, 90 min. and 200 W. Under these conditions, the *E. tirucalli* leaf extract yielded 2.93 mg GAE/g FW of TPC and exhibited potent antioxidant capacity. These conditions can be utilised for further isolation and purification of phenolic compounds from *E. tirucalli* leaf.

Keywords: antioxidant; *Euphorbia tirucalli*; ultrasonic-assisted extraction; optimization; phenolic compounds; response surface methodology

1. Introduction

Euphorbia tirucalli (*E. tirucalli*) is native to Madagascar and Africa, but it is now widespread around the world because of its tolerance to a wide range of climatic conditions [1,2]. *E. tirucalli* has been used as folk medicines in the Middle East, India, Africa and South America for the treatment of a range of ailments including syphilis, asthma, cancer, colic, intestinal parasites and leprosy [3–5]. Recently, it has been linked to other benefits including hepatoprotective, antimicrobial, antioxidant, insecticidal, larvicidal, molluscicide and antiarthritic activities [6], which have resulted in significant scientific interest in the phytochemical profile of the plant [1].

Phenolic and terpenoid compounds have been identified in the phytochemical profile of *E. tirucalli*, and extracts have been shown to possess potent antioxidant properties [7,8]. Phenolic compounds are major bioactive compounds in medicinal plants and have been reported as powerful antioxidants and health promoters. The phenolic profile and antioxidant properties of *E. tirucalli* have been reported in a previous study, which found that acetone extracts yielded a higher concentration of phenolics than more polar solvent systems (80% aqueous methanol) [8]. However, optimal extraction conditions were not investigated and further study is required to fully characterise the phenolic profile.

Ultrasonic-assisted extraction (UAE) has been shown to be a fast and effective technique for extracting phytochemicals from plant materials that is easily up-scaleable [9]. Ultrasonic parameters such as temperature, time and power have been reported to exert significant impact on the extraction yield of plant phytochemicals and antioxidants [10–12]. A mixture of ethyl acetate: ethanol (4:1 v/v) was reported to efficiently extract triterpenoids from the root of *Euphorbia pekinensis* Rupr [13]. Therefore, this solvent mixture was used in this study and it was hypothesised that UAE temperature, time and power had significant effects on extraction efficiency of total phenolic compounds (TPC) and total antioxidant capacity (TAC) of the extracts from *E. tirucalli* leaf and the optimal extraction conditions could be established using response surface methodology (RSM).

The current study aimed to optimise the UAE parameters of temperature, time and power for the extraction of phenolics from *E. tirucalli*. These optimal conditions can be applied for further isolation and purification of phenolic compounds from *E. tirucalli*.

2. Experimental Section

2.1. Plant Materials

The leaf of the *Euphorbia tirucalli* tree (phylloclades) was collected on July 16, 2013 from a property located in Saratoga, NSW, Australia (33.47° S, 151.35° E). The leaf was then immediately transferred to the laboratory and stored at −20 °C to minimise phenolic degradation. Before commencing experiments, the leaf was immersed in liquid nitrogen, then particulated using a commercial blender. The fresh ground leaf was then stored at −20 °C until required.

2.2. Ultrasound-Assisted Extraction (UAE)

A mixture of ethyl acetate: ethanol 4:1 (v/v) was utilized as the solvent system for optimisation of UAE conditions and was applied at a solvent-to-sample ratio of 100:32 mL/g of fresh leaf weight. The ground *E. tirucalli* leaf was placed in the extraction chamber, and filled with extraction solvent. The extraction chamber was completely immersed into an ultrasonic bath (Soniclean, 220 V, 50 Hz and 250 W, Soniclean Pty Ltd., Thebarton, Australia) with pre-set conditions for temperature, time and power as designed by response surface methodology software. When the ultrasonic extraction was completed, the extracts were immediately cooled on ice to room temperature, filtered using a 5 mL syringe fitted with a 0.45 μm cellulose syringe filter (Phenomenex Australia Pty. Ltd., Lane Cove, Australia) and diluted to the required volume for quantitative analysis.

2.3. Response Surface Methodology (RSM)

A response surface methodology (RSM) approach with a Box-Behnken design was employed to design experimental conditions to investigate the influence of the three independent ultrasonic parameters: temperature (30, 45, and 60 °C), time (30, 45, and 60 min) and power (60%, 80%, and 100% or 150, 200, and 250 W).

The independent variables and their code variable levels are shown in Table 1. To express the level of total phenolic compounds (TPC) and total antioxidant capacity (TAC) as a function of the independent variables, a second-order polynomial equation was used as follows [14]:

$$Y = \beta_o + \sum_{i=1}^{k} \beta_i X_i + \sum_{\substack{i=1 \\ i<j}}^{k-1} \sum_{j=2}^{k} \beta_{ij} X_i X_j + \sum_{i=1}^{k} \beta_{ii} X_i^2 \quad (1)$$

where various X_i values are independent variables affecting the responses Y; β_0, β_i, β_{ii} *and* β_{ij} are the regression coefficients for intercept, linear, quadratic, and interaction terms, respectively; and k is the number of variables.

The three independent ultrasonic parameters were assigned as; X_1 (temperature, °C), X_2 (time, min.) and X_3 (power, %). Thus, the function containing these three independent variables is expressed as follows:

$$Y = \beta_0 + \beta_1 X_1 + \beta_2 X_2 + \beta_3 X_3 + \beta_{12} X_1 X_2 + \beta_{13} X_1 X_3 + \beta_{23} X_2 X_3 + \beta_{11} X_1^2 + \beta_{22} X_2^2 + \beta_{33} X_3^2 \quad (2)$$

2.4. Determination of Total Phenolic Content (TPC)

The extract was diluted 20× to fit within the optimal absorbance range for colorimetric assessment of total phenolic compounds (TPC), which was determined according to the method of Vuong *et al.* [15]. Gallic acid was used as the standard for the construction of a calibration curve, with the results expressed as mg of gallic acid equivalents per gram of fresh weight (FW) (mg GAE/g).

Table 1. Box-Behnken design and observed responses

Run	Ultrasonic Conditions			Experimental Values (n = 3)			
					Antioxidant Capacity		
	Temperature (°C)	Time (min)	Power (%) *	TPC (mg GAE/g)	ABTS (%)	DPPH (%)	CUPRAC (mM TE/g)
1	30	30	80	2.99	42.81	17.80	37.07
2	30	60	60	2.05	56.31	21.94	42.74
3	30	60	100	2.40	50.20	19.22	41.01
4	30	90	80	2.34	52.59	18.12	36.61
5	45	30	60	2.20	74.88	25.17	56.66
6	45	30	100	2.99	74.01	27.32	67.63
7	45	60	80	2.71	66.07	30.25	55.67
8	45	60	80	3.11	46.91	18.58	38.56
9	45	60	80	3.51	74.52	25.17	66.72
10	45	90	60	2.63	64.23	23.43	46.81
11	45	90	100	3.34	74.27	30.28	67.00
12	60	30	80	2.05	74.52	20.90	71.70
13	60	60	60	2.39	53.82	47.46	51.95
14	60	60	100	2.83	69.13	43.27	57.17
15	60	90	80	3.12	62.22	39.66	48.13

* 60%, 80% and 100% power were equivalent to 150, 200 and 250 W.

2.5. Determination of Antioxidant Capacity

ABTS total antioxidant capacity: The extract was diluted 40× to fit within the optimal absorbance range for colorimetric assessment. Total antioxidant capacity (TAC) was measured using 2,2′-azino-bis-3-ethylbenzothiazoline-6-sulphonic acid (ABTS) assay as described by Thaipong *et al.* [16]. Results were expressed as percentage of inhibition and were calculated using the formula:

$$\text{TAC (\%)} = (Abs_{control} - Abs_{sample}) \times 100/Abs_{control} \qquad (3)$$

where $Abs_{control}$ = control absorbance and Abs_{sample} = sample absorbance.

Free radical scavenging capacity: The extract was diluted 40× and analyzed using 1,1-diphenyl-2-picrylhydrazyl (DPPH) assay as described by Vuong *et al.* [15] with results expressed as percentage of inhibition, calculated according to Equation 3.

Cupric reducing antioxidant capacity (CUPRAC): The extract was diluted 40× and its iron chelating capacity analyzed using cupric ion reducing antioxidant capacity (CUPRAC) assay as described by Apak *et al.* [17]. Trolox (6-hydroxy-2,5,7,8-tetramethylchroman-2-carboxylic acid) was used as the calibration standard, with results expressed as mM of trolox equivalents per g of fresh weight (mM TE/g).

2.6. Statistical Analysis

RSM experimental design and analysis were conducted using JMP software (Version 11, SAS, Cary, NC, USA). The software was also used to establish the model equation to graph the 3D- and 2D-contour plots of variable responses, and to predict optimum values for the three response variables. The Student's *T*-test (conducted using the SPSS statistical software version 20, IBM, Armonk, NY, USA) was used for comparison of the means analysis. Differences between the mean levels in the different experiments were taken to be statistically significant at $p < 0.05$.

3. Results and Discussion

3.1. Fitting of the Models for Prediction of Total Phenolic Content and Total Antioxidant Capacity

It is necessary to test the reliability of the RSM mathematical model in predicting optimal variances and accurately representing the real interrelationships between the selected parameters. Therefore, fitting of the models for total phenolic content and antioxidant capacity of the euphorbia extracts was undertaken. Results of analysis of variances of the Box-Behnken design are shown in Figure 1 and Table 2. Figure 1 revealed a correlation between the predicted and experimental values, while Table 2 presents the summary of variance analysis.

Table 2. Analysis of variance for determination of model fitting.

Sources of Variation	TPC	Antioxidant Capacity		
		ABTS	DPPH	CUPRAC
Lack of fit	0.77	0.0007 *	0.13	0.0025 *
R^2	0.83	0.84	0.88	0.87
Adjusted R^2	0.53	0.54	0.67	0.65
PRESS	3.73	4661.69	2121.07	4042.87
F Ratio of Model	2.73	2.81	4.23	3.88
p of Model > F	0.14	0.13	0.06	0.07

* Significantly difference with $p < 0.05$.

Figure 1A showed that the model TPC outputs did not differ significantly from the experimental values ($p > 0.05$). Furthermore, the coefficient of determination (R^2) of the model was 0.83, indicating that 83% of the experimental data can be predictively matched against the model data for TPC. Table 2 also showed that the p value for "lack of fit" was 0.77, indicating that the lack of fit was not significant ($p > 0.05$). In addition, the Predicted Residual Sum of Square (PRESS) for the model (a measure of how well the predictive model fits each point in the design) [12], was 3.73 and the F value of the model was 2.73, further revealing that the mathematical model was adequate for prediction of TPC and was fitted to the following second-order polynomial formula:

$$Y_{TPC} = 3.1067 + 0.0754X_1 + 0.1503X_2 + 0.2863X_3 + 0.4284X_1X_2 + 0.0224X_1X_3 - 0.0157X_2X_3 - 0.4273X_1^2 - 0.0556X_2^2 - 0.2621X_3^2 \quad (4)$$

Fitting of the models for three different antioxidant properties including total antioxidant capacity (ABTS), DPPH free radical scavenging capacity and cupric reducing antioxidant capacity (CUPRAC) were also tested. The results (Figure 1B–D) revealed p values for ABTS, DPPH and CUPRAC of 0.13, 0.06 and 0.07, respectively, indicating that there was no significant difference between the predicted values and experimental values ($p > 0.05$). Coefficient of determination (R^2) for the ABTS, DPPH and CUPRAC models (Table 2) were determined to be 0.84, 0.88 and 0.87, respectively, revealing a close correlation between the predicted values and experimental values, with at least 84% of data matching.

PRESS values (4661, 2121 and 4042) and F values (2.81, 4.23 and 3.88) revealed that these mathematical models were reliable predictors of antioxidant capacity and could be fitted to the following second-order polynomial formulas:

$$Y_{ABTS} = 74.27 + 7.22X_1 + 2.13X_2 + 3.59X_3 - 0.42X_1X_2 - 3.95X_1X_3 - 2.13X_2X_3 - 10.94X_1^2 - 0.19X_2^2 - 11.06X_3^2 \quad (5)$$

$$Y_{ABTS} = 74.27 + 7.22X_1 + 2.13X_2 + 3.59X_3 - 0.42X_1X_2 - 3.95X_1X_3 - 2.13X_2X_3 - 10.94X_1^2 - 0.19X_2^2 - 11.06X_3^2 \quad (6)$$

$$Y_{ABTS} = 74.27 + 7.22X_1 + 2.13X_2 + 3.59X_3 - 0.42X_1X_2 - 3.95X_1X_3 - 2.13X_2X_3 - 10.94X_1^2 - 0.19X_2^2 - 11.06X_3^2 \quad (7)$$

Figure 1. Correlations between predicted and experimental total phenolic content and antioxidant capacity. (**A**) Phenolic content; (**B**) 2,2′-azino-bis-3-ethylbenzothiazoline-6-sulphonic acid (ABTS) antioxidant capacity; (**C**) 1,1-diphenyl-2-picrylhydrazyl (DPPH) free radical scavenging capacity; and (**D**) Cupric reducing antioxidant power (CUPRAC).

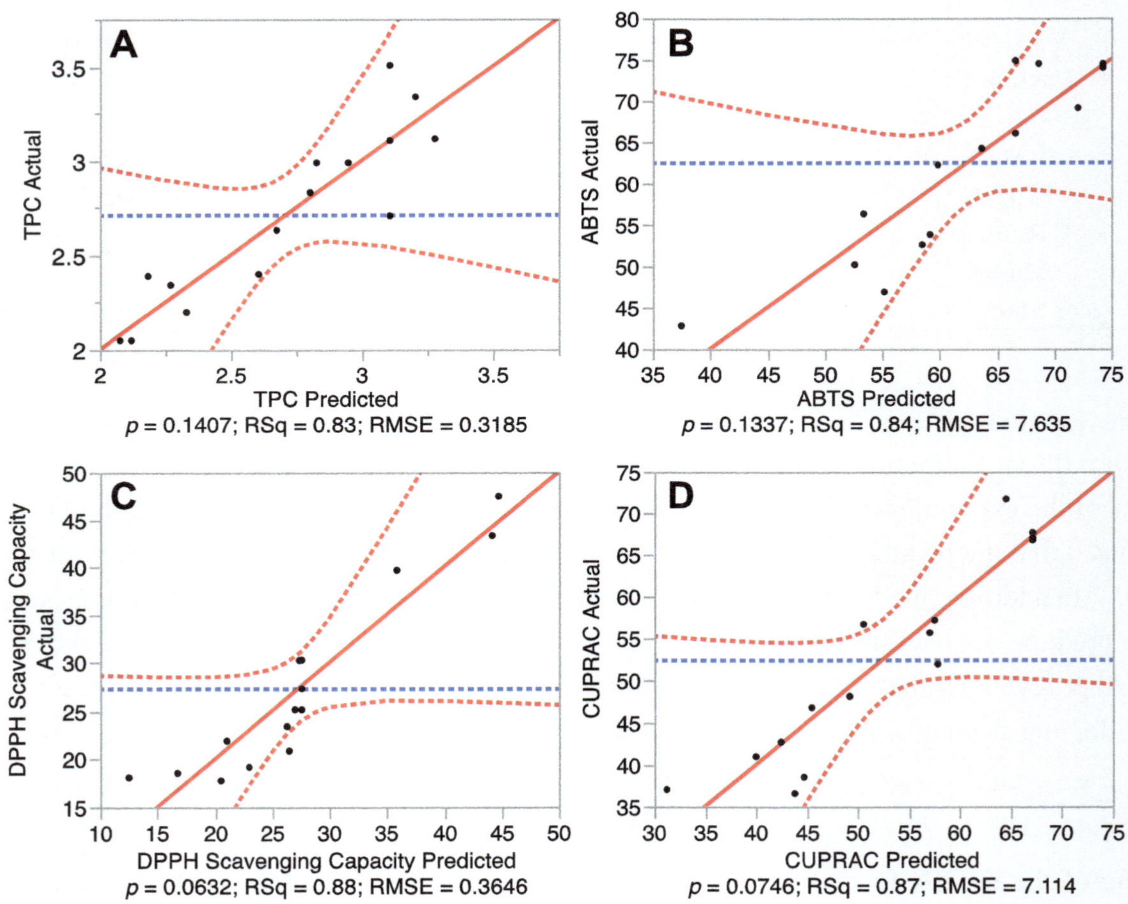

3.2. Effects of Ultrasonic Variables on Total Phenolic Content of E. tirucalli Extracts

Our data showed that the extraction efficiency of TPC had a positive correlation to the three experimental variables; bath temperature (30–50 °C), sonication time (30–90 min.) and sonication power (60%–80%; 150–200 W). Levels of TPC increased steadily when ultrasonic temperature increased from

30 °C to 50 °C; however, the levels of TPC decreased when temperature exceeded 55 °C (Figure 2). Levels of TPC also increased when ultrasonic time increased to 90 min. However, both ultrasonic temperature and time did not significantly affect levels of TPC ($p > 0.05$; Table 3), indicating that these two factors had the least impact on extraction efficiency of TPC. This demonstrated that ultrasonic power was the only parameter to significantly influence the extraction efficiency of TPC from *E. tirucalli* leaf ($p < 0.05$; Table 3). Levels of TPC plateaued when ultrasonic power exceeded 200 W (80%) (Figure 2). Therefore, the maximum TPC could be obtained at ultrasonic-assisted extraction conditions of 50 °C, 90 min and 200 W.

Figure 2. Impact of ultrasonic temperature (30–50 °C), time (30–90 min) and power (60%–100% or 150–250 W) on total phenolic compounds. The 2D impact of temperature, time and power were expressed in Figure 2A–C; while their 3D effects were shown in Figure 2D–F.

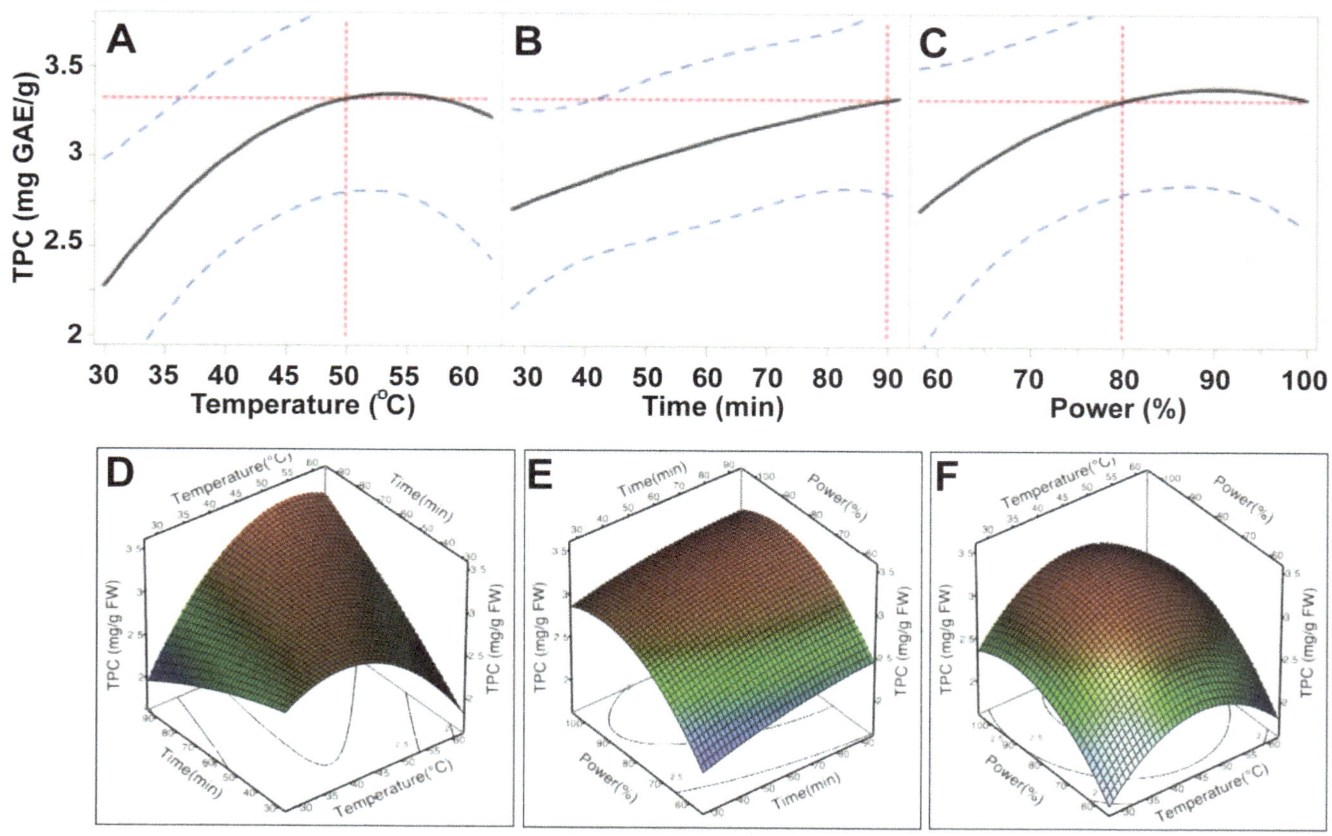

The impact of ultrasonic parameters on profile of the TPC extraction curve was similar to findings in previous studies examining seed cake extracts [10], olive pomace [12] and procyanidins removal from *Larix gmelinii* bark [18], which reported that the general application of higher temperatures, longer extraction times and/or higher sonication power increased TPC yields. The rising profile may be explained by two distinct processes; namely, a fast extraction of phenolics from cells close to the surface of the plant material, which are quickly solubilised, and slower diffusion and osmosis-based processes (known as "slow extraction") involving the liberation of more deeply embedded compounds [12].

3.3. Effects of Ultrasonic Conditions on Antioxidant Capacity of *E. tirucalli*

As the antioxidant activities of a sample could vary depending on the efficiency of antioxidant assays used [16], the impact of UAE conditions on antioxidant capacity of *E. tirucalli* was determined using three antioxidant assays; ABTS, DPPH and CUPRAC. Analysis of the ABTS assays of the extracts revealed that antioxidant capacity was influenced by all three ultrasound bath variables, however, only ultrasonic temperature significantly affected antioxidant capacity ($p < 0.05$; Table 3). These data indicated that ultrasonic temperature was the major factor influencing ABTS antioxidant capacity, whereas, ultrasonic time and power had least impact on ABTS antioxidant capacity.

Table 3. Analysis of variance for the experimental results.

Parameter	DF	TPC		Antioxidant Capacity					
				ABTS		DPPH		CUPRAC	
		F	*p > F*	*F*	*p > F*	*F*	*p > F*	*F*	*p > F*
β_0	1	16.90	<0.01 *	16.85	<0.01 *	8.91	<0.01 *	16.34	<0.01 *
β_1	1	0.45	0.53	7.16	0.04 *	23.92	0.00 *	12.63	0.02 *
β_2	1	1.78	0.24	0.62	0.47	1.46	0.28	0.32	0.59
β_3	1	6.47	0.05 *	1.78	0.24	2.22	0.20	2.98	0.15
β_{12}	1	7.24	0.04 *	0.01	0.92	5.96	0.06	0.35	0.58
β_{13}	1	0.02	0.89	1.07	0.35	0.35	0.58	0.00	0.99
β_{23}	1	0.02	0.90	0.31	0.60	0.86	0.40	0.26	0.63
β_{11}	1	6.65	0.05 *	7.59	0.04 *	0.85	0.40	7.26	0.04 *
β_{22}	1	0.11	0.75	0.00	0.96	2.17	0.20	1.89	0.23
β_{33}	1	2.50	0.17	7.75	0.04 *	0.10	0.77	11.59	0.02 *

* Significantly different at $p < 0.05$; β_0: Intercept; β_1, β_2, and β_3: Linear regression coefficients for temperature, time and power; β_{12}, β_{13}, and β_{23}: Regression coefficients for interaction between temperature × time, temperature × power and time × power; β_{11}, β_{22}, and β_{33}: Quadratic regression coefficients for temperature × temperature, time × time and power × power.

Table 3 indicates that the magnitude of the effect of the ultrasonic variables for ABTS antioxidant capacity was: temperature > power > time. ABTS antioxidant capacity increased when increasing the ultrasonic temperature from 30 °C to 50 °C and power from 150 W to 200 W. However, antioxidant capacity likely decreased when ultrasonic temperatures and ultrasonic power exceeded 50 °C and 200 W, respectively (Figure 3). Results from the ABTS assay revealed that the optimal conditions for maximum extraction of TPC could result in the highest antioxidant capacity. These findings can be explained by the high correlation between TPC and antioxidant capacity [15].

Figure 3. Impact of ultrasonic temperature (30–50 °C), time (30–90 min) and power (60%–100% or 150–250 W) on ABTS antioxidant capacity. The 2D impact of temperature, time and power were expressed in Figure 3A–C; while their 3D effects were shown in Figure 3D–F.

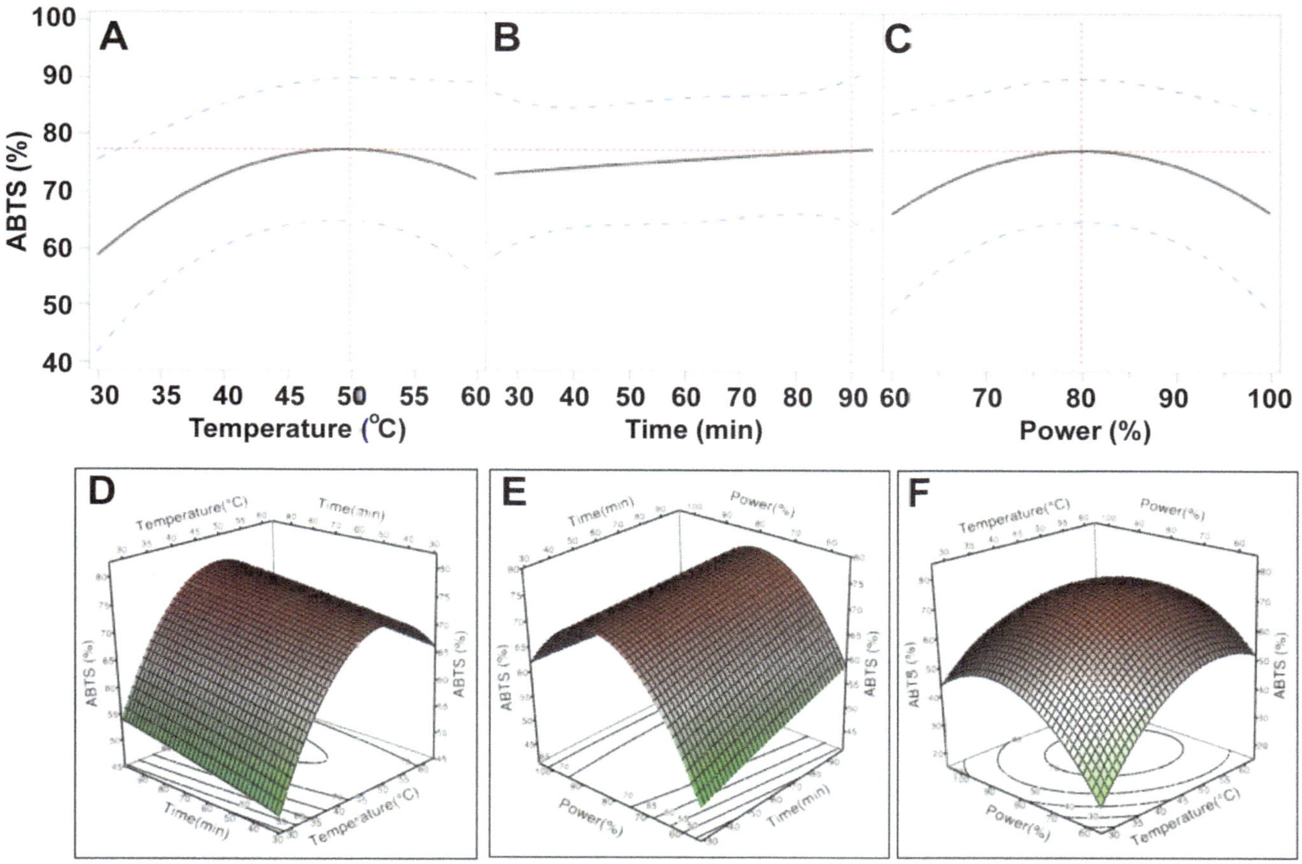

Data from the DPPH assay also indicated that free radical scavenging capacity of *E. tirucalli* extracts varied with the application of different ultrasonic temperature, time and power conditions; however, only temperature was reported to significantly affect free radical scavenging capacity ($p < 0.05$; Table 3). Based on the p values, the order of the influence was also found to be similar to ABTS: temperature > power > time. Free radical scavenging capacity of *E. tirucalli* extract increased steadily when ultrasonic temperature increased from 30 °C to 60 °C; whereas, its free radical scavenging capacity increased slightly with increasing power (150–250 W) and time (30–80 min; Figure 4). These data revealed that the highest DPPH free radical scavenging capacity of the extract was obtained at extraction conditions of 60 °C, 80 min and 250 W. At the optimal conditions for TPC (50 °C, 90 min and 200 W), only 66.5% of the maximum DPPH antioxidant value could be obtained.

The results from the CUPRAC assay further confirmed that ultrasonic temperature had a significant impact on cupric reducing antioxidant capacity (CUPRAC) of the antioxidant capacity ($p < 0.05$). Ultrasonic time and power affected, but not significantly, the CUPRAC of the *E. tirucalli* extract ($p > 0.05$; Table 3). Based on the p values, the order of the effects was similar to those of ABTS and

DPPH assays (temperature > power > time; Table 3). CUPRAC was observed to increase when increasing temperature from 30 °C to 50 °C, time from 30 min to 60 min and power from 150 W to 200 W; however, when ultrasonic temperature, time and power exceeded 50, 60 and 200 W, respectively, the CUPRAC of *E. tirucalli* extract decreased (Figure 5). These findings further confirmed that optimal extraction conditions for TPC could obtain maximum cupric reducing antioxidant capacity from *E. tirucalli* leaf.

Figure 4. Impact of ultrasonic temperature (30–50 °C), time (30–90 min) and power (60%–100% or 150–250 W) on DPPH free radical scavenging capacity. The 2D impact of temperature, time and power were expressed in Figure 4A–C; while their 3D effects were shown in Figure 4D–F.

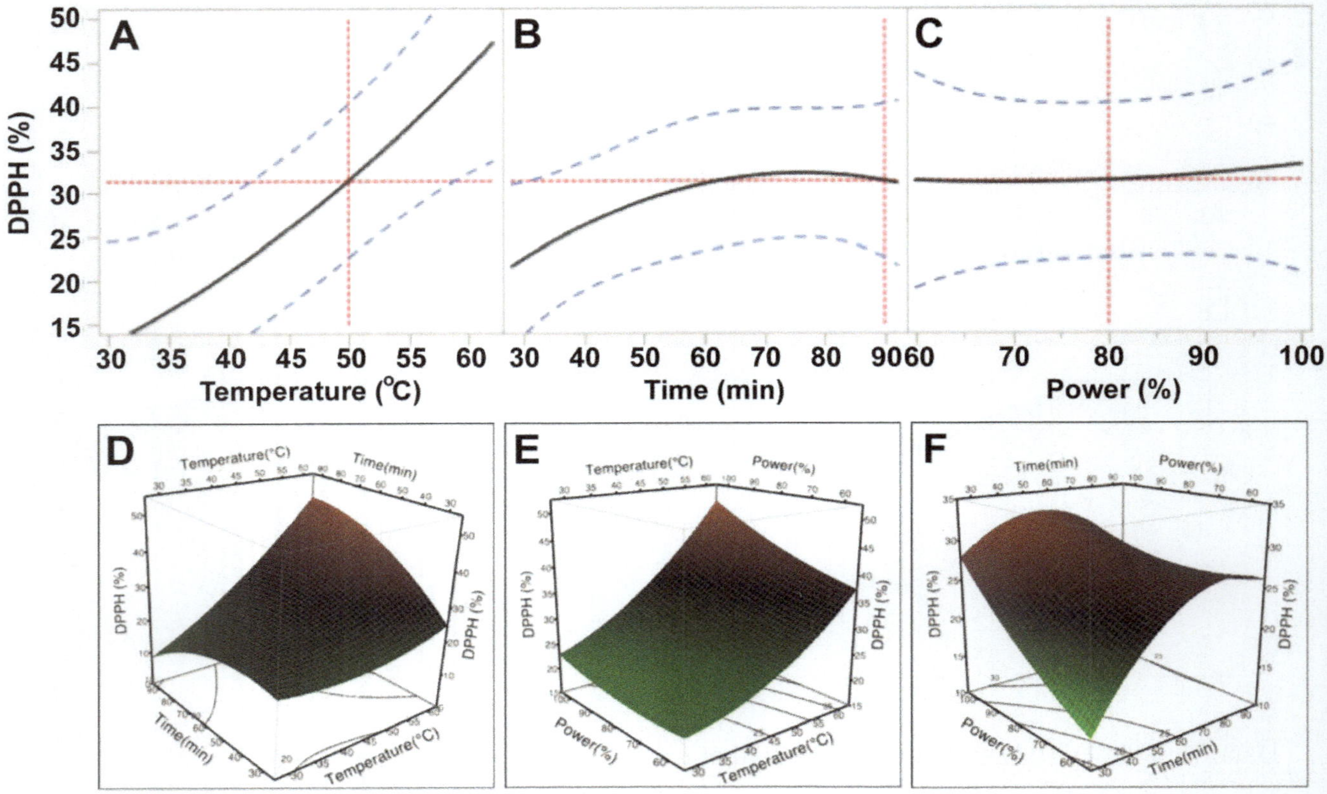

The current findings showed that ultrasonic temperature, time and power affected the antioxidant capacity of the *E. tirucalli* extract; however temperature had the highest impact, followed by power, while time had the least impact on antioxidant capacity of the *E. tirucalli* extract. Sahin *et al.* [12] also found that ultrasonic temperature and time affected antioxidant capacity of an *Artemisia absinthium* extract and generally, antioxidant capacity increased when the time increased, but decreased when temperature exceeded 50 °C. Teh *et al.* [10] also reported that ultrasonic temperature and time influenced antioxidant capacity of extract from defatted hemp, flax and canola seed cakes. The impact of ultrasonic conditions on antioxidant capacity can be explained by the influence on the total phenolic compounds, which were found to contribute significantly to the antioxidant capacity of plant extracts [19–21].

Figure 5. Impact of ultrasonic temperature (30–50 °C), time (30–90 min) and power (60%–100% or 150–250 W) on cupric reducing antioxidant capacity. The 2D impact of temperature, time and power were expressed in Figure 5A–C; while their 3D effects were shown in Figure 5D–F.

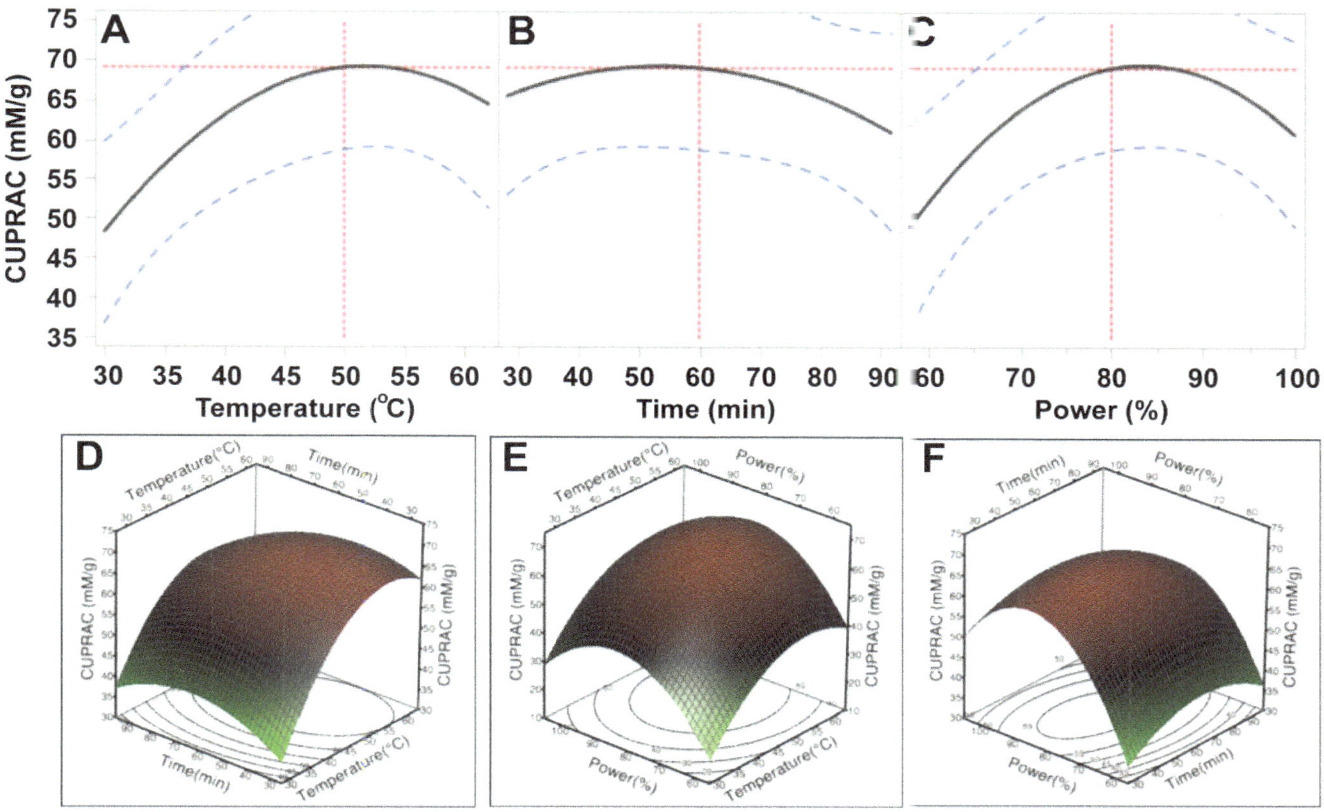

3.4. Optimisation of Ultrasonic Extraction Conditions for Total Phenolic Content and Antioxidant Capacity of E. tirucalli

Previous epidemiological studies have established links between the consumption of foods containing high concentrations of phenolic and antioxidant compounds and a lower incidence of cardiovascular diseases and certain types of cancer [22–24]. An understanding of the factors affecting the extraction efficiency of phenolics and/or antioxidant compounds from plant sources is therefore important.

Based on the predictive models and values shown in Figures 2–5, the optimum UAE conditions for the extraction of total phenolics, ABTS and CUPRAC from *E. tirucalli* leaf were determined to be: temperature = 50 °C, time = 90 min and power = 200 W; whereas, the optimum conditions for DPPH free radical scavenging capacity were: temperature = 60 °C, time = 80 min and power = 250 W. Of note, extraction under optimum conditions for TPC, ABTS and CUPRAC could obtain 66.5% of the maximum DPPH antioxidant value under its optimum conditions (60 °C, 80 min and 250 W). Therefore, the conditions of 50 °C, 90 min and 200 W were selected as optimal conditions for extraction of TPC and enhanced antioxidant capacity.

To validate the optimum conditions predicted by the models, *E. tirucalli* leaf was extracted under UAE conditions of 50 °C, 90 min and 200 W and the results showed that the predicted values of TPC and three antioxidant assays were similar to those of the experimental values ($p > 0.05$; Table 4). Therefore, these conditions were suggested for use to extract TPC and antioxidants from *E. tirucalli* leaf for further isolation and utilisation. In addition, these findings further confirmed the appropriateness of the models used for optimising the extraction conditions using UAE, and also revealed that response surface methodology was an effective technique for designing and optimising the extraction conditions.

Table 4. Validation of the predicted values for total phenolic content (TPC) and antioxidant capacity.

Variables	Values of TPC and Antioxidant Capacity	
	Predicted	Experimental ($n = 4$)
TPC (mg GAE/g FW)	3.32 ± 0.74 [a]	2.93 ± 0.14 [a]
ABTS (%)	77.26 ± 17.73 [a]	71.50 ± 1.06 [a]
DPPH (%)	31.33 ± 12.47 [a]	35.24 ± 0.66 [a]
CUPRAC (mM TAE/g FW)	61.77 ± 16.53 [a]	54.03 ± 3.53 [a]

All the values are means ± standard deviations and those in the same row not sharing the same superscript letter are significantly different from each other ($p < 0.05$).

4. Conclusions

As hypothesised, ultrasonic temperature, time and power had effects on extraction efficiency of total phenolic content and antioxidant capacity of the extracts from *E. tirucalli* leaf; however, the effects varied. Ultrasonic power had the highest impact on TPC; whereas, temperature had the strongest influence on antioxidant capacity. Levels of TPC and antioxidant capacity increased when ultrasonic temperature, time and power increased to 50 °C, 90 min and 200 W, respectively. Therefore, the optimum ultrasonic-assisted extraction conditions for TPC and antioxidant capacity from *E. tirucalli* leaf were: temperature of 50 °C, time of 90 min and power of 200 W. These conditions can be applied for further isolation and purification of phenolic compounds from the *E. tirucalli* leaf.

Acknowledgments

The authors would like to acknowledge the following funding support: Ramaciotti Foundation (ES2012/0104); Cancer Australia and Cure Cancer Australia Foundation (1033781). The authors also kindly thank the Vietnamese Government through the Vietnam International Education Development - Ministry of Education and Training (Project 911) and the University of Newcastle for awarding a VIED-TUIT scholarship to VTN and TTD.

Author Contributions

Quan V. Vuong, Chloe D. Goldsmith, Trung Thanh Dang, Van Tang Nguyen, Deep Jyoti Bhuyan and Christopher J. Scarlett designed the study. Quan V. Vuong, Chloe D. Goldsmith, Elham Sadeqzadeh, Christopher J. Scarlett and Michael C. Bowyer analysed and interpreted the results. All Authors prepared and approved the final version of the manuscript.

Conflicts of Interest

The authors declare no conflict of interest.

References

1. Mwine, J.T.; Damme P.V. Why do Euphorbiaceae tick as medicinal plants? A review of Euphorbiaceae family and its medicinal features. *J. Med. Plants Res.* **2011**, *5*, 652–662.
2. Hassall, D.C. The genus Euphorbia in Australia. *Aust. J. Bot.* **1977**, *25*, 429–453.
3. Gupta, N.; Vishnoi, G.; Wal, A.; Wal, P. Medicinal Value of *Euphorbia tirucalli*. *Res. Rev. J. Pharmacogn. Phytochem.* **2013**, *1*, 16–25.
4. Cataluna, P.; Rates, S. The traditional use of the latex from *Euphorbia tirucalli* Linnaeus (Euphorbiaceae) in the treatment of cancer in South Brazil. *Acta Hortic.* **1997**, *501*, 289–296.
5. Oliver-Bever, B. *Medicinal Plants in Tropical West Africa*; Cambridge University Press: Cambridge, UK, 1986.
6. Priya, C.L.; Rao, K.V.B. A review on phytochemical and pharmacological profile of *Euphorbia tirucalli*. *Pharmacologyonline* **2011**, *2*, 384–390.
7. Zhang, L.; Gao, L.; Li, Z.; Yan, X.; Yang, Y.; Tang, Y.; Cao, Y.; Ding, A. Bio-guided isolation of the cytotoxic terpenoids from the roots of *Euphorbia kansui* against human normal cell lines L-O2 and GES-1. *Int. J. Mol. Sci.* **2012**, *13*, 11247–11259.
8. De Araújo, K.; de Lima, A.; Silva, J.; Rodrigues, L.; Amorim, A ; Quelemes, P.; dos Santos, R.; Rocha, J.; de Andrades, É.; Leite, J.; Mancini-Filho, J.; da Trindade, R. Identification of phenolic compounds and evaluation of antioxidant and antimicrobial properties of *Euphorbia tirucalli* L. *Antioxidants* **2014**, *3*, 159–175.
9. Vinatoru, M. An overview of the ultrasonically assisted extraction of bioactive principles from herbs. *Ultrason. Sonochem.* **2001**, *8*, 303–313.
10. Teh, S.S.; Birch, E.J. Effect of ultrasonic treatment on the polyphenol content and antioxidant capacity of extract from defatted hemp, flax and canola seed cakes. *Ultrason. Sonochem.* **2014**, *21*, 346–353.
11. Prakash Maran, J.; Manikandan, S.; Vigna Nivetha, C.; Dinesh, R. Ultrasound assisted extraction of bioactive compounds from *Nephelium lappaceum* L. fruit peel using central composite face centered response surface design. *Arabian J. Chem.* **2013**, doi:10.1016/j.arabjc.2013.02.007.
12. Şahin, S.; Şamlı, R. Optimization of olive leaf extract obtained by ultrasound-assisted extraction with response surface methodology. *Ultrason. Sonochem.* **2013**, *20*, 595–602.
13. Zhang, P.; Jin, Y.; Chen, J.; Yao, H.; Zhang, H.; Yu, A.; Li, X. Ultrasonic-assisted nebulization extraction coupled with SPE and HPLC for the determination of triterpenoids in root of *Euphorbia pekinensis* Rupr. *Chromatographia* **2013**, *76*, 967–974.
14. Vuong, Q.V.; Stathopoulos, C.E.; Golding, J.B.; Nguyen, M.H.; Roach, P.D. Optimum conditions for the water extraction of L-theanine from green tea. *J. Sep. Sci.* **2011**, *34*, 2468–2474.
15. Vuong, Q.V.; Hirun, S.; Roach, P.D.; Bowyer, M.C.; Phillips, P.A.; Scarlett, C.J. Effect of extraction conditions on total phenolic compounds and antioxidant activities of *Carica papaya* leaf aqueous extracts. *J. Herbal Med.* **2013**, *3*, 104–111.

16. Thaipong, K.; Boonprakob, U.; Crosby, K.; Cisneros-Zevallos, L.; Hawkins Byrne, D. Comparison of ABTS, DPPH, FRAP, and ORAC assays for estimating antioxidant activity from guava fruit extracts. *J. Food Compos. Anal.* **2006,** *19*, 669–675.
17. Apak, R.; Güçlü, K.; Özyürek, M.; Karademir, S.E. Novel total antioxidant capacity index for dietary polyphenols and vitamins C and E, using their cupric ion reducing capability in the presence of neocuproine: CUPRAC method. *J. Agric. Food Chem.* **2004**, *52*, 7970–7981.
18. Sun, X.; Jin, Z.; Yang, L.; Hao, J.; Zu, Y.; Wang, W.; Liu, W. Ultrasonic-assisted extraction of procyanidins using ionic liquid solution from *Larix gmelinii* bark. *J. Chem.* **2013**, *2013*, 1–9.
19. Pinelo, M.; Rubilar, M.; Jerez, M.; Sineiro, J.; Nunez, M.J. Effect of solvent, temperature, and solvent-to-solid ratio on the total phenolic content and antiradical activity of extracts from different components of grape pomace. *J. Agric. Food Chem.* **2005**, *53*, 2111–2117.
20. Alu'datt, M.H.; Alli, I.; Ereifej, K.; Alhamad, M.N.; Alsaad, A.; Rababeh, T. Optimisation and characterisation of various extraction conditions of phenolic compounds and antioxidant activity in olive seeds. *Nat. Prod. Res.* **2011**, *25*, 876–889.
21. Li, Y.; Guo, C.; Yang, J.; Wei, J.; Xu, J.; Cheng, S. Evaluation of antioxidant properties of pomegranate peel extract in comparison with pomegranate pulp extract. *Food Chem.* **2006**, *96*, 254–260.
22. Johnsen, S.; Overvad, K.; Stripp, C.; Tjonneland, A.; Husted, S.E.; Sorensen, H.T. Intake of fruit and vegetables and the risk of ischemic stroke in a cohort of Danish men and women. *Am. J. Clin. Nutr.* **2003**, *78*, 57–64.
23. Temple, N.J.; Gladwin, K.K. Fruit, vegetable, and the prevention of cancer: Research challenges. *Nutrition* **2003**, *19*, 467–470.
24. Vuong, Q.V. Epidemiological Evidence Linking Tea Consumption to Human Health: A Review. *Crit. Rev. Food Sci. Nutr.* **2014**, *54*, 523–536.

7

Assessing Antioxidant Capacity in Brain Tissue: Methodologies and Limitations in Neuroprotective Strategies

Jennifer E. Slemmer [1] and John T. Weber [2,*]

[1] Bioscience Technology, Holland College, 140 Weymouth Street, Charlottetown, PE, C1A 4Z1, Canada; E-Mail: jeslemmer@hollandcollege.com

[2] School of Pharmacy, Memorial University of Newfoundland, 300 Prince Philip Drive, St. John's, NL, A1B 3V6, Canada

* Author to whom correspondence should be addressed; E-Mail: jweber@mun.ca

External Editor: Wenlan Liu

Abstract: The number of putative neuroprotective compounds with antioxidant activity described in the literature continues to grow. Although these compounds are validated using a variety of *in vivo* and *in vitro* techniques, they are often evaluated initially using *in vitro* cell culture techniques in order to establish toxicity and effective concentrations. Both *in vivo* and *in vitro* methodologies have their respective advantages and disadvantages, including, but not limited to, cost, time, use of resources and technical limitations. This review expands on the inherent benefits and drawbacks of *in vitro* and *in vivo* methods for assessing neuroprotection, especially in light of proper evaluation of compound efficacy and neural bioavailability. For example, *in vivo* studies can better evaluate the effects of protective compounds and/or its metabolites on various tissues, including the brain, in the whole animal, whereas *in vitro* studies can better discern the cellular and/or mechanistic effects of compounds. In particular, we aim to address the question of appropriate and accurate extrapolation of findings from *in vitro* experiment-where compounds are often directly applied to cellular extracts, potentially at higher concentrations than would ever cross the blood-brain barrier—to the more complex scenario of neuroprotection due to pharmacodynamics *in vivo*.

Keywords: antioxidant; bioavailability; cell culture; neuroprotection

1. Introduction

The present review focuses on the relative advantages, disadvantages, and methodological concerns when assessing antioxidant compounds for the treatment of various health conditions, particularly related to the nervous system. Our analysis of the literature, including our own work using neuroprotective compounds, indicates that extrapolating findings from *in vitro* experiments to neuroprotection *in vivo* requires appropriate methodological choices, as well as recognition of the limitations of *in vitro* experiments. Some of these methodologies involve examining the structure-function relationships of successful neuroprotective compounds; for this reason, we describe some specific molecules, such as various polyphenols, which have been successful *in vivo*, in both rodents and humans, in enhancing cognitive function, and compare them to some molecules that possessed promise on paper, but did not perform well in human clinical trials.

Initial findings and studies are almost always conducted using *in vitro* techniques, with either cell lines or primary cell cultures, before moving successful compounds into the whole animal. As described in detail in future sections, the use of *in vitro* experimentation is a faster, more cost-effective manner to screen compounds from a diverse panel of candidates. Many of the compounds that we describe in this review are antioxidants, and for this reason, we focus on the effects of oxidative stress on brain tissue, and the treatment of various conditions, such as stroke, with antioxidant compounds. Again, the choice of methodology is critical when investigating a compound's neuroprotective capacity. Is the compound a true antioxidant, in that it is capable of neutralizing oxidizing molecules that could damage cell membranes and/or DNA, or does it have a different mechanism of action? If the experimental design does not allow for several possibilities, then a potentially beneficial compound may be rejected for failing to provide direct neuronal protection *in vitro*. Our aim is to shed light on the relative advantages and disadvantages of *in vitro* and *in vivo* methodologies for assessing potential neuroprotective, antioxidant compounds, and to provide guidance for studies using these compounds in the future.

2. Cellular Mechanisms of Protection to the Brain Due to Antioxidant Activity

2.1. Redox Homeostasis and Oxidative Stress

Oxidative stress has been purported to be a common underlying mechanism behind many human health conditions, such as stroke, traumatic brain injury, and aging [1]. Briefly, oxidative stress is the intracellular overproduction of reactive oxygen species (ROS), such as superoxide ($O_2^{\bullet -}$) and hydroxyl radicals ($^{\bullet}OH$). Nitrosative stress is a related process, involving the overproduction of reactive nitrogen species (RNS), such as nitric oxide ($NO^{\bullet}$) [1,2]. Unlike free radicals, which are chemicals with one or more unpaired electrons, other compounds, such as hydrogen peroxide (H_2O_2) and peroxynitrite ($ONOO^-$), are non-radicals, but are still capable of causing extensive cellular damage.

The investigation of ROS and RNS, and strategies to block their cellular effects, or their generation in the first place, has been the focus of many reviews and books to date [1–4]. All cells—whether *in vitro* or *in vivo*—which utilize oxygen for aerobic respiration must maintain a delicate homeostasis between the generation and the subsequent removal of ROS and RNS. Normal, healthy cells are capable of performing adequate reduction/oxidation (redox) homeostasis. Neuronal cells in particular, however, have been found to be vulnerable to oxidative stress, partly due to their intense levels of oxidative respiration. Multiple forms of neural tissue can experience long-term degeneration, including retinal tissue in conditions such as age-related macular degeneration and diabetic retinopathy. Retinal tissue consumes a lot of oxygen, and thus the production of ROS through cellular respiration is also quite high [5]. In addition, this tissue is high in fatty acids, a common target of ROS. Therefore, there is considerable interest in antioxidant treatment for delaying or preventing retinal neurodegeneration. Most data surrounding the effects of oxidative stress in the nervous system, therefore, have focused on finding treatments that will delay or prevent neuronal cell loss rather than other cell types.

One of the major tenets of oxidative stress is that endogenous cellular detoxification systems can only handle a finite ROS/RNS load. Because oxidative stress has been linked to many neuropathological and neuropsychiatric conditions, many compounds have been developed that attempt to reduce the cellular load of ROS or RNS [1,6]. Of course, ROS and RNS are normally produced during cellular respiration, and cells have developed endogenous mechanisms of neutralizing these compounds. These endogenous systems are either enzymatic, such as superoxide dismutase (SOD), catalase or glutathione peroxidase, or non-enzymatic, such as the tripeptide glutathione. Because many of the endogenous systems are enzymatic, increasing the amount of intracellular SOD, for example, requires either delayed SOD degradation, or enhanced SOD gene expression and subsequent increased SOD protein production. A potentially easier route could be the addition of exogenous compounds in the diet, the so-called "free radical scavengers" which are, in essence, antioxidants because of their ability to return cells to their normal redox homeostasis. This class of compounds includes commonly known antioxidants, such as vitamin E (tocopherol), vitamin C (ascorbic acid), carotenoids, and polyphenols (Figure 1) [7,8].

These types of dietary molecules are often referred to as nutraceuticals, which are compounds believed to exert a positive effect on health. Plant-derived polyphenols in particular have received a lot of attention for their potential health benefits. For example, the high quantities of polyphenolic compounds found in some species of berries (e.g., *Vaccinium* species such as blueberries and lingonberries), and their reported antioxidant properties, may be beneficial for neurological disorders and processes, such as brain aging [9,10]. Given the idea that increased oxidative stress may be a major contributor to several neurological diseases and brain aging, the ingestion of berries or dietary supplements containing their constituents may have a positive effect on brain health [1,10]. The potential neuroprotective effects of berry-derived polyphenols are discussed in more detail in Section 4.

2.2. Structure-Function Relationships of Antioxidant Compounds

The number of people affected by neurological and neurodegenerative diseases continues to rise, which has led to an increased need for new antioxidant, neuroprotective compounds. Much literature has been dedicated to unraveling the mechanisms behind neuroprotective compounds, with the aim of reducing or prohibiting neural loss [11,12]. Like most drug discovery methods, this is a black-box process, in which a definitive cause-effect relationship must be obtained for proof-of-concept. In addition, understanding the relationship between a compound's structure and its cellular function allows for top-down drug design to improve bioavailability, increase efficacy and reduce toxicity. In general, the efficacy of many of these compounds derives from their structure, and, as seen in Figure 1, antioxidant compounds often have structural similarities that enable them to trap excess electrons from oxidizing compounds. Interestingly, these compounds themselves are capable of being oxidized, and thus require their own neutralization pathways.

Figure 1. Structures of various antioxidant compounds. **A**: vitamin E (tocopherol); constituents at the R_1 and R_2 positions are either –H or $–CH_3$; **B**: beta-carotene, a member of the carotenoid family; **C**: vitamin C (ascorbic acid); **D**: anthocyanin; constituents at the R_1 and R_2 positions are –H, –OH or $–OCH_3$, and the sugar is glucose, galactose or arabinose; **E**: resveratrol; **F**: oxyresveratrol; note the additional OH group as compared to resveratrol.

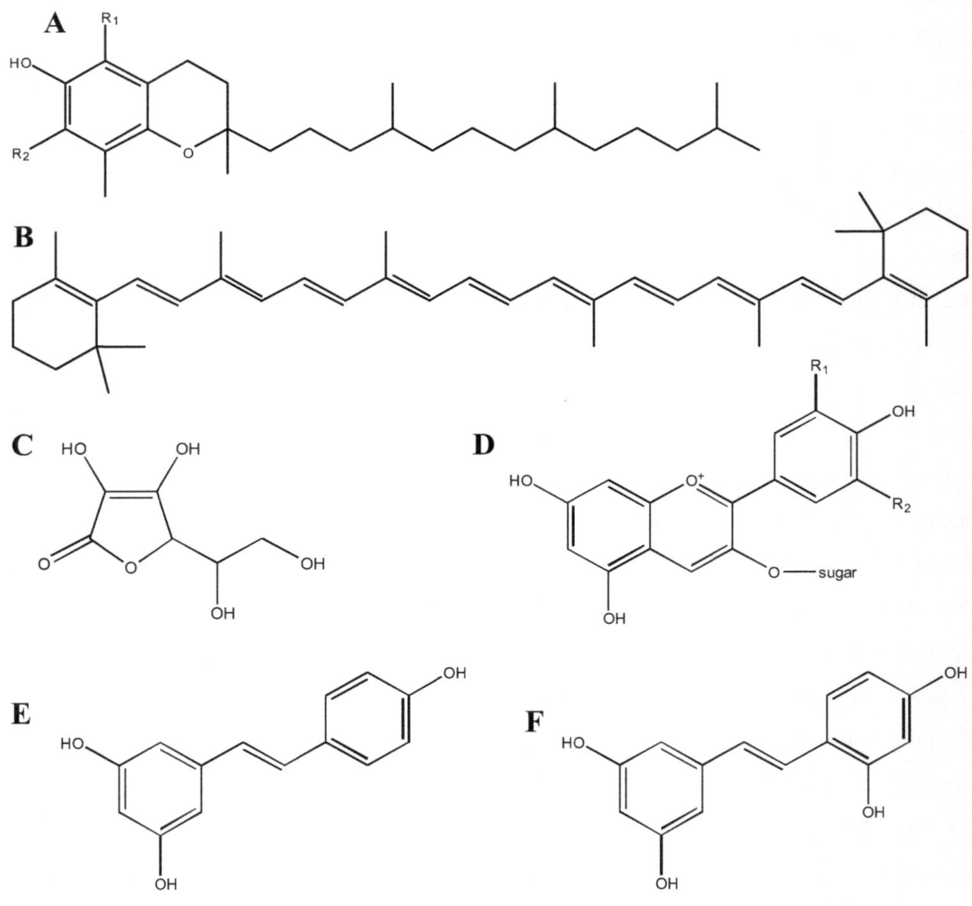

The fact that molecules, such as polyphenols, are purported to exert their antioxidant capability by neutralizing unpaired electrons, is given credence by comparing two similar chemicals: resveratrol and oxyresveratrol (Figure 1). Oxyresveratrol is a compound very similar to resveratrol, an antioxidant polyphenol found in the seeds and skins of red grapes. These molecules are identical, other than the addition of another –OH substituent on one of the phenol rings in oxyresveratrol; this additional group may make this compound a stronger antioxidant than resveratrol, in that it can more easily neutralize unpaired electrons. As we describe later, however, this explanation may be too simple, and may downplay the complexity of compounds in brain tissue. For example, one compound that failed to provide reproducible results in two clinical trials for patients with acute ischemic stroke (NXY-059;

chemical name: disodium 2,4-disulfophenyl-N-tert-butylnitrone) did not demonstrate protective effects against H_2O_2-induced oxidative stress in neuroblastoma cells *in vitro*. However, this compound may have exerted its protective effects by acting as an NO• mimetic [1,13].

Interestingly, one of the reported misconceptions about antioxidants is that, since they perform the same basic function, they are all the same and thus interchangeable [14]. However, that is clearly not the case. For example, an appropriate antioxidant for retinal tissue could preferentially target free radicals and ROS that damage fatty acids due to the high amount of these chemical compounds in this type of tissue. Many research teams believe that anthocyanins found in fruits, such as blueberries and bilberries, could be the answer for protecting this tissue from oxidative stress.

3. Screening of Antioxidants Using *in Vitro* Approaches

3.1. Cell Lines versus Primary Cultures

Determination of compound efficacy-before the initiation of animal experiments *in vivo* or human clinical trials-requires extensive testing *in vitro* to establish critical parameters, such as toxicity. In many situations, *in vitro* testing is used as a high-throughput screening method for compounds developed via bottom-up molecular synthesis. This type of screening is fast, inexpensive and relatively reliable. Drug screening *in vitro*, in which confounding variables can be controlled for, and cause-effect relationships can be more easily discerned, are often both useful and necessary for elucidating cellular and/or mechanistic effects of compounds.

The use of cell lines and/or primary cell cultures to devise and test neuroprotective compounds is a widely accepted strategy, and one that is necessary for various regulatory bodies. Cell lines are cells that have become "immortalized", usually through mutation, and continue to divide, as long as their growth and nutritional requirements are met [15,16]. Many mammalian cell lines are derived from biopsies of cancerous tissue, and often long outlive their original host. Two of the main advantages of using cell lines are their ease of use, and their low cost. A particular cell line can be purchased and maintained almost indefinitely in-house, and requires only a basic cell culture facility. Since the cells have already been removed from their host by the production facility, dissections are not required, and researchers do not require direct access to an animal facility. In addition, the number of human-derived cell lines currently available is extremely diverse, making it easy to compare the effects of one antioxidant compound on a variety of tissue types, including neuronal and glial tissue. In our opinion, this is one of the main strengths of using cell lines for mechanistic studies, as a particular compound may not be efficacious in the brain, but may instead exert its effects on other tissue types.

Of course, cell lines have distinct disadvantages when used to study the antioxidant capability of various compounds. The fact that many cell lines are cancerous makes it difficult to study the effects of compounds on "normal" tissue. Additionally, cell lines are notorious for becoming contaminated with other cancerous cell types: for example, it has been estimated that 29% of cell line stocks are contaminated with HeLa cells [17]. These issues can be avoided when using primary cell cultures, which are derived directly from the host animal through dissection. In the case of experiments analyzing neuroprotection *in vitro*, these cultures are typically derived from embryonic or neonatal brains of mice or rats [18–20]. However, these cultures are accompanied by their own specific set of disadvantages when it comes to their use for screening potential antioxidant compounds. Specifically, establishing primary cultures are more expensive, more heavily regulated, requires an animal care facility, animal care protocols, more time, and continuous maintenance.

3.2. Rationale for in Vitro Testing of Antioxidants

Cells derived from immortal cell lines or from primary sources are cultured either in suspension (where cells are freely floating in media) or as adherent monolayers on a substrate (usually plastic or glass). The bulk of our experimental work has used adherent cells, and their ability to form a monolayer makes it very easy to visualize cells under a microscope, to perform immunocytochemistry, and so on [18–20]. Our aim in this review is to indicate various caveats one should consider with regards to demonstrating neuroprotective compound efficacy *in vitro*. Indeed, we believe that *in vitro* screening can be viewed as a very reliable technique as long as the correct approach is used. The beautiful complexity of the brain, however, could be its own downfall, with regards to *in vitro* testing, as cultures do not maintain the exact cellular architecture of an intact brain, making it difficult to appropriately and accurately extrapolate findings from *in vitro* experiments to the more complex scenario of neuroprotection *in vivo*. The use of isolated cells *in vitro* is a necessary stepping-stone to demonstrating proof-of-concept for neuroprotective compounds. Various studies in our own laboratories have been conducted solely *in vitro*, with recommendations that compounds be further tested *in vivo* [18,19].

Most *in vitro* experiments, using adherent cells, apply compounds (in various doses) directly to cells, in order to generate a dose-response relationship. The assumptions made here are that the negative control treatment will not exert any effects, that there will be an effective dose, and that at high enough concentrations, the compound will kill cells. Of course, these high concentrations do provide critical information about toxicity, but the fear is that the effective dose is higher than what would ever cross the blood-brain barrier (BBB). However, the BBB is often damaged or weakened after various insults, such as stroke or traumatic brain injury, which could allow compounds to cross more easily, and at higher concentrations than in people with normal, undamaged brains. For example, oxyresveratrol was unable to effectively cross the BBB in healthy animals, but was found in much higher concentrations after experimental stroke [21]. A similar rationale was proposed for NXY-059, in that this compound is water-soluble and does not easily cross an intact BBB [1,22]. In this way, *in vitro* experimentation using adherent cells could replicate the situation of compounds crossing the BBB, and provides a rational explanation for continuing to test compound efficacy in this manner.

There is a second major issue that must be considered when gathering data about a compound *in vitro*. The direct application of compounds to cells (including, but not limited to neurons and glia) eliminates any of the changes that are made to those compounds through standard xenobiotic metabolism. In this way, the critical issue of bioavailability is improperly addressed, as unmetabolized antioxidant compounds could likely not reach the brain at the concentration, or in the time-window, required for effective treatment. Again though, a damaged or weakened BBB may assist in timely delivery to neural tissue. It is also possible that metabolites of various compounds may have antioxidant activity as well, which would not typically be captured with *in vitro* approaches. In the last sections of this review, we focus on the use of compounds administered *in vivo*, and how we can use these methodological caveats to improve our findings *in vitro*. In particular, we examine some positive evidence for neuroprotection *in vivo* using berry-derived polyphenolic compounds.

4. *In Vivo* Studies with Antioxidants

4.1. Berry-Derived Polyphenolics

The potential of various berries to protect the brain from aging and neurodegenerative disorders has gained increased attention in recent years, in large part due to their high polyphenol content and antioxidant capacity [9,10]. Many studies using whole animals, usually rodents, have been conducted recently in order to evaluate the effects of berries on the nervous system. For example, dietary supplementation with high amounts of blueberries can decrease age-related behavioral deficits in rats [23]. In a recent study conducted using a mouse model of Alzheimer's disease, treatment with bilberries, which are rich in polyphenols, decreased the extent of behavioral abnormalities associated with the disease [24]. Another study demonstrated that rats fed a diet enriched with blueberries can protect the brain against oxidative stress and associated learning deficits [25]. Perhaps most surprisingly, diets enriched with blueberries over the course of several weeks have been shown to protect animals from damage induced by insults as severe as ischemic stroke [26,27].

Some *in vivo* studies have specifically investigated the protective effects of polyphenols against retinal damage. In one such study mice were treated prophylactically with bilberry extract, which was quantified and found to contain about 39% anthocyanins, after which they were subjected to retinal inflammation [28]. The findings suggested that the high levels of anthocyanins in bilberry extract were able to directly scavenge ROS produced via inflammation, and provide substantial neuroprotection to retinal tissue. In another study, rats were fed blueberries by oral gavage prophylactically for two or seven weeks before being subjected to light-induced retinopathy, and both groups experienced significant retinal neuroprotection [29].

These types of *in vivo* experimental approaches offer several advantages over cell-based models. For example, *in vivo* studies are more realistic in the sense that animals must ingest a diet containing berries or their extracts, as would humans. Animals can also be fed for various periods of time (e.g., a single day *versus* many weeks), and with different percentages of berries constituting the diet. Several different behavioral tests can be administered in animals to measure motor and/or cognitive functions, and the results can be compared to animals treated with a non-berry enriched diet. In addition, at the end of behavioral testing, several other analyses can be conducted, such as immunocytochemical and histological analysis of various brain areas and other parts of the body, including the liver, heart, and kidneys. Additionally, as mentioned above, the effects of various berries or extracts can be tested in genetic rodent models for various diseases, such as Alzheimer's disease [24].

Despite the many inherent advantages of *in vivo* approaches, there are also some drawbacks. These types of experiments can be financially expensive, especially when considering the cost of maintenance of many animals over the course of several weeks or months. *In vivo* experimentation is not a method that can easily be justified for compound screening, due to the cost, time, and number of animals needed to observe an effect. For this reason, *in vitro* tests must be rigorous and well defined, so that promising compounds are then explored *in vivo*. As with *in vitro* approaches, animals often receive a high amount of berries or extracts in their diets that may not be realistically achieved with humans in order to see a definitive effect. Lastly, many studies do not analyze the extent to which berry-derived polyphenols have entered the brain, making it difficult to determine a mechanism by which a positive effect may have occurred.

4.2. Polyphenolic Bioavailability

There is now substantial evidence suggesting that the ingestion of diets high in berries can have positive effects on the brain, not just in rodents, but also in the human population [30,31]. However, the data remain inconclusive as to whether this is due to direct or indirect effects on nervous system tissue. Some recent research has demonstrated that dietary polyphenols can cross the BBB [30], and anthocyanin compounds specifically have been detected in brain tissue after oral administration to rodents [32–34] as well as pigs [35,36]. Some estimates of specific anthocyanins in brain tissue are in the sub-nanomolar range (0.2–0.25 nmol/g tissue) [33,34], whereas some others are as low as the femtomolar range [36]. Although it cannot be expected that every research group conducting *in vitro* experiments on brain cells, or other *in vivo* tests, measure polyphenol levels in brain tissue of berry-fed animals, it is important to utilize data from bioavailability studies in order to test concentrations of antioxidant compounds that would reach the brain. In some of the previous *in vitro* work that we have conducted, we found that the final concentration of blueberry and lingonberry extracts that we tested in cell cultures was 0.833 μg/ml of fruit extract and 0.083 μg/ml of leaf extract [19]. In other previous work we conducted chemical analysis of commercially available lingonberry extracts and found that these extracts contain an estimated 63.7 mg of cyanidin-3-galactoside per 100 mg of fresh extract weight (unpublished data). If our fresh lingonberry extracts tested *in vitro* contained a similar amount of this compound, this would translate to the cultured cells being exposed to approximately a 10 nM concentration of fruit extract and 1 nM in leaf extract. Talavera *et al.* [33] detected a level of another cyanidin compound (cyanidin-3-glucoside) of 0.25 nmol equivalent per g of tissue. Therefore, the amount of extract that we tested for neuroprotective effects in cultures is most likely somewhat higher than what might be achieved in the brain after oral administration. The amount we added to cultures is also much higher than femtomolar estimates in pigs that had ingested polyphenols orally [36]. However, the polyphenol measurements occurred 18 h postprandial in these latter studies, so it is possible that higher polyphenol levels may have been detected in the brain if measurements had occurred earlier. Most studies in whole animals also feed animals berry-rich diets for several weeks. However, the extent to which berry-derived polyphenols enter the brain from short periods of ingestion (e.g., a day or a week), or how long these constituents stay present in the brain, is not known.

A recent review highlighted ten common misconceptions about antioxidants, including the purported ability of these compounds to cure any disease, or to increase one's lifespan [14]. In addition, the authors point out that a "true" antioxidant should be efficacious at its target (e.g., DNA) at relatively low concentrations, repudiating the notion that "the more antioxidant, the better" when it comes to administration. In relation to this, some researchers have suggested that tissue storage of anthocyanins may become saturated after several weeks (four to eight) of supplementation in the diet [37], which would therefore limit availability to the brain. Recently, it was demonstrated that tissue saturation with antioxidants need not occur in order to provide a neuroprotective effect [29]. We feel that this is a critical finding, in that low compound bioavailability may still provide marked neuroprotection.

Another important consideration in study design using berries and their constituents is that polyphenolic compounds contained in extracts that are tested *in vitro* may not be the predominate forms that would actually enter the brain. In fact, some recent studies have found that although anthocyanins have a fairly high bioavailability, they also undergo significant metabolism, producing diverse metabolites [38,39]. Some experimental evidence suggests that certain polyphenolic compounds are maintained in their natural glycosylated form [32,33]. Xenobiotic metabolism also most likely contributes to the amounts and different forms of polyphenols that cross the BBB, as additional evidence has demonstrated that glucuronide forms of anthocyanins can be detected in the brain [36]. A significant amount of additional research is needed in order to determine the specific types of polyphenolic compounds that can enter the brain, and to what extent.

5. Other Potential Mechanisms of Protection of Natural Compounds

Due to the extensive amount of information suggesting that oxidative stress can contribute to a variety of disease states, including neurological disorders, the ability of polyphenolic compounds to act as antioxidants has arguably received the most attention as far as their mechanism of protection. Although polyphenols such as anthocyanins and flavonols may exert some of their neuroprotective effects by acting directly as antioxidants, they likely have other important effects, such as scavenging reactive nitrogen species, activating protective cell signaling pathways, or altering the expression of various proteins [30,31,40,41]. This suggestion is strengthened by evidence that the bioavailability of these compounds in the brain is much lower than the levels of endogenous antioxidant compounds [41]. The compound resveratrol was initially believed to exert positive health benefits by acting as an antioxidant compound. However, recently it has been found that resveratrol exhibits its potential anti-aging effects by acting primarily as a phosphodiesterase inhibitor [42]. Although oxyresveratrol has indeed been shown to exert antioxidant effects [43], due to its similarity in structure to resveratrol, it is possible that it also has varied mechanisms of action resulting in neuroprotection.

One possibility is that polyphenols exert beneficial properties through purported hormetic effects. One example of such a mechanism is that low levels of these compounds appear to activate the transcription factor Nrf2, which can induce the production of endogenous antioxidant enzymes and other related protective compounds [30,41]. Polyphenolic compounds can also decrease the level of pro-inflammatory mediators in the brain, such as tumor necrosis factor-α and a variety of interleukins [31]. The anti-nitrosative properties of polyphenols may also contribute significantly to protecting the brain from damage compared to antioxidant effects, by scavenging excessive damaging compounds, such as peroxynitrite. It can also not be ruled out that polyphenols have an indirect effect on the brain that leads to beneficial effects. For example, antioxidant effects could be positive for the cardiovascular system, which may lead to an increase in blood flow to the brain. This secondary effect could improve cognitive function both in experimental animals and in humans. These latter biological effects of polyphenols in the brain are poorly understood and warrant further investigation.

6. Conclusions

Oxidative stress is believed to contribute to a wide variety of nervous system disorders, including neurodegenerative diseases, brain aging, and insults such as traumatic brain injury and stroke. Therefore, antioxidant compounds have received significant attention as potential treatments for a variety of brain abnormalities, and evidence suggests that antioxidant compounds can be beneficial for the nervous system. Assessment of antioxidant compounds is typically conducted using a variety of *in vitro* and *in vivo* techniques. In this review, we have illustrated many of the advantages and disadvantages of both approaches. For example, although *in vitro* cell culture systems are quite useful for screening antioxidant compounds for neuroprotective potential, cell lines and cells directly isolated from brain tissue do not maintain the exact properties of an intact brain. Although it is generally acceptable to add a high concentration of a compound in order to determine if there are any potential protective effects, the level that an antioxidant compound may achieve in the brain is impossible to determine without *in vivo* animal studies. More studies are currently needed to determine the bioavailability of compounds with high antioxidant capacity, such as polyphenols or similar substances. Although these latter types of studies primarily need to be conducted using *in vivo* experimentation, complimentary *in vitro* studies will continue to significantly aid in deciphering the cellular mechanisms by which antioxidants are truly beneficial, as neuroprotection may be mediated through other mechanisms that are unrelated to alleviating or preventing oxidative stress. At this point however, it is sufficient to say that, although *in vitro* studies provide a wealth of information on various intrinsic compound parameters, we feel that it is highly likely that many compounds incorrectly enter animal trials, with no subsequent success *in vivo*, and that many putative neuroprotective compounds never enter animal trials because of the means used to evaluate their potential protective efficacy *in vitro*. A careful use of both *in vitro* and *in vivo* approaches is necessary in order to lead to the development of antioxidant therapeutic compounds for the human population.

Acknowledgements

Some of the work reviewed in this article was supported through grants from the Canada Foundation for Innovation and the Natural Sciences and Engineering Research Council to John T. Weber.

Author Contributions

The authors contributed equally to the writing of this manuscript and approve of the final version.

Conflicts of Interest

The authors declare no conflict of interest.

References

1. Slemmer, J.E.; Shacka, J.J.; Sweeney, M.I.; Weber, J.T. Antioxidants and free radical scavengers for the treatment of stroke, traumatic brain injury and aging. *Curr. Med. Chem.* **2008**, *15*, 404–414.
2. Martinez, M.C.; Andriantsitohaina, R. Reactive nitrogen species: Molecular mechanisms and potential significance in health and disease. *Antioxid. Redox Signal* **2009**, *11*, 669–702.
3. Halliwell, B. Oxidative stress and neurodegeneration: Where are we now? *J. Neurochem.* **2006**, *97*, 1634–1658.

4. Halliwell, B.; Gutteridge, J.M.C. *Free Radicals in Biology and Medicine*, 4th ed.; Oxford University Press: New York, NY, USA, 2007.
5. Panfoli, I. Beneficial effect of antioxidants in retinopathies: A new hypothesis. *Med. Hypothesis Discov. Innov. Ophthalmol.* **2012**, *1*, 76–79.
6. Pandya, C.D.; Howell, K.R.; Pillai, A. Antioxidants as potential therapeutics for neuropsychiatric disorders. *Prog. Neuropsychopharmacol. Biol. Psychiatry* **2013**, *46*, 214–223.
7. Valko, M.; Leibfritz, D.; Moncol, J.; Cronin, M.T.; Mazur, M.; Telser, J. Free radicals and antioxidants in normal physiological functions and human disease. *Int. J. Biochem. Cell Biol.* **2007**, *39*, 44–84.
8. Droge, W. Free radicals in the physiological control of cell function. *Physiol. Rev.* **2002**, *82*, 47–95.
9. Lau, F.C.; Shukitt-Hale, B.; Joseph, J.A. The beneficial effects of fruit polyphenols on brain aging. *Neurobiol. Aging* **2005**, *26*, S128–S132.
10. Gao, X.; Cassidy, A.; Schwarzschild, M.A.; Rimm, E.B.; Ascherio, A. Habitual intake of dietary flavonoids and risk of Parkinson disease. *Neurology* **2012**, *78*, 1138–1145.
11. Aboul-Enein, H.Y.; Berczyńsk, P.; Kruk, I. Phenolic compounds: The role of redox regulation in neurodegenerative disease and cancer. *Mini Rev. Med. Chem.* **2013**, *13*, 385–398.
12. Panickar, K.S.; Jang, S. Dietary and plant polyphenols exert neuroprotective effects and improve cognitive function in cerebral ischemia. *Rec. Pat. Food Nutr. Agric.* **2013**, *5*, 128–143.
13. Hainsworth, A.H.; Bhuiyan, N.; Green, A.R. The nitrone disodium 2,4-sulphophenyl-*N-tert*-butylnitrone is without cytoprotective effect on sodium nitroprusside-induced cell death in N1E-115 neuroblastoma cells *in vitro*. *J. Cereb. Blood Flow Metab.* **2008**, *28*, 24–28.
14. Bast, A.; Haenen, G.R.M.M. Ten misconceptions about antioxidants. *Trends Pharmacol. Sci.* **2013**, *34*, 430–436.
15. Masters, J.R.W. Human cancer cell lines: Fact and fantasy. *Nat. Rev. Mol. Cell Biol.* **2000**, *1*, 233–236.
16. Gillet, J.P.; Varma, S.; Gottesman, M.M. The clinical relevance of cancer cell lines. *J. Natl. Cancer Inst.* **2013**, *105*, 452–458.
17. Capes-Davis, A.; Theodosopoulos, G.; Atkin, I.; Drexler, H.G.; Kohara, A.; MacLeod, R.A.; Masters, J.R.; Nakamura, Y.; Reid, Y.A.; Reddel, R.R.; *et al.* Check your cultures! A list of cross-contaminated or misidentified cell lines. *Int. J. Cancer* **2010**, *127*, 1–8.
18. Weber, J.T.; Lamont, M.; Chibrikova, L.; Vlug, A.S.; Fekkes, D.; Lorenz, P.; Kreutzmann, P.; Slemmer, J.E. Potential protective effects of oxyresveratrol against traumatic injury. *Eur. J. Pharm.* **2012**, *680*, 55–62.
19. Vyas, P.; Kalidindi, S.; Chibrikova, L.; Igamberdiev, A.U.; Weber, J.T. Chemical analysis and effect of blueberry and lingonberry fruits and leaves against glutamate-mediated excitotoxicity in rat brain cultures. *J. Agric. Food Chem.* **2013**, *61*, 7769–7776.
20. Engel, D.C.; Slemmer, J.E.; Vlug, A.S.; Maas, A.I.R.; Weber, J.T. Combined effects of mechanical and ischemic injury to cortical cells: Secondary ischemia increases damage and decreases effects of neuroprotective agents. *Neuropharmacology* **2005**, *49*, 985–995.
21. Breuer, C.; Wolf, G.; Andrabi, S.A.; Lorenz, P.; Horn, T.F. Blood-brain barrier permeability to the neuroprotectant oxyresveratrol. *Neurosci. Lett.* **2006**, *393*, 113–118.

22. Feuerstein, G.Z.; Zaleska, M.M.; Krams, M.; Wang, X.; Day, M.; Rutkowski, J.L.; Finklestein, S.P.; Pangalos, M.N.; Poole, M.; Stiles, G.L.; *et al.* Missing steps in the STAIR case: A Translational Medicine perspective on the development of NXY-059 for treatment of acute ischemic stroke. *J. Cereb. Blood Flow Metab.* **2008**, *28*, 217–219.
23. Shukitt-Hale, B.; Galli, R.L.; Meterko, V.; Carey, A.; Bielinski, D.F.; McGhie, T.; Joseph, J.A. Dietary supplementation with fruit polyphenolics ameliorates age-related deficits in behavior and neuronal markers of inflammation and oxidative stress. *Age* **2005**, *27*, 49–57.
24. Vepsäläinen, S.; Koivisto, H.; Pekkarinen, E.; Mäkinen, P.; Dobson, G.; McDougall, G.J.; Stewart, D.; Haapasalo, A.; Karjalainen, R.O.; Tanila, H.; *et al.* Anthocyanin-enriched bilberry and blackcurrant extracts modulate amyloid precursor protein processing and alleviate behavioral abnormalities in the APP/PS1 mouse model of Alzheimer's disease. *J. Nutr. Biochem.* **2013**, *24*, 360–370.
25. Duffy, K.B.; Spangler, E.L.; Devan, B.D.; Guo, Z.; Bowker, J.L.; Janas, A.M.; Hagepanos, A.; Minor, R.K.; DeCabo, R.; Mouton, P.R.; *et al.* A blueberry-enriched diet provides cellular protection against oxidative stress and reduces a kainate-induced learning impairment in rats. *Neurobiol. Aging* **2008**, *29*, 1680–1689.
26. Sweeney, M.I.; Kalt, W.; MacKinnon, S.L.; Ashby, J.; Gottschall-Pass, K.T. Feeding rats diets enriched in lowbush blueberries for six weeks decreases ischemia-induced brain damage. *Nutr. Neurosci.* **2002**, *5*, 427–431.
27. Wang, Y.; Chang, C.F.; Chou, J.; Chen, H.L.; Deng, X.; Harvey, B.K.; Cadet, J.L.; Bickford, P.C. Dietary supplementation with blueberries, spinach, or spirulina reduces ischemic brain damage. *Exp. Neurol.* **2005**, *193*, 75–84.
28. Miyake, S.; Takahashi, N.; Sasaki, M.; Kobayashi, S.; Tsubota, K.; Ozawa, Y. Vision preservation during retinal inflammation by anthocyanin-rich bilberry extract: Cellular and molecular mechanism. *Lab. Investig.* **2012**, *92*, 102–109.
29. Tremblay, F.; Waterhouse, J.; Nason, J.; Kalt, W. Prophylactic neuroprotection by blueberry-enriched diet in a rat model of light-induced retinopathy. *J. Nutr. Biochem.* **2013**, *24*, 647–655.
30. Vauzour, D. Dietary polyphenols as modulators of brain functions: Biological actions and molecular mechanisms underpinning their beneficial effects. *Oxid. Med. Cell Longev.* **2012**, *2012*, doi:10.1155/2012/914273.
31. Miller, M.G.; Shukitt-Hale, B. Berry fruit enhances beneficial signaling in the brain. *J. Agric. Food Chem.* **2012**, *60*, 5709–5715.
32. Andres-Lacueva, C.; Shukitt-Hale, B.; Galli, R.L.; Jauregui, O.; Lamuela-Raventos, R.M.; Joseph, J.A. Anthocyanins in aged blueberry-fed rats are found centrally and may enhance memory. *Nutr. Neurosci.* **2005**, *8*, 111–120.
33. Talavéra, S.; Felgines, C.; Texier, O.; Besson, C.; Gil-Izquierdo, A.; Lamaison, J.L.; Rémésy, C. Anthocyanin metabolism in rats and their distribution to digestive area, kidney, and brain. *J. Agric. Food Chem.* **2005**, *53*, 3902–3908.
34. El Mohsen, M.A.; Marks, J.; Kuhnle, G.; Moore, K.; Debnam, E.; Kaila Srai, S.; Rice-Evans, C.; Spencer, J.P. Absorption, tissue distribution and excretion of pelargonidin and its metabolites following oral administration to rats. *Br. J. Nutr.* **2006**, *95*, 51–58.

35. Kalt, W.; Blumberg, J.B.; McDonald, J.E.; Vinqvist-Tymchuk, M.R.; Fillmore, S.A.; Graf, B.A.; O'Leary, J.M.; Milbury, P.E. Identification of anthocyanins in the liver, eye, and brain of blueberry-fed pigs. *J. Agric. Food Chem.* **2008**, *56*, 705–712.
36. Milbury, P.E.; Kalt, W. Xenobiotic metabolism and berry flavonoid transport across the blood-brain barrier. *J. Agric. Food Chem.* **2010**, *58*, 3950–3956.
37. Del Bò, C.; Ciappellano, S.; Klimis-Zacas, D.; Martini, D.; Gardana, C.; Riso, P.; Porrini, M. Anthocyanin absorption, metabolism, and distribution from a wild blueberry-enriched diet (*Vaccinium angustifolium*) is affected by diet duration in the Sprague—Dawley rat. *J. Agric. Food Chem.* **2010**, *58*, 2491–2497.
38. Czank, C.; Cassidy, A.; Zhang, Q.; Morrison, D.J.; Preston, T.; Kroon, P.A.; Botting, N.P.; Kay, C.D. Human metabolism and elimination of the anthocyanin, cyanidin-3-glucoside: A ^{13}C-tracer study. *Am. J. Clin. Nutr.* **2013**, *97*, 995–1003.
39. Kalt, W.; Liu, Y.; McDonald, J.E.; Vinqvist-Tymchuk, M.R.; Fillmore, S.A. Anthocyanin metabolites are abundant and persistent in human urine. *J. Agric. Food Chem.* **2014**, *62*, 3926-3934.
40. Doré, S. Unique properties of polyphenol stilbenes in the brain: More than direct antioxidant actions; gene/protein regulatory activity. *Neurosignals* **2005**, *14*, 61–70.
41. Schaffer, S.; Halliwell, B. Do polyphenols enter the brain and does it matter? Some theoretical and practical considerations. *Genes Nutr.* **2012**, *7*, 99–109.
42. Park, S.J.; Ahmad, F.; Philp, A.; Baar, K.; Williams, T.; Luo, H.; Ke, H.; Rehmann, H.; Taussig, R.; Brown, A.L.; *et al.* Resveratrol ameliorates aging-related metabolic phenotypes by inhibiting cAMP phosphodiesterases. *Cell* **2012**, *148*, 421–433.
43. Lorenz, P.; Roychowdhury, S.; Engelmann, M.; Wolf, G.; Horn, T.F. Oxyresveratrol and resveratrol are potent antioxidants and free radical scavengers: Effect on nitrosative and oxidative stress derived from microglial cells. *Nitric Oxide* **2003**, *9*, 64–76.

8

Antioxidant Capacity, Cytotoxicity and Antimycobacterial Activity of Madeira Archipelago Endemic *Helichrysum* Dietary and Medicinal Plants

Sandra C. Gouveia-Figueira [1,2,3,*], Carla A. Gouveia [1], Maria J. Carvalho [1], Ana I. Rodrigues [4], Malin L. Nording [2] and Paula C. Castilho [1]

[1] Centro de Química da Madeira, CCCEE, Universidade da Madeira, Campus Universitário da Penteada, piso 0, Funchal 9000-390, Portugal; E-Mails: carlaapgouveia@gmail.com (C.A.G.); mariajmcarvalho@hotmail.com (M.J.C.); castilho@uma.pt (P.C.C.)

[2] Department of Chemistry, Umeå University, Umeå SE-901 87, Sweden; E-Mail: malin.nording@chem.umu.se

[3] Department of Pharmacology and Clinical Neuroscience, Umeå University, Umeå SE-901 87, Sweden

[4] Unidade de Geologia Marinha, Laboratório Nacional de Energia e Geologia, I.P., Estrada da Portela, Zambujal—Alfragide Apartado 7586, Amadoram 2720-866, Portugal; E-Mail: ana.rodrigues@lneg.pt

* Author to whom correspondence should be addressed; E-Mail: sandra.gouveia@chem.umu.se

External Editors: Maria G. Migue and João Rocha

Abstract: The potential bioactivity of dietary and medicinal endemic *Helichrysum* plants from Madeira Archipelago was explored, for the first time, in order to supply new information for the general consumer. *In vitro* antioxidant properties were investigated using DPPH, $ABTS^{\bullet+}$, FRAP and β-Carotene assays, and the total phenolic content (TPC) and total flavonoid content (TFC) were also determined. Although the results generally showed a large variation among the three analyzed plants, the methanolic extracts showed the highest antioxidant capacity. Exception is made for *H. devium n*-hexane extract that showed good radical scavenger capacity associated to compounds with good reducing properties. In the *Artemia salina* toxicity assay and antimycobaterial activity, *H. devium* was the most potent plant with the lowest LD_{50} at 216.7 ± 10.4 and MIC ≤ 50 μg·mL^{-1}. Chemometric evaluation

(Principal Component Analysis—PCA) showed close interdependence between the ABTS, TPC and TFC methods and allowed to group *H. devium* samples.

Keywords: antioxidant; antimycobacterial; *Artemia salina*; *Helichrysum*; chemometrics

1. Introduction

There is a growing effort in the search for natural compounds displaying biological activities associated with low cytotoxicity.

High levels of free radicals and reactive oxygen species (ROS) such as superoxide anion ($O_2^{\bullet-}$), hydroxyl radical ($OH^{\bullet}$) and peroxyl radical ($ROO^{\bullet}$) produced *in vivo* are extremely reactive. Those species have been associated with severe pathological processes such as cancer, atherosclerosis, neurodegenerative and cardiovascular diseases, inflammation and aging, as well as to food deterioration [1,2].

Edible plants have been described in traditional medicines to treat several diseases and conditions. Many of these plants have an important antioxidant effect without some of the disadvantages presented by the synthetic antioxidants [3].

A large number of antioxidants isolated from higher plants are secondary metabolites, such as phenolic compounds [4].

Tuberculosis is caused by *Mycobacterium tuberculosis* (MBT) and, to a low level, by *Mycobacterium bovis* and *Mycobacterium africanum.* Tuberculosis is a leading cause of mortality worldwide, infecting about nine million people and killing about two million people annually [5]. The new infections and reactivation of latent tuberculosis is rising mainly in individuals with compromised immune systems, such as cases of HIV-positive individuals [6].

Natural purified compounds and extracts from plants, microorganisms and marine organisms with high antioxidant capacity have been described as inhibiting *Mycobacterium tuberculosis* (MBT). In the last decades, several literature reviews have been reported regarding natural compounds active against MBT [6–12].

Plants of the genus *Helichrysum* Mill. belong to the Asteraceae family and comprise more than 500 species [13]. They are normally used as herbal infusions and are associated with numerous biological activities such as antioxidant, antimicrobial, anti-inflammatory, anti-allergic, in addition to relief of abdominal pain, heart burn, cough, cold and wounds [14,15].

In Madeira Archipelago (Portugal), there are four endemic species of *Helichrysum* and three (*Helichrysum devium*, *Helichrysum melaleucum* and *Helichrysum obconicum*) are reported as being largely used in the local traditional medicine and diet [16].

Helichrysum devium Johns. and *Helichrysum melaleucum* Rchb. ex. Holl. are used against respiratory diseases, such as bronchitis and pharyngitis and also as a cough relief. *Helichrysum obconicum* DC. is used in infusions as a digestive, to relieve stomachic pain, as well as for intestinal diseases [16].

In our previous work [13,17,18], characterization and quantification of the phenolic compounds of these three species by HPLC-DAD-ESI/MS^n was reported. Phenolic compounds, namely flavonoids and hydroxycinnamic acids, were found to be the major components.

To the best of our knowledge, this paper is the first study of the antioxidant capacity (DPPH, $ABTS^{\bullet+}$, FRAP and β-Carotene), cytotoxicity and antimicrobial activity of these three *Helichrysum* dietary medicinal plants.

The interrelations between these parameters were studied using chemometric methods (PCA analysis) for data evaluation.

2. Materials and Methods

2.1. Chemicals

The following reagents were purchased from Merck (Darmstadt, Germany): potassium persulfate (99%), sodium chloride (99.5%), disodium phosphate dodecahydrated (99%), glacial acetic acid (100%), sodium carbonate (p.a.), and ferrous sulfate heptahydrate (99%), from Fluka (Lisbon, Portugal), 2,2-diphenyl-1-picrylhydrazyl (DPPH) (>95%), Trolox (≥99.8%), 2,2′-azinobis-(3-ethylbenzthiazoline-6-sulfonic acid) (ABTS) (≥99%), 2,4,6-tri(2-pyridyl)-*s*-triazine (TPTZ) (≥99.0%), β-Carotene (≥97%, UV), Tween 40 and Folin–Ciocalteu's phenol reagent were purchased from Fluka (Lisbon, Portugal). Potassium chloride (>99.5%), gallic acid (99%), rutin (≥98%, HPLC) and ferric chloride hexahydrated (97%–102%) were purchased from Panreac (Barcelona, Spain); potassium dihydrogen phosphate (99.5%), aluminum chloride (98%), sodium acetate trihydrate (pure) and dimethylsulfoxide (97%) were purchased from Riedel-de Haën (Hanover, Germany). Alamar Blue solution was purchased from Trek Diagnostics (Westlake, OH, USA).

All solvents for plant extraction were AR grade, from Fisher (Lisbon, Portugal). Water was purified by a Milli-Q Gradient system (Millipore, Milford, MA, USA).

2.2. Instruments

Spectrophotometric measurements were performed on a Perkin Elmer UV-Vis spectrometer Lambda 2 (Perkin Elmer, Ueberlingen, Germany) equipped with a water thermostatic cell holder with glass cells of 1 cm optical path. The UV-Vis measurements in the β-Carotene method were performed using a model Victor3 microtiter reader (Perkin–Elmer, Ueberlingen, Germany).

Fluorescence was measured in a plate fluorometer (Fluoroskan Ascent FL, Thermo, Finland) at an excitation wavelength of 490 nm and an emission wavelength of 540 nm, and relative fluorescence units (*rfu*) were recorded.

2.3. Plant Material

Specimens of three endemic species of *Helichrysum* were collected during May and June from the northern coast of Madeira Island. They were identified by taxonomist Fátima Rocha and vouchers were deposited in the Madeira Botanical Garden Herbarium collection. The total aerial parts were dried at room temperature (protected from direct sunlight) and ground into a fine powder by a mechanical grinder.

Each sample (100 $g \cdot plant \cdot L^{-1}$ of solvent) was extracted through sequential maceration with four organic solvents of increasing polarity (*n*-hexane, chloroform, ethyl acetate and methanol), at room temperature for 24 h. The extracts were filtered and evaporated to dryness under reduced pressure in a rotary evaporator, at 40 °C.

For the *Mycobacterium tuberculosis* studies, crude methanolic extracts were obtained by plant maceration for 48 h followed by filtration and concentration to dryness.

2.4. Antimycobacterial Activity

2.4.1. *Mycobacterium* Strains

The following *Mycobacterium* species was obtained from the American Type Culture Collection (ATCC): *Mycobacterium tuberculosis* H37Rv (27294).

2.4.2. Inoculum Preparation for Biological Assays

The strain was cultured at 37 °C in Middlebrook 7H9 broth (7H9), supplemented with 0.2% glycerol and 10% OADC enrichment (oleic acid, albumin, dextrose, catalase; Difco) until *log* phase growth was achieved. The inocula for microcolorimetric assay was prepared by diluting *log* phase growth cultures with sterile 7H9 to the McFarland No. 1 turbidity standard, and were then further diluted 1:20 in 7H9. The working suspension was prepared just prior to inoculation of the microplate.

2.4.3. Antimycobacterial Screening by Microplate Alamar Blue Assay

The methodology used was based on that described by Jimenez-Arellanes *et al.* [19].

Stock solutions of each sample were prepared in DMSO at a concentration of 20 $g \cdot L^{-1}$. Serial dilutions of each sample were prepared; final concentrations ranged from 50 to 200 $mg \cdot L^{-1}$. Duplicates of each sample were made per plate and each experiment was repeated at least twice. Bacterial suspension (100 μL) was added to test wells and to controls. A 1:10 diluted control was included in each plate, representing the growth of 10% of the bacterial population tested (10% control). The plates were incubated at 37 °C for 5 days and after that they were developed by adding 20 μL of Alamar Blue solution (Trek Diagnostics, Westlake, OH, USA) to each well. The plates were reincubated, at 37 °C, for 24 h. Fluorescence was measured in a plate fluorometer (Fluoroskan Ascent FL, Thermo, Finland) at an excitation wavelength of 490 nm and an emission wavelength of 540 nm, and relative fluorescence units (*rfu*) were recorded. Wells with a well-defined pink color were scored as positive for growth.

The minimal inhibitory concentration (MIC) was defined as the lowest sample concentrations that prevent a color change to pink and that presented *rfu* values lower than those presented by the 10% growth control.

Extracts were considered active if they gave a MIC < 200 $\mu g \cdot mL^{-1}$. Extracts active at concentrations lower than 50 $\mu g \cdot mL^{-1}$ were further tested at lower concentrations (down to 6.25 $\mu g \cdot mL^{-1}$).

2.5. Artemia Salina Toxicity Evaluation

The brine shrimp toxicity assay was adapted from the method reported by Dey and Harborne [20].

Filtered seawater was added to a small tank and air was bubbled through it, using an aquarium pump; shrimp eggs were added to the aired water and left to incubate at room temperature for 48 h; fully developed shrimp larvae were collected at this point and immediately used.

For each sample, stock solutions were prepared in DMSO with a concentration (m/v) of 20 mg·mL^{-1}. The tested solutions presented the following concentrations: 5 mg·mL^{-1}; 1 mg·mL^{-1}; 0.5 mg·mL^{-1} and 0.1 mg·mL^{-1}. 5 mL of seawater, 50 µL of each sample and 10 shrimp larvae (30 per dilution) were added to each vial. The percentage of larvae deaths was calculated after 24 h of incubation. The LD_{50} was calculated using a linear regression equation. When high mortality was observed, intermediary concentrations were tested (3.5 and 2.5 mg·mL^{-1}). For each experiment a control was performed consisting of adding 50 µL of DMSO.

2.6. Determination of Total Phenolic Content (TPC)

Total phenolic contents were determined by the Folin–Ciocalteu method described by Zheng and Wang [21] with some modifications. Plant extracts were dissolved in methanol to yield a final concentration (w/v) of 10 mg·mL^{-1}. Of each diluted extract, 50 µL was mixed with 1.25 mL of Folin–Ciocalteau reagent (diluted 1:10 fold) and 1 mL of 7.5% sodium carbonate solution. The mixture was incubated for 30 min, at room temperature, and then absorbance was measured at 765 nm. The TPC was expressed as gallic acid equivalents per 100 g of dried plant (mg GAE 100 g^{-1}).

2.7. Determination of Total Flavonoid Content (TFC)

Total flavonoid content was measured using a colorimetric aluminum chloride method [22]. Ten mg of each extract was dissolved in 5 mL of methanol and 0.5 mL of this diluted extract was mixed with 1.5 mL of methanol, 2.8 mL of water, 0.1 mL of potassium acetate (1 M) and 0.1 mL of aluminum chloride (10% in methanol). After incubation for 30 min, the decrease in absorbance was measured at 415 nm. The TFC was calculated using a standard calibration curve of rutin solutions (12.5 to 100 µg·mL^{-1}), and expressed as milligrams of rutin equivalents per 100 g of dried sample (mg RUE 100 g^{-1}).

2.8. Antioxidant Assays

2.8.1. 2,2-Diphenyl-1-Picrylhydrazyl (DPPH) Radical Scavenging Activity

The DPPH assay was executed according to [23] with minor modifications. One hundred µL of extract solution (10 mg·mL^{-1}) was added to 3.5 mL of a 0.06 mM methanol DPPH radical solution. The decrease in absorbance at 516 nm was measured every minute during a 30 min period, in the dark. The DPPH radical scavenging activity was expressed based on the Trolox calibration curve as µmol Trolox equivalent per 100 g of dried plant (µmol eq. Trolox 100 g^{-1} dried plant).

2.8.2. 2,2′-Azinobis-(3-Ethylbenzthiazoline-6-Sulfonic Acid) ($ABTS^{\bullet+}$) Radical Scavenging Activity

A modified method, initially reported by [24] was used for the determination of the antioxidant activity by the method of decolorization of free radical $ABTS^{\bullet+}$. The $ABTS^{\bullet+}$ radical was prepared by reacting 50 mL of 2 mM $ABTS^{\bullet+}$ aqueous solution with 200 µL of 70 mM $K_2S_2O_8$ solution.

This mixture was kept in the dark for 16 h, at room temperature. Before each experiment, the $ABTS^{\bullet+}$ solution was diluted with pH 7.4 phosphate buffered saline (PBS) solution to an initial absorbance of 0.700 ± 0.021 at 734 nm.

Briefly, an aliquot of 100 µL of extract solution (10 $mg \cdot mL^{-1}$) was added to 1.8 mL of $ABTS^{\bullet+}$ solution and the absorbance at 734 nm was recorded during 6 min. Results were expressed in terms of µmol Trolox equivalent per 100 g of dried plant antioxidant capacity (µmol eq. Trolox 100 g^{-1} dried plant).

2.8.3. Ferric Reducing Activity (FRAP Assay)

The ferric reducing activity of the plant extracts was estimated based on the FRAP assay [25]. At low pH, the ferric-tripyridyltriazine (Fe^{3+}-TPTZ) orange complex is reduced to a blue-colored ferrous complex (Fe^{2+}-TPTZ) by the action of electron-donating antioxidants. This reaction was followed with an increase in absorbance at 593 nm. FRAP reagent was prepared daily by mixing 2.5 mL of solution $FeCl_3 \cdot 6H_2O$ (20 mM), 2.5 mL of solution TPTZ (10 mM in 40 mM of HCl) and 25 mL of acetate buffer 0.3 M (pH 3.6) and was incubated at 37 °C. For each analysis, 30 µL of solution (1 $mg \cdot mL^{-1}$) was added to 180 µL of distilled water and 1.8 mL of FRAP solution. The variance absorbance of the reaction mixture was recorded at 593 nm in 15 s intervals, during 30 min against methanol as blank. Methanolic solutions of known Fe (II) concentration, in the range of 2.00–500 mM ($FeSO_4 \cdot 7H_2O$) were used to prepare the calibration curve. The FRAP results were expressed as mmol $FeSO_4 \cdot 7H_2O$ per mg of dried plant (mmol Fe(II) mg^{-1}).

2.8.4. β-Carotene (BC) Bleaching Assay

This method was based on that described by Siddhuraju and Becker [26]. Briefly, 2 mL of β-Carotene solution 0.2 $mg \cdot mL^{-1}$ in chloroform was added to a round-bottom flask (250 mL) containing 0.04 mL of linoleic acid and 200 mg of Tween 40. The chloroform was completely evaporated using nitrogen and then 50 mL of oxygenated ultra-pure water, obtained by bubbling air through the water for 15 min was added, and the mixture was vigorously shaken. The resulting emulsion was freshly prepared before each experiment. Stock solutions of the extracts were prepared in ethanol (1 $mg \cdot mL^{-1}$). An aliquot of 250 µL of the β-Carotene/linoleic acid emulsion was distributed in each of the wells of the 96-well microtiter plates and 30 µL of the sample solutions were added. An equal amount of ethanol was used for the control sample. The samples were then subjected to thermal autoxidation at 45 °C for 210 min. The absorbance of the solution was measured at 490 nm by taking measurements at 15 min intervals. The antioxidant activity (AA) of each sample was evaluated in terms of the bleaching of β-Carotene using the following equation: $AA (\%) = (1 - (A_0 - A_t/A'_0 - A'_t)) \times 100$, where A_0 and A'_0 are the absorbance values measured at zero incubation time for the test and control respectively and A_t and A'_t are the corresponding absorbance values measured after incubation for 210 min. All samples were assayed in triplicate.

2.9. Statistical Analysis

All measurements were performed in triplicate and results are expressed as mean ± SD.

Significant differences in antioxidant activity and total phenolic content of the different extracts were determined using one-way ANOVA. The Pearson correlation coefficients were determined using SPSS. The statistical probability was considered to be significantly different at the level of $p < 0.05$.

Principal components analysis (PCA) was done on the results of TPC, TFC, DPPH, ABTS, FRAP, BC and *Artemia salina* of the total aerial parts extracts of *Helichrysum* plants using SIMCA software v.13 (Umetrics AB, Umeå, Sweden).

3. Results and Discussion

3.1. Extraction Yield

The percentage yields of all analyzed extracts of *Helichrysum* species are presented in Table 1. Yields ranged from 0.18% (*H. melaleucum*, ethyl acetate) to 15.0% (*H. obconicum*, methanol), and extraction with methanol was the most efficient presenting a higher yield.

3.2. Antimycobacterial Activity

Given the traditional uses of *Helichrysum* plants in Madeira against respiratory problems such as bronchitis and pharyngitis, preliminary studies over *Mycobacterium tuberculosis* were performed. The methanolic crude extracts of *H. devium*, *H. melaleucum* and *H. obconicum* were evaluated for their activity against *M. tuberculosis* H37Rv and the results are shown in Figure 1. *H. devium* was very potent against *M. tuberculosis* with a MIC equal to 50 $\mu g \cdot mL^{-1}$ and *H. melaleucum* gave a moderate activity with 100 $\mu g \cdot mL^{-1}$, while *H. obconicum* presented low activity, with a MIC of 200 $\mu g \cdot mL^{-1}$.

Figure 1. Antimycobacterial activity of methanolic crude extracts of *Helichrysum* plants.

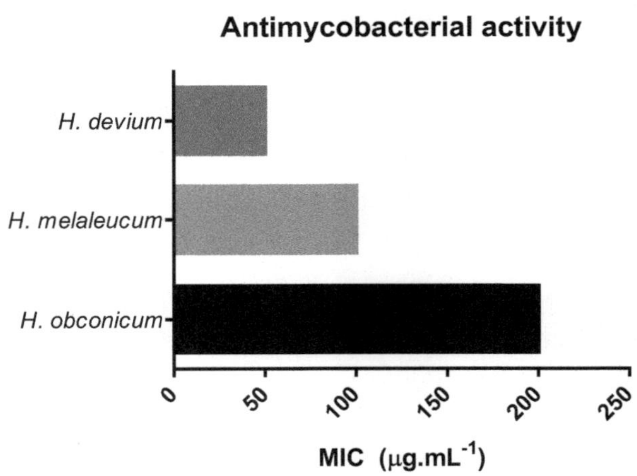

Others have studied the antimycobacterial activity of other *Helichrysum* species. *Helichrysum melanacme* ethanolic extract showed a MIC of 500 $\mu g \cdot mL^{-1}$ against *M. tuberculosis* H37Rv. Biofractionation of this extract led to isolation of two chlacones with MIC of 50 $\mu g \cdot mL^{-1}$ [27].

Table 1. Experimental determinations of total phenolic (TPC), flavonoid content (TFC), antioxidant capacity (DPPH, ABTS, FRAP and β-Carotene) and toxicity activity (mean ± SD) from total aerial parts of *Helichrysum* species extracts.

Plant Extracts		TPC (mg GAE 100 g^{-1})	TFC (mg RUE 100 g^{-1})	DPPH μmol eq. Trolox 100 g^{-1}	ABTS μmol eq. Trolox 100 g^{-1}	FRAP mmol Fe(II) mg^{-1}	BC (%)	Toxicity Activity LD_{50} (μg mL^{-1})	Extraction Yield (%)
H. devium	*n*-Hexane	221.4 ± 1.72 ^{c}	44.95 ± 0.193 ^{d}	289.7 ± 1.03 ^{e}	116.4 ± 0.434 ^{f}	694.9 ± 3.89 ^{b}	62.82 ± 1.58 ^{f}	2.36 ^{d}	216.7 ± 10.4
	Chloroform	234.6 ± 3.61 ^{d}	40.27 ± 0.429 ^{c}	234.8 ± 1.09 ^{d}	84.57 ± 0.0700 ^{d}	852.4 ± 11.1 ^{e}	60.62 ± 2.25 ^{f}	3.63 ^{e}	5025 ± 63.2
	Ethyl acetate	312.7 ± 1.73 ^{f}	180.3 ± 10.6 ^{f}	236.4 ± 4.41 ^{d}	86.12 ± 0.0707 ^{d}	2140.0 ± 14.6 ^{g}	52.34 ± 1.53 ^{d}	3.61 ^{e}	*
	Methanol	399.6 ± 1.52 ^{g}	302.8 ± 1.19 ^{g}	235.4 ± 1.63 ^{d}	107.1 ± 0.0706 ^{e}	2431.8 ± 12.9 ^{h}	46.82 ± 1.75 ^{c}	4.85 ^{f}	479.0 ± 8.20
H. melaleucum	*n*-Hexane	258.9 ± 0.631 ^{e}	46.26 ± 0.477 ^{d}	137.6 ± 2.66 ^{c}	56.94 ± 0.0658 ^{b}	354.8 ± 1.35 ^{a}	61.02 ± 1.45 ^{f}	1.14 ^{c}	322.9 ± 11.9
	Chloroform	106.5 ± 0.373 ^{b}	56.61 ± 0.663 ^{e}	119.2 ± 0.691 ^{b}	71.97 ± 0.0348 ^{c}	831.0 ± 3.09 ^{d}	56.06 ± 1.29 ^{e}	1.35 ^{c}	752.0 ± 36.6
	Ethyl acetate	NA	NA	NA	NA	NA	NA	0.18 ^{a}	3349 ± 102.3
	Methanol	1214 ± 2.11 ^{i}	816.9 ± 1.96 ^{i}	812.9 ± 1.65 ^{g}	286.9 ± 1.28 ^{g}	1581.7 ± 7.71 ^{f}	22.85 ± 0.29 ^{a}	7.64 ^{g}	*
H. obconicum	Hexane	39.75 ± 0.214 ^{a}	19.20 ± 0.251 ^{a}	NI	NI	NI	NI	1.23 ^{c}	934.5 ± 56.2
	Chloroform	NA	NA	NA	NA	NA	NA	NA	NA
	Ethyl acetate	42.05 ± 0.134 ^{a}	23.61 ± 0.195 ^{b}	23.78 ± 0.754 ^{a}	5.780 ± 0.031 ^{a}	741.08 ± 19.9 ^{c}	36.43 ± 0.58 ^{b}	0.57 ^{b}	2,410 ± 88.3
	Methanol	773.4 ± 14.3 ^{h}	703.03 ± 2.98 ^{h}	638.8 ± 1.50 ^{f}	687.9 ± 7.25 ^{h}	19,918.3 ± 75.4 ^{i}	37.96 ± 0.59 ^{b}	15.0 ^{h}	1075 ± 71.5

* Values represented as mean ± SD ($n = 3$); Means not sharing the same letter in the same column are significantly different at $p < 0.05$ probability level; NA—Not Analyzed; NI—No Inhibition.

3.3. *Artemia Salina* Toxicity

Naturally occurring compounds can show the therapeutic effect by exhibiting toxicity to the pernicious cells or materials. Regarding the safety of the *Helichrysum* medicinal and dietary plants, evaluation of toxicity was performed *in vitro* with the *Artemia salina* toxicity assay.

The results were expressed as LD_{50} values (concentration able to kill 50% of the brine shrimp larvae). These values were calculated by linear regression using the least squares method. Samples with values of LD_{50} higher than 1,000 $\mu g \cdot mL^{-1}$ were considered non-toxic [28].

The LD_{50} results obtained for *H. devium*, *melaleucum* and *obconicum* extracts are shown in Table 1.

The *n*-hexane extracts of *H. devium* and *H. melaleucum* presented toxicity on *Artemia salina* with values of 216.7 ± 10.4 and 322.9 ± 11.9 $\mu g \cdot mL^{-1}$, respectively. The methanolic extract of *H. devium* gave a low LD_{50} value at 479.0 ± 8.20 $\mu g \cdot mL^{-1}$, suggesting a moderate toxicity capacity.

H. obconicum extracts were considered almost non-toxic, the *n*-hexane extract is on the limit with a LD_{50} value of 934.5 ± 56.2 $\mu g \cdot mL^{-1}$.

Samples rich in flavonoids are known to possess low LD_{50} values against *Artemia salina* [29,30]. Several flavonoids were identified in *H. devium* [13] and *H. melaleucum* [17], while *H. obconicum* was rich in quinic acid derivatives [18]. These differences in the composition can contribute to the different toxicity of each plant.

The higher toxicity of the *n*-hexane extracts can be attributed to the presence of non-polar compounds, such as terpenes, also known for being toxic to *Artemia salina* larvae [28], or other non-identified hexane soluble substances.

3.4. Total Phenolic Content (TPC) and Total Flavonoid Content (TFC)

Plant secondary metabolites (phenolics and/or polyphenolics compounds) are known for their antioxidant activity. In this study, therefore, endemic *Helichrysum* species from Madeira Archipelago were evaluated for TPC and TFC (Table 1).

Results showed that TPC and TFC varied considerably for each plant. TFC was 10 times higher for the methanolic extract and *H. melaleucum* gave the biggest amount followed by *H. obconicum* and *H. devium*.

TPC values ranged from 39.75 ± 0.214 to 1214 ± 2.11 mg GAE 100 g^{-1} found in *H. obconicum* *n*-hexanic and *H. melaleucum* methanolic extracts, respectively. For all three species, methanolic extracts showed the highest TPC, and the *n*-hexane extracts of *H. devium* and *H. obconicum* presented the lowest, while for *H. melaleucum* the lowest TPC was for chloroform extract. The TFC varied from 19.20 ± 0.251 to 703.03 ± 2.98 mg RUE 100 g^{-1} (Table 1).

Albayrak *et al.* [31] reported the composition and antioxidant activity of 16 *Helichrysum* species from Turkey. The TPC values (66–160 $mg \cdot GAE \cdot g^{-1}$) were higher than the values that we found for Madeira *Helichrysum* species. However, they also detected different TPC values for different species mainly associated to plant origin.

An exploratory study with *Helichrysum graveolens* [32] showed that ethyl acetate extracts have higher TPC and antioxidant capacity when compared with hexane or methanol extracts. Apigenin was the major component of the most active fraction.

Phenolic compounds are polar, thus normally extracted from plants by polar solvents. The observed high value of phenolic content in non-polar solvents, such as *n*-hexane extracts, is not expected but can be tentatively explained. As stated by Huang *et al.* [33], the Folin–Ciocalteu reagent can also react with other reducing compounds rather than phenolic compounds, such as sugars, amino acids or ascorbic acid, and the final results obtained by this method take into account more than the contribution of the phenolic compounds of the sample. Hence, special attention must be given to the results obtained by this method and whenever possible compare them with HPLC quantification of each individual compound and/or other spectrophotometric methods that can give more information to the type of compounds present in the extract.

3.5. Antioxidant Assays

The antioxidant capacity of a complex matrix, such as a plant extract, is attributed to the presence of several components from different classes of compounds. The determination of each individual component contribution to the total antioxidant activity is very demanding and time consuming. Therefore, there are several methods reported for the determination of the whole extract antioxidant capacity. These methods are based on two main mechanisms: single electron transfer (ET) and hydrogen atom transfer (HAT). In HAT assays, the antioxidant and the sample compete for the generated peroxyl radicals. ET-based assays measure the capacity of an antioxidant to reduce an oxidant which changes color when reduced. DPPH, ABTS and FRAP belong to the ET methods [33].

A special remark must be made regarding the comparison of antioxidant assays results with those published in the literature since small variations on the experimental conditions can affect, to a large extent, the results obtained.

3.5.1. DPPH$^{\bullet}$ Radical Scavenging Activity

Antioxidant properties of *Helichrysum* endemic species were first analyzed by the TLC-DPPH screening method. The TLC plate was spotted with the crude extract, developed and dried. The TLC plate was then sprayed with a DPPH methanolic solution (0.2%) and incubated in the dark during 30 min. After this period, the active components appeared as yellow spots against a purple background. All extracts of *Helichrysum* showed at least one yellow spot indicating the presence of antioxidant components.

The spectrophotometric DPPH assay results are usually expressed as the efficient concentration (EC_{50}) that corresponds to the amount of antioxidant necessary to decrease by 50% the initial DPPH radical concentration. However, this calculation is dependent on the specific conditions used in the assay, chiefly the initial DPPH concentration. Therefore, the construction of a calibration curve of a strong standard antioxidant compound like Trolox or ascorbic acid allows for the interpolation of the values of absorbance variation and the results are expressed as equivalent concentration.

The results obtained for DPPH assay are given in Table 1. A large range of activity was detected, from 23.78 ± 0.75 μmol eq. Trolox 100 g^{-1} (*H. obconicum*, ethyl acetate) to 812.95 ± 1.65 μmol eq. Trolox 100 g^{-1} (*H. melaleucum*, methanol).

With the exception of the *n*-hexane extract, the *H. devium* extracts did not show significant difference ($p < 0.05$).

H. melaleucum and *H. obconicum* showed a similar order of activity concerning the solvent polarity, *i.e.*, methanolic extracts gave the highest value followed by *n*-hexane, chloroform and ethyl acetate. Nevertheless, extracts with the solvent of extraction in common gave significantly different ($p > 0.05$) values.

3.5.2. ABTS$^{•+}$ Radical Scavenging Activity

The ABTS assay is based on the neutralization of a radical cation, ABTS$^{•+}$, formed by a single-electron oxidation process [34]. In the presence of electron/hydrogen donors, the ABTS solution turns colorless and this reaction can be accompanied by measuring the decrease in absorbance over time.

As observed in the DPPH method, for *H. devium* samples the *n*-hexane extract presented the highest value of activity of decoloration of ABTS solution (116.4 ± 0.434 μmol eq. Trolox 100 g^{-1}) (Table 1).

In general, the values obtained in the ABTS assay are lower than those obtained for the same sample by the DPPH method. This fact can possibly be explained by the presence of compounds with maximum absorptions wavelengths near the working wavelength in the ABTS method ($\lambda = 734$ nm).

The presence of tannins, which can react with ABTS better than with DPPH [35] could be a plausible explanation. However, this hypothesis is excluded based on our recent studies [13,17,18] where the polar extracts of *H. devium*, *melaleucum* and *obconicum* were analyzed by HPLC-DAD-ESI/MS^n and the major compounds identified were hydroxycinnamic acids, mainly quinic acid derivatives, and flavonoids normally in their *O*-glycosilated form, and no high molecular weight compounds were discovered.

3.5.3. Ferric Reducing Activity (FRAP Assay)

FRAP assay measures the antioxidant capacity of a sample based on its reducing capacity.

The reducing capacity of *Helichrysum* samples varied markedly, with values between 354.8 ± 1.35 mmol Fe (II) mg^{-1} (*H. melaleucum*, hexane) to 19,918 ± 75.4 mmol Fe (II) mg^{-1} (*H. obconicum*, methanol) (Table 1).

For the three species, the highest reducing capacity values were obtained for the methanolic extracts, although with significantly difference between them ($p < 0.05$).

3.5.4. β-Carotene (BC) Bleaching Assay

The evaluation of the antioxidant activity by the β-Carotene assay is based on the fact that the free radical linoleic acid attacks the highly unsaturated β-Carotene; the presence of compounds with antioxidant properties delays the β-Carotene oxidation by neutralizing the free radicals in the medium [22].

In order to compare the percentage of antioxidant activity (AA) of each sample, the same sample concentration was used (1 $mg \cdot mL^{-1}$). At this concentration, none of the samples fully inhibited the β-Carotene oxidation. Nevertheless, all samples prevented, to some extent, the β-Carotene complete oxidation. The registered AA values varied from 22.85% ± 0.29% (*H. melaleucum*, methanol) to 62.82% ± 1.58% (*H. devium*, *n*-hexane) (Table 1).

The methanolic extracts, in general, were less effective in contrast to the results obtained by the other methods, whereas they showed great ability in radical scavenging or reducing properties.

From the three *Helichrysum* species, *H. devium* was the one causing the highest inhibition of β-Carotene oxidation and *H. obconicum* exhibited the lowest capacity to prevent β-Carotene bleaching.

The fact that this method is carried out in emulsion makes its matrix closer to that of real food, but the obtained data are dependent on the polarity of the compounds and, consequently, on their partition between the two phases (aqueous and lipidic). Global results are more sensitive to specific individual components than the other assays. The extracts with a higher AA value contain compounds with high capacity of preventing the oxidation of lipids and could be used as preservatives to delay or limit lipid oxidation.

3.5.5. Correlations between Antioxidant Assays

Table 2a shows the Pearson correlations between TPC and DPPH, ABTS, FRAP and β-Carotene data obtained for *H. devium* and *H. melaleucum*. For *H. obconicum,* these correlations were not established since only two points were measured (*n*-hexane extract did not showed any activity and the yield of chloroform extraction was very low to establish its antioxidant activity).

The correlations between TPC and antioxidant assays obtained for *H. melaleucum* extracts were good ($R^2 > 0.867$). These results are in good agreement with the fact that samples with high levels of phenolic compounds possess, normally, high antioxidant capacity.

In contrast, *H. devium* samples showed a very poor correlation between TPC concerning the DPPH and ABTS assay ($R^2 < 0.140$). This information suggests that the large percentage of compounds responsible for the antioxidant activity of *H. devium* does not belong to the phenolic type. However, *H. devium* extracts gave a very good correlation between the TPC and the FRAP and β-Carotene results. This behavior was expected due to the fact that the Folin–Ciocalteu method has a mechanism based on the reducing properties of phenolic compounds. It is also possible to infer that the phenolic compounds responsible for the high antiradical scavenging capacity of *H. devium* do not possess an effective reducing capacity.

The correlation between the TPC and β-Carotene values was very good for both plants. These results indicate a great influence of the phenolic components of these two samples in the inhibition of β-Carotene oxidation.

The data obtained by the four methods of antioxidant assays were also correlated using Pearson's correlation shown in Table 2b.

An excellent correlation between the DPPH and ABTS values was found for *H. melaleucum* ($R^2 = 0.997$), confirming the same type of reaction involved in the antioxidant measurement. However, for *H. devium,* the correlation was weaker with a $R^2 = 0.755$. A weak correlation between two mechanistically similar methods, such as ABTS and DPPH, is mainly related to the composition of the sample. Therefore, it is possible to infer that *H. devium* has within its composition compounds with different abilities for scavenging DPPH and ABTS.

Table 2. (**a**) The Pearson correlation coefficients between the total phenolic content (TPC) and the antioxidant assays data (DPPH, ABTS, FRAP and BC); (**b**) the Pearson's correlation coefficients between antioxidant assays data.

	R^2	DPPH			ABTS		FRAP	BC
(a)	*H. devium*	0.140			0.054		0.952	0.980
	H. melalecum	0.995			0.983		0.867	0.970
(b)	R^2	DPPH			ABTS		FRAP	
		ABTS	*FRAP*	*BC*	*FRAP*	*BC*	*BC*	
	H. devium	0.755	0.380	0.036	0.891	0.068	−0.984	
	H. melaleucum	0.997	0.914	0.990	0.994	0.998	0.926	

The FRAP values showed good correlations against DPPH and ABTS for *H. melaleucum* ($R^2 > 0.914$). A weak correlation between the DPPH and FRAP data for *H. devium* ($R^2 < 0.38$) was obtained. This fact is linked to the behavior of the *n*-hexane extract in the FRAP method that is opposite to what was observed for the DPPH and ABTS assays where the *n*-hexane extract displayed an antioxidant activity at the same level of the methanol extract. Once more, the reducing properties of the components present in the *H. devium n*-hexane extract are evidenced.

The correlations between BC and DPPH/ABTS results were very good for *H. melaleucum* and no correlation was found in *H. devium* sample. In contrast, the FRAP results correlated very well with those of the BC method for *H. devium* and *H. melaleucum.*

3.6. Principal Component Analysis (PCA)

PCA was applied to the data set of antioxidant capacity methods, TPC, TFC and *Artemia salina* assays extracts after standardization (the mean of the values for each variable was subtracted from each variable value and the result was divided by the standard deviation of the values for each variable). After standardization, each parameter contributed equally to the data set variance and carried equal weight in principal component calculation.

The loadings, eigenvalues, percentage of cumulative variance (R^2) and cumulative predictive variance (Q^2) are shown in Table 3. The high dimensionality of the data was reduced to two principal components (PC1 and PC2), totaling 98% of the variance and a very good R^2 (cum) was achieved (0.945), in addition to a good Q^2 (cum) of (0.397).

PC1 is the component that best approximates the data in the least square sense.

The scores and loading plots of PC1 *vs.* PC2 are shown in Figure 2. The loading plot displays the relationship between all variables. Variables grouped together are positively correlated like the ABTS, TPC, TFC, FRAP and, to some extent, like DPPH, which is also in good agreement with Pearson's correlation.

Artemia salina and BC are located far from the origin and are the variables with major impact on the model. These variables have a higher impact in separating *H. obconicum* and *H. melaleucum* samples.

The PCA plot segregates *H. devium* on the basis of the FRAP, ABTS, TPC and TFC values. The other two plant extracts are also grouped, with the exception of the methanol extracts that present a deviant behavior due to influence of the *A. salina* variable.

Table 3. Loadings, eigenvalues and percentage of cumulative variance for the first three principal components of the data from the *Helichrysum* samples.

Variable	PC1	PC2
TPC	0.01524	0.4357
TFC	−0.00098	0.4327
DPPH	0.03629	0.4742
ABTS	0.00767	0.4315
FRAP	−0.00560	0.34415
BC	0.1924	0.29152
A. salina	0.1924	0.03366
R^2 (cum)	0.879	0.945
eigenvalue	5.07	1.63
Q^2 (Cum)	0.214	0.397

Figure 2. PCA plot of the scores (**a**) and loadings (**b**) of the *Helichrysum* samples.

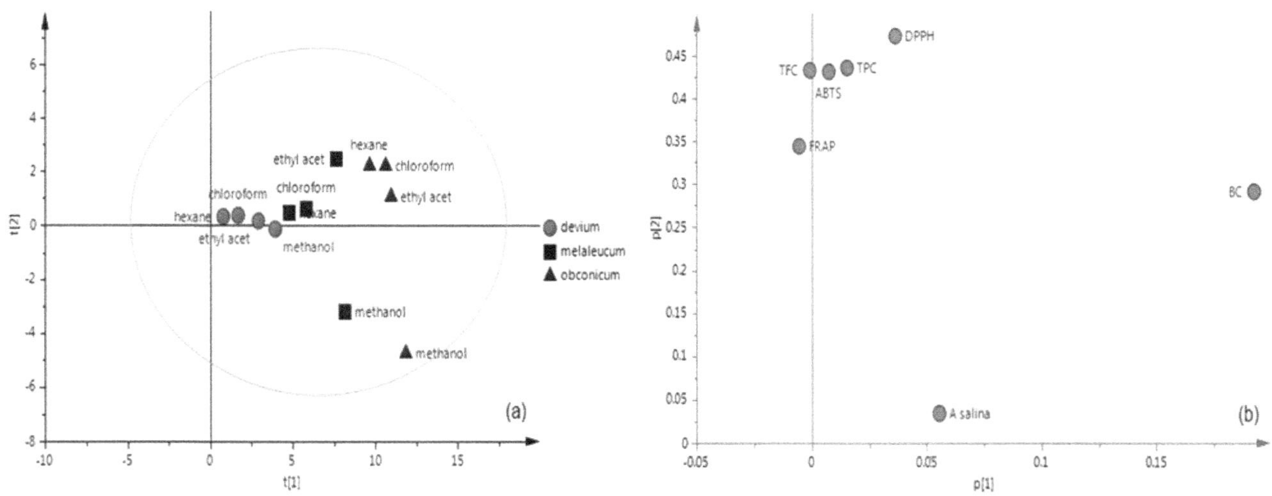

4. Conclusions

In the present study, three endemic *Helichrysum* plants used in diet and folk medicine of Madeira Archipelago were analyzed in terms of their antioxidant capacity, toxicity and antimycobacterial power.

Statistically significant differences were observed among the different samples in the different antioxidant assays. For *H. melaleucum* and *H. obconicum,* the methanolic extracts showed the highest antioxidant capacity, whereas the phenolic and flavonoid compounds played an important role in the antioxidant capacity (evidenced by an excellent correlation). For *H. devium,* it is possible to conclude that phenolic compounds are not the only ones responsible for the antioxidant properties since the *n*-hexane extract gave similar or even slightly higher antioxidant values than the methanolic extract.

The PCA analysis allowed the grouping of *H. devium* samples based on the TPC, TFC, ABTS and FRAP variables.

H. devium was revealed to be toxic towards *Artemia salina* larvae and to *Mycobacterium tuberculosis*. Further studies with these plant extracts to identify the bioactive compounds and further *in vivo* studies of inhibition are therefore warranted.

Acknowledgments

Sandra C. Gouveia is grateful to Fundação para a Ciência e Tecnologia (FCT) for a Ph.D. grant SFRH/BD/24227/2005. This research was supported by FCT with funds from the Portuguese Government (Project PEst-OE/QUI/UI0674/2011). The authors wish to thank to Doctor Julieta Luna-Herrera (Departamento de Inmunología, Escuela Nacional de Ciencias Biológicas, México) for the MBT analysis.

Author Contributions

Sandra C. Gouveia-Figueira, Ana I. Rodrigues and Paula C. Castilho conceived and designed the experiments; Sandra C. Gouveia-Figueira and Carla A. Gouveia performed the antioxidant assays; Maria J. Carvalho performed the Artemia Salina assay; Sandra C. Gouveia-Figueira and Maria J. Carvalho analyzed the data; Malin L. Nording performed multivariate analysis. Sandra C. Gouveia-Figueira wrote the paper.

Conflicts of Interest

The authors declare no conflict of interest.

References

1. Tsao, R.; Deng, Z. Separation Procedures for Naturally Occurring Antioxidant Phytochemicals. *J. Chromatogr. B* **2004**, *812*, 85–99.
2. Fu, L.; Xu, B.-T.; Xu, X.-R.; Gan, R.-Y.; Zhang, Y.; Xia, E.-Q.; Li, H.-B. Antioxidant capacities and total phenolic contents of 62 fruits. *Food Chem.* **2011**, *129*, 345–350.
3. Michiels, J.A.; Kevers, C.; Pincemailc, J.; Defraignec, J.O.; Dommesb, J. Extraction conditions can greatly influence antioxidant capacity assays in plant food matrices. *Food Chem.* **2012**, *130*, 986–993.
4. Atoui, A.K.; Atoui, A.K.; Mansouri, A.; Boskou, G.; Kefalas, P. Tea and herbal infusions: Their antioxidant activity and phenolic profile. *Food Chem.* **2005**, *89*, 27–36.
5. McGaw, L.J.; Lallb, N.; Meyer, J.J.M.; Eloff, J.N. The potential of South African plants against Mycobacterium infections. *J. Ethnopharmacol.* **2008**, *119*, 482–500.
6. Copp, B.R. Antimycobacterial natural products. *Nat. Prod. Rep.* **2003**, *20*, 535–557.
7. Okunade, A.L.; Elvin-Lewis, M.P.F.; Lewis, W.H. Natural antimycobacterial metabolites: Current status. *Phytochemistry* **2004**, *65*, 1017–1032.
8. Gibbons, S. Plants as a source of bacterial resistance modulators and anti-infective agents. *Phytochem. Rev.* **2005**, *4*, 63–78.
9. Pauli, G.F.; Case, R.J.; Inui, T.; Wang, Y.; Cho, S.; Fischer, N.H.; Franzblau, S.G. New perspectives on natural products in TB drug research. *Life Sci.* **2005**, *78*, 485–494.

10. Frothingham, R.; Stout, J.E.; Hamilton, C.D. Current issues in global tuberculosis control. *Int. J. Infect. Dis.* **2005**, *9*, 297–311.
11. Newton, S.M.; Lau, C.; Wright, C.W. A review of antimycobacterial natural products. *Phytother. Res.* **2000**, *14*, 303–322.
12. Newton, S.M.; Lau, C.; Gurcha, S.S.; Besra, G.S.; Wright, C.W. The evaluation of forty-three plant species for *in vitro* antimycobacterial activities; isolation of active constituents from *Psoralea corylifolia* and *Sanguinaria canadensis*. *J. Ethnopharmacol.* **2002**, *79*, 57–67.
13. Gouveia, S.C.; Castilho, P.C. Analysis of phenolic compounds from different morphological parts of *Helichrysum devium* by liquid chromatography with on-line UV and electrospray ionization mass spectrometric detection. *Rapid Commun. Mass Spectrom.* **2009**, *23*, 3939–3953.
14. Carini, M.; Aldini, G.; Furlanetto, S.; Stefani, R.; Facino, R.M. LC coupled to ion-trap MS for the rapid screening and detection of polyphenol antioxidants from *Helichrysum stoechas*. *J. Pharm. Biomed. Anal.* **2001**, *24*, 517–526.
15. Matic, I.; Aljančić, I.; Žižak, Ž.; Vajs, V.; Jadranin, M.; Milosavljević, S.; Juranić, Z.D. *In vitro* antitumor actions of extracts from endemic plant *Helichrysum zivojinii*. *BMC Complement. Altern. Med.* **2013**, *13*, 36.
16. Rivera, D.; Obón, C. The ethnopharmacology of Madeira and Porto Santo Islands, a review. *J. Ethnopharmacol.* **1995**, *46*, 73–93.
17. Gouveia, S.C.; Castilho, P.C. Characterization of phenolic compounds in *Helichrysum melaleucum* by high-performance liquid chromatography with on-line ultraviolet and mass spectrometry detection. *Rapid Commun. Mass Spectrom.* **2010**, *24*, 1851–1868.
18. Gouveia, S.C.; Castilho, P.C. Characterisation of phenolic acid derivatives and flavonoids from different morphological parts of *Helichrysum obconicum* by a RP-HPLC-DAD-(-)-ESI-MS^n method. *Food Chem.* **2011**, *129*, 333–344.
19. Jimenez-Arellanes, A.; Meckes, M.; Ramirez, R.; Torres, J.; Luna-Herrera, J. Activity against multidrug-resistant *Mycobacterium tuberculosis* in Mexican plants used to treat respiratory diseases. *Phytother. Res.* **2003**, *17*, 903–908.
20. Hostettmann, K. *Methods In Plant Biochemistry—Assays For Bioactivity*; Academic Press: London, UK, 1991; Volume 6.
21. Zheng, W.; Wang, S.Y. Antioxidant activity and phenolic compounds in selected herbs. *J. Agric. Food Chem.* **2001**, *49*, 5165–5170.
22. Gouveia, S.C.; Castilho, P.C. *Helichrysum monizii* Lowe: Phenolic composition and antioxidant potential. *Phytochem. Anal.* **2012**, *23*, 72–83.
23. Gordon, M.H.; Paiva-Martins, F.; Almeida, M. Antioxidant activity of hydroxytyrosol acetate compared with that of other olive oil polyphenols. *J. Agric. Food Chem.* **2001**, *49*, 2480–2485.
24. Re, R.; Pellegrini, N.; Proteggente, A.; Pannala, A.; Yang, M.; Rice-Evans, C. Antioxidant activity applying an improved ABTS radical cation decolorization assay. *Free Radic. Biol. Med.* **1999**, *26*, 1231–1237.
25. Gouveia, S.C.; Castilho, P.C. Antioxidant potential of *Artemisia argentea* L'Hér alcoholic extract and its relation with the phenolic composition. *Food Res. Int.* **2011**, *44*, 1620–1631.

26. Siddhuraju, P.; Becker, K. Studies on antioxidant activities of mucuna seed (*Mucuna pruriens* var utilis) extract and various non-protein amino/imino acids through *in vitro* models. *J. Sci. Food Agric.* **2003**, *83*, 1517–1524.
27. Lall, N.; Hussein, A.A.; Meyer, J.J.M. Antiviral and antituberculous activity of *Helichrysum melanacme* constituents. *Fitoterapia* **2006**, *77*, 230–232.
28. Leite, A.M.; de O. Lima, E.; de Souza, E.L.; de F.F.M. Diniz, M.; Leite, S.P.; Xavier, A.L.; de Medeiros, I.A. Preliminary study of the molluscicidal and larvicidal properties of some essential oils and phytochemicals from medicinal plants. *Rev. Bras. Farmacogn.* **2009**, *19*, 842–846.
29. Santos Pimenta, L.P.; Pinto, G.B.; Takahashi, J.A.; e Silva, L.G.; Boaventura, M.A. Biological screening of annonaceous brazilian medicinal plants using *Artemia salina* (Brine shrimp test). *Phytomedicine* **2003**, *10*, 209–212.
30. Cuadra, P.; Furrianca, M.; Oyarzún, A.; Yáñez, E.; Gallardo, A.; Fajardo, V. Biological activity of some Patagonian plants. *Fitoterapia* **2005**, *76*, 718–721.
31. Albayrak, S.; Aksoy, A.; Sagdic, O.; Hamzaoglu, E. Compositions, antioxidant and antimicrobial activities of *Helichrysum* (Asteraceae) species collected from Turkey. *Food Chem.* **2010**, *119*, 114–122.
32. Süntar, I.; Küpeli Akkol, E.; Keles, H.; Yesilada, E.; Sarker, S.D. Exploration of the wound healing potential of *Helichrysum graveolens* (Bieb.) Sweet: Isolation of apigenin as an active component. *J. Ethnopharmacol.* **2013**, *149*, 103–110.
33. Huang, D.; Ou, B.; Prior, R.L. The Chemistry behind Antioxidant Capacity Assays. *J. Agric. Food Chem.* **2005**, *53*, 1841–1856.
34. Stratil, P.; Klejdus, B.; Kubáň, V. Determination of total content of phenolic compounds and their antioxidant activity in vegetables evaluation of spectrophotometric methods. *J. Agric. Food Chem.* **2006**, *54*, 607–616.
35. Siddhuraju, P. Antioxidant activity of polyphenolic compounds extracted from defatted raw and dry heated *Tamarindus indica* seed coat. *LWT Food Sci. Technol.* **2007**, *40*, 982–990.

9

Role of Oxidative Stress in HIV-1-Associated Neurocognitive Disorder and Protection by Gene Delivery of Antioxidant Enzymes

Jean-Pierre Louboutin * and David Strayer

Department of Pathology, Anatomy and Cell Biology, Thomas Jefferson University, 1020 Locust street, Philadelphia, PA 19107, USA; E-Mail: David.Strayer@jefferson.edu

* Author to whom correspondence should be addressed; E-Mail: jplouboutin@hotmail.com

External Editor: Wenlan Liu

Abstract: HIV encephalopathy covers a range of HIV-1-related brain dysfunction. In the Central Nervous System (CNS), it is largely impervious to Highly Active AntiRetroviral Therapy (HAART). As survival with chronic HIV-1 infection improves, the number of people harboring the virus in their CNS increases. Neurodegenerative and neuroinflammatory changes may continue despite the use of HAART. Neurons themselves are rarely infected by HIV-1, but HIV-1 infects resident microglia, periventricular macrophages, leading to increased production of cytokines and to release of HIV-1 proteins, the most likely neurotoxins, among which are the envelope glycoprotein gp120 and HIV-1 *trans*-acting protein Tat. Gp120 and Tat induce oxidative stress in the brain, leading to neuronal apoptosis/death. We review here the role of oxidative stress in animal models of HIV-1 Associated Neurocognitive Disorder (HAND) and in patients with HAND. Different therapeutic approaches, including clinical trials, have been used to mitigate oxidative stress in HAND. We used SV40 vectors for gene delivery of antioxidant enzymes, Cu/Zn superoxide dismutase (SOD1), or glutathione peroxidase (GPx1) into the rat caudate putamen (CP). Intracerebral injection of SV (SOD1) or SV (GPx1) protects neurons from apoptosis caused by subsequent inoculation of gp120 and Tat at the same location. Vector administration into the lateral ventricle or cisterna magna protects from intra-CP gp120-induced neurotoxicity comparably to intra-CP vector administration. These models should provide a better understanding of the pathogenesis of HIV-1 in the brain as well as offer new therapeutic avenues.

Keywords: HIV-1; gene therapy; dementia; oxidative stress; neuroinflammation; antioxidant enzymes

---

1. Clinical Presentation of HIV-1-Associated Neurocognitive Disorder

HIV-1 enters the Central Nervous System (CNS) soon after it enters the body. There, it is largely impervious to highly active anti-retroviral therapeutic drugs (HAART). Human immunodeficiency virus (HIV-1) encephalopathy covers a range of HIV-related CNS dysfunction. Advances in the treatment of HIV-1 have dramatically improved survival rates over the past 10 years, but HIV-associated neurocognitive disorders (HAND) remain highly prevalent and continue to represent a significant public health problem, partly because HAART penetrate the CNS poorly. In early 1990s, the neurologic complications of HIV-1 infection were classified into two levels of disturbance: (1) HIV-associated dementia (HAD) with motor, behavioral/psychosocial, or combined features; and (2) minor cognitive motor disorder (MCMD). HAD was considered as the most common cause of dementia in adults under 40 [1] and was estimated to affect as many as 30% of patients with advanced AIDS [1], but has become less common since HAART was introduced [2]. This reduction probably reflects better control of HIV in the periphery, since antiretroviral drugs penetrate the CNS poorly. Before the introduction of HAART, most neuroAIDS patients showed subcortical dementia, with predominant basal ganglia involvement, manifesting as psychomotor slowing, Parkinsonism, behavioral abnormalities and cognitive difficulties [3]. MCMD described a less severe presentation of HIV-associated neurocognitive impairment that did not meet criteria for HAD.

More recently, in light of the changing epidemiology of HIV infection, the need to update and further structure the diagnostic criteria for HAND has been recognized [4]. There are several reasons for this update. First, the applicability of the old criteria appears limited in the present age of HAART. Prior to the advent of HAART, a diagnosis of HAD was associated strongly with high viral loads, low T-cell counts, and opportunistic infections. With HAART limiting viral severity, patients with HIV typically live longer with milder medical symptoms. Secondly, guidelines regarding possible neurocognitive impairment due to comorbid conditions with CNS effects (e.g., substance use disorders) were not precisely described in the previous diagnostic scheme. This limitation is particularly important in the era of HAART as those infected with HIV-1 live longer with a host of CNS risk factors, including substance abuse disorders (e.g., methamphetamine dependence), medical conditions associated with HAART treatment (e.g., hyperlipidemia) and comorbid infectious diseases (e.g., hepatitis C virus) [5].

Thus, the newly redefined criteria allow for three possible research diagnoses: (1) asymptomatic neurocognitive impairment (ANI); (2) HIV-associated mild neurocognitive disorder (MND); and (3) HAD. In this classification, the diagnosis of HAND must be determined by assessing at least five areas of neurocognitive functioning known to be affected by HIV infection (e.g., attention/working memory, executive functions, speed of information processing, episodic memory, motor skills, language, and sensoriperception) [4].

However, if there are currently less cases of HAD as survival with chronic HIV-1 infection improves, the number of people harboring the virus in their CNS increases, leading to new HIV-1-related neurological manifestations. The prevalence of HAND therefore continues to rise, and less fulminant forms of HAND have become more common than their more severe predecessors [4,5]. HAND remains a significant independent risk factor for AIDS mortality [2,4–9]. Incident cases of HAND are accelerating fastest among drug users, ethnic minorities, and women [6–9]. The number of HIV-infected individuals over 50 years of age is rapidly growing, including patients taking HAART [9]. It has been suggested that in 10 years, 50% of AIDS patients in the United States will be over the age of 50. Moreover, it is becoming clear that the brain is an important reservoir for the virus, and that neurodegenerative and neuroinflammatory changes may continue despite HAART [8].

2. Neuropathogenesis of HAND

2.1. Role of HIV-1 Proteins in Neuronal Damage

The principal manifestations of central nervous system in HIV infection result from neuronal injury and loss and from extensive damage to the dendritic and synaptic structures in the absence of neuronal loss. Neurons themselves are rarely infected by HIV-1, and neuronal damage is felt to be mainly indirect. In fact, the pathogenesis of HAND largely reflects the neurotoxicity of HIV-1 proteins [10]. HIV-1 infects resident microglia, periventricular macrophages and some astrocytes [11], leading to increased production of cytokines and to release of HIV-1 proteins, the most likely neurotoxins, among which are the envelope (Env) proteins gp120 and gp41 and the nonstructural proteins Nef, Rev, Vpr and Tat [9,12,13].

2.1.1. Trans-Acting Protein Tat

The HIV-1 *trans*-acting protein Tat, an essential protein for viral replication, is a key mediator of neurotoxicity. Brain areas that are particularly susceptible to Tat toxicity include the CA3 region and the dentate gyrus of the hippocampus and the striatum. Tat is internalized by neurons primarily through lipoprotein related protein receptor (LRP) and by activation of *N*-methyl-D-aspartate (NMDA) receptor [14,15]. It also interacts with several cell membrane receptors, including integrins, VEGF receptor in endothelial cells and possibly CXCR4 [16].

Tat can directly depolarize neuron membranes, independently of Na^+ flux [17] and may potentiate glutamate- and *N*-methyl-D-aspartate (NMDA)-triggered calcium fluxes and neurotoxicity [17]. It promotes excitotoxic neuron apoptosis [18,19] by activating endoplasmic reticulum pathways to release intracellular calcium ((Ca^{2+})i). Consequent dysregulation of calcium homeostasis [18,20–22] leads to mitochondrial calcium uptake, caspase activation and, finally, neuronal death. Tat also increases levels of lipid peroxidation [23] by generating the reactive oxygen species (ROS) superoxide (O_2^-) and hydrogen peroxide (H_2O_2). It activates inducible nitric oxide synthase (iNOS) to produce nitric oxide (NO), which binds superoxide anion to form the highly reactive peroxynitrite (ONOO) [24].

Tat neurotoxicity has been reported in cultured cells, but fewer studies have demonstrated its neurotoxic properties *in vivo* [25–29]. Despite evidence that Tat has been detected in the striatum of patients with HIV encephalitis [30,31], it is difficult to know the exact levels of Tat generated. Although mRNA for Tat was detected by RT-PCR in brain extracts from half [31] or more [30] of patients with HIV encephalitis, protein levels could not be measured by ELISA [31]. There are important differences between the situation in the striatum of patients with AIDS and models where Tat is directly injected into the CP. In these models, Tat is localized initially in extracellular space following intra-CP injection, then it is internalized in neurons and in some microglial cells, while the sites of production are focal in patients with HAND (*i.e.*, microglial cells and infected macrophages). Direct injection of Tat results in acute injury, while production of Tat is more protracted in the brain of patients with HAND. The lesions of HAND reflect chronic injury caused by ongoing production of Tat, as well as other susbstances, by HIV-1-infected cells.

2.1.2. Envelope Glycoprotein gp120

The HIV-1 *env* gene codes for gp120 which is cleaved into two major envelope glycoproteins, gp120 and gp41. Soluble gp120 can induce apoptosis in a wide variety of cells including lymphocytes, cardiomyocytes and neurons [32,33]. HIV-1 gp120 may be directly neurotoxic at high concentrations [34]. Gp120-induced apoptosis has been demonstrated in studies in cortical cell cultures, in rat hippocampal slices and by intracerebral injections *in vivo* [35]. Gp120 binds neuron cell membrane co-receptors (CCR3, CCR5 and CXCR4) and elicits apoptosis, apparently via G-protein-coupled pathways [21,36]. Soluble gp120 also increases glial cell release of arachidonate, which impairs neuron and astrocyte reuptake of glutamate [37], leading to prolonged activation of NMDA receptor with consequent disruption of cellular Ca^{2+} homeostasis [38]. This process involves generation of superoxide and peroxide species, with resultant oxidative stress, and leads to neuron cell death after mitochondrial permeabilization, cytochrome c release and activation of caspases and endonucleases [2].

2.1.3. Other HIV-1 Proteins

The trans-membrane protein gp41 is elevated in patients with HAD. *In vitro*, gp41 can induce neuronal death in the nanomolar range, requires the presence of astrocytes, suggesting indirect mechanisms, involving iNOS, NO formation, depletion of glutathione and disruption of mitochondrial function [39,40].

Other HIV-1 proteins (Vpr, Nef, Rev) are also involved in HAND neuropathogenesis. HIV-1 viral protein r (Vpr) is thought to be important for effective viral replication in the early stages of the infection. Vpr is present as a soluble protein within the blood serum and the CSF of patients infected with HIV-1 [41,42] and accumulates within these compartments to increasing concentrations as disease progresses toward the later stages of disease. As an extracellular protein, HIV-1 Vpr has been shown to negatively affect the survival of brain-resident cells, especially neurons and astrocytes, which are the cell types most sensitive to local insult; they become dysfunctional and are gradually lost as patients infected with HIV-1 advance towards AIDS. Some studies have shown that Vpr can directly induce neuronal apoptosis [43], and that Vpr can deregulate calcium secretion in neural cells [44].

The non-structural protein Nef is required for the proper budding of virions from HIV-infected cells. *In vitro*, Nef can be lethal for astrocytes and neurons and can increase the expression of matrix metalloproteinases (MMPs) [45]. Abundant Nef expression has been shown in astrocytes of HIV-1-infected patients with neuronal damage [46].

The HIV-1 phosphoprotein Rev is involved in the nuclear export of unspliced viral mRNAs. Extracellular Rev has neurotoxic properties. These ones have been demonstrated in rodents by intracerebroventricular injection of a synthetic peptide spanning the basic region of Rev causing neuronal death [47].

2.2. HIV-1 Proteins and Astrocytes

Astrocytes have a role in HAND [48]. Several HIV-1 proteins can influence the role of astrocytes in HAND. Astroglial infection is characterized by an initial small burst in viral production followed by a state of persistent infection with the presence of multiple spliced short transcripts (encoding primarily the Nef protein), inefficient translation of structural proteins (gag and env), and almost undetectable levels of viral genomic transcripts [49]. Astrocytes could represent a reservoir for HIV-1. During late stage HIV-1 disease, an increased frequency of infiltrating monocytes and CD4+ T cells may deliver neurotoxic factors, such as chemokines and viral proteins (Tat, Vpr, gp120, and Nef) [50], which stimulates astroglia to secrete an elevated amount of glutamate, increasing the overall level of excitotoxicity. This sequence of events could play a significant role in astrocytic and neuronal dysregulation, leading to mild to severe neurocognitive impairment. Tat also induces NOS in human astroglia [51] and monocyte chemoattractant protein-1 (MCP-1) is induced in HIV-1 Tat-stimulated astrocytes [52]. Tat expression in astrocytes leads to astrocytes activation and neuronal death [53].

3. Oxidative Stress in HAND

3.1. Role of Oxidative Stress in HAND

Oxygen is vital for all living cells whether neuronal or not, but on the other hand it is potentially dangerous in excess. Oxygen has a role in glucose breakdown in mitochondria through oxidative phosphorylation and generates energy currency of cell, *i.e.*, ATP [54]. Under physiologic normal conditions, ROS, which include superoxide (O_2^-), hydrogen peroxide (H_2O_2) and hydroxyl radical (OH–), are generated at low levels and play important roles in signaling and metabolic pathways [55]. Oxidative stress arises due to the disturbances of the balance in pro-oxidant/antioxidant homeostasis that further causes the generation of ROS which are potentially toxic for neurons. Reactive oxygen and nitrogen species (ROS/RNS) change cellular responses through diverse mechanisms. Oxidative damage and the associated mitochondrial dysfunction may result in energy depletion, accumulation of cytotoxic mediators and cell death. There are several reasons why the brain is more susceptible to ROS. Glial cells require more oxygen and glucose consumption to generate continuous ATP pool *in vivo* for normal functioning of the brain as it is one of the busiest organs, making them more susceptible to oxygen overload, and thus to free radicals generation [54]. Neurons are particularly susceptible to ROS because of their biochemical composition: brain contains high levels of fatty acids, which are particularly susceptible to peroxidation and oxidative modification. Double bonds of unsaturated fatty acids are hot spots for attack by free radicals that initiate cascade to damage neighboring unsaturated fatty acids [56]. Membrane lipids can undergo oxidation, producing cytotoxic lipid peroxidation products like malondialdehyde (MDA) and 4-hydroxynonenal (4-HNE). Finally, brain has less antioxidant activity compared to other tissues and has higher levels of iron in some areas [54].

Organisms respond to oxidative injury by orchestrating a stress response to prevent further damage. An increase in the intracellular levels of antioxidant agents, and at the same time the removal of already damaged components, are both part of the oxidative stress response. ROS levels are controlled by endogenous antioxidants such as superoxide dismutases (SOD), glutathione peroxidase (GPx1), glutathione and catalase. The tripeptide glutathione (γ-L-glutamyl-L-cysteinylglycine, GSH) is the key low molecular thiol antioxidant involved in the defense of brain cells against oxidative stress. A decrease in GSH levels has been connected to physiological processes such as aging and neurological disorders like Alzheimer's disease (AD), epilepsy, and Parkinson's disease [57]. Although GSH is the primary molecule involved in detoxification of ROS in the body, antioxidant enzymes like GPx1, are also known to play a role in this process [58]. During detoxification of peroxides, the enzyme GPx1 converts GSH to GSSG (glutathione disulphide).

Interaction of ROS with other tissue components produces a variety of other radicals: following activation of iNOS, NO can bind superoxide anion to form the highly reactive peroxynitrite [24]. The latter may attack lipids, proteins and DNA, to enhance oxidant-related injury. Mitochondria are the primary source of ROS involved in many brain tissue injuries (*i.e.*, hypoxia, excitotoxicity). Once generated, mitochondrial ROS influence the release of cytochrome c and other apoptotic proteins from the mitochondria into the neuronal cytosol, which leads to apoptosis [55]. For example, once released into the cytosol, cytochrome c forms a complex referred to as an apoptosome with procaspase-9, apoptotic protease activating factor 1 (APAF-1) and dATP. The formation of the apoptosome activates caspase-9 which then cleaves other procaspases. The activation of caspase-3 by this process, among other effectors, has multiple effects including proteolysis of an inhibitor of the caspase-activated DNase [59]. Thus, a link between oxidative stress and activation of some caspases seems highly probable.

Abnormalities in oxidative metabolism have been reported in many nervous system diseases. These include neurodegenerative diseases (Parkinson's disease, AD, Huntington's disease, amyotrophic lateral sclerosis and cerebellar degeneration) [60–63], vascular diseases (ischemia-reperfusion) [64] or toxic reactions (chronic alcoholism) [65], as well as aging [66].

Oxidative stress, accumulation of protein aggregates, impaired mitochondrial function, and autophagic stress are common in many pathologies, including neurodegenerative diseases. The highly abundant mitochondria in brain cells are a major site of generation and action of ROS/RNS. Lipid peroxidation is a consistent feature of neurodegenerative diseases and biologically active reactive lipid species, such as HNE, accumulates in brains individuals with Parkinson's disease, AD, and HIV-1-associated neurocognitive disorder. Mechanisms of protein oxidation are NO-dependent, through generation of ONOO−, or *S*-nitrosylation. These changes have been reported in a broad range of pathologies, including Parkinson's disease, which is associated with both nitrated α-synuclein and *S*-nitrosated parkin. Likewise, ONOO−-dependent modifications of proteins are widespread in brains of individuals with AD. The cross-talk between autophagy, oxidative stress and mitochondrial dysfunction is not well understood, particularly in neurodegenerative diseases.

Oxidative stress plays a role in the development of HAND as well [67,68]. Oxidative stress in HIV-1 dementia has been documented by analyses of brain tissue, including increased levels of lipid peroxidation product (*i.e.*, HNE) and the presence of oxidized proteins. Serum levels of GSH and GPx1 are decreased in HIV-1 patients while MDA levels are increased [58]. A characteristic of patients infected with HIV-1 in late stage disease is diffuse intracellular oxidation in the form of decreased availability of GSH, the main cellular antioxidant and redox buffer, and augmented lipid oxidation, which triggers a cascade of downstream signaling events.

Membrane-associated oxidative stress correlates with HIV-1 dementia pathogenesis and cognitive impairment [9]. HNE-positive neurons have been demonstrated in the brains of patients with HIV-1 encephalitis [23,68,69]. In the case of HIV-1 infection, Tat and gp120 can elicit such oxidative stress [9,70]. Such oxidative stress can induce apoptosis in cultured neurons [71]. It can also damage neurons and cause cognitive dysfunction *in vivo* [72]. Tat and gp120 induce ceramide production in cultured neurons by triggering sphingomyelinase activity via a mechanism that involves induction of oxidative stress by CXCR4 activation [9]. Oxidative stress can play a role in HAND in other ways. Circulating toxins in the CSF, derived from HIV-1-infected cells, may damage mitochondria, leading to release of cytochrome c and then to a cascade of events leading to apoptosis [67,68]. HIV-1 gp120 and Tat can cause free radical production, possibly as part of the signal-transduction pathways they activate [9,70].

It is still unclear whether oxidative stress is the primary initiating event associated with neurodegeneration. However, a growing body of evidence implicates it as being involved in at least the propagation of cellular injury that leads to neuron death. Earlier reports support the hypothesis that oxidative modifications of macromolecular cell components (lipids, proteins and nucleic acids) may be an early step in the mechanism of Tat and gp120 neurotoxicity [27,28].

3.2. Oxidative Stress Associated with Tat

Tat-induced protein oxidation is well documented [27,28] and its effects on lipid peroxidation have also been reported. We recently demonstrated that Tat activates multiple signaling pathways. In one of these, Tat-induced superoxide acts as an intermediate, while the other utilizes peroxide as a signal transducer [70].

Tat-mediated neurotoxicity may be associated with increased oxidative modifications of proteins [27]. For example, increased protein carbonyl formation, a well-known marker of protein oxidative damage, occurred early after Tat injection and coincided with the earliest changes in the amount of degenerating striatal neurons [28]. When the number of degenerating neurons reaches its peak 1 day after Tat administration, protein oxidation in striatal extracts decreased back to control levels, probably because oxidized proteins are prone to proteolytic degradation [28]. There was a later increase in protein carbonyl levels 7 days after Tat injection, possibly caused by Tat-induced compromise astrocytic functions [28]. However, astrocytosis and associated changes in protein oxidation were not sufficient to cause an additional neuronal cell death [28]. Tat increase in levels of protein oxidation may result from Tat-mediated increase of the production of prooxidants, as Tat can trigger the production of inflammatory products, which, in turn, may cause an excess of ROS [28,73].

Tat can also mediate neurotoxicity through lipid peroxidation. There are few reports concerning MDA levels in the brain after Tat injection, and there are no data concerning late time points after inoculation. In one study, repeated intravenous injection of 50 ng Tat during 5 days decreases brain levels of GSH and GPx1 and increases levels of MDA [57]. Pretreatment of the animals with thiol antioxidant *N*-acetylcysteine amide (NACA) increased the GSH levels significantly, indicating that the antioxidant NACA was able to partially abrogate oxidative stress induced damage in these animals. A significant decrease in the activity of GPx1 was observed in animals treated with Tat, as compared to the controls, indicating that the overwhelming oxidative stress induced by these toxins depletes the antioxidant enzyme in the brain. Animals pretreated with NACA had GPx-1 levels similar to that of the control.

In one study, we injected Tat into the striatum. We observed elevated MDA levels persisting one week after Tat administration [74]. The sustained MDA levels might be due to the longterm neuroinflammation, because it is known that increased production of inflammatory products induced by Tat may cause an excess formation of ROS [28]. However, persisting elevated MDA levels were not associated with continuing apoptosis. These data resemble to the ones observed when an increase in protein carbonyl levels seen 7 days after Tat injection was not accompanied by neuron death [28].

Tat is also known to trigger an increased production of inflammatory products, which in turn, may cause an excess formation of ROS [73,75]. Tat may induce superoxide and nitrite release in a microglial cell line [73]. An exposure of macrophages and astrocytes to Tat for few minutes *in vitro* is sufficient for sustained release of cytokines for several hours [75]. Thus, Tat might promote oxidative stress and its consequences (*i.e.*, neuron death) through activation of proinflammatory responses.

Numerous neurotoxic effects of Tat injection can be transient and can be observed only at early time points after its administration. Tat can decrease levels of GSH available to relieve oxidant stress [57]. The presence of Tat in the striatum is short-lived after its injection. It is thus possible that after degradation of Tat, the levels of GSH are restored to normal levels. GSH could then protect neurons against ROS directly and indirectly, and could bind to lipid peroxidation products such as HNE, thereby providing neuroprotection [58]. Tat can also induce a lipid imbalance in neurons, resulting in an overproduction of sphingomyelin and ceramide, followed by increased levels of HNE [58]. Once Tat is degraded, the levels of ceramide and sphingomyelin return to control levels, limiting cellular dysfunction and death due to lipid imbalance. Tat can also trigger the expression of iNOS, leading to the overproduction of NO, which can react with superoxide anion to form peroxynitrite, a neurotoxic compound. NO can increase glutamate release from astrocytes, enhancing NMDA excitotoxicity [58]. If NO production can be increased shortly after Tat treatment, NO levels would decrease once Tat is degraded. Thus, if persisting increased MDA levels are observed one week after injection (possibly linked to continued neuroinflammation), they might not be enough, by themselves, to induce neuronal death at that time, because: (1) there is no direct interaction of Tat with neurons and no Tat-mediated dysregulation of calcium homeostasis one week after the injection; (2) some protective mechanisms (*i.e.*, GSH) are probably restored at that time; (3) neurotoxic compounds like NO and peroxynitrite are probably not present at that time.

Oxidative stress is intimately linked with an integrated series of cellular phenomena, which all seem to contribute to neuronal death. Interaction between these various components is not necessarily a cascade but might be a cycle of events, of which oxidative stress is a major component [76].

Consequently, if one of the events, besides oxidative stress, is missing, neuronal death might be limited or not occur. Inhibition of oxidative stress therapeutically might act to 'break the cycle' of cell death. It might also suggest that a direct interaction of Tat with neurons is necessary for inducing early neuron death. However, it is difficult to directly answer the question whether Tat directly induces oxidative stress in neurons or promotes it through activation of proinflammatory responses. It remains plausible that direct interactions of Tat with neurons play the role of a triggering mechanism in the process of the development of oxidative stress and neurodegeneration [28].

3.3. Gp120-Induced Oxidative Stress

It has been previously shown that HIV-1 gp120 can cause lipid peroxidation and production of hydroxynonenal esters [69], which can mediate oxidative stress-induced apoptosis of cultured neurons [77] and can damage neurons and cause cognitive dysfunction *in vivo* [72]. Recently, cytochrome P-450, in association with NADPH oxidase, has been implicated in gp120-induced oxidative stress and apoptosis in astrocytes [78].

We reported that direct injection of recombinant gp120 into the striatum can induce lipid peroxidation attested by the measurement of MDA and the production of HNE [79]. HNE was localized, not only in neurons, but also in endothelial cells and in astrocytes.

Experimental systems for studying the effects of gp120 and other HIV proteins on the brain have been limited to the acute effects of recombinant proteins *in vitro* or *in vivo*, or in chronic situation like simian immunodeficiency virus-infected monkeys. We described an experimental rodent model of ongoing gp120-induced neurotoxicity in which HIV-1 envelope gp120 is expressed in the brain using an SV40-derived gene delivery vector, SV(gp120) [80]. We previously demonstrated that SV40-derived vectors deliver long-term transgene expression to brain neurons and microglia, when administered by several different routes. rSV40s were employed in the current study because they transduce a wide range of cell types from humans and other mammals and deliver genes to cells in Go efficiently, including neurons, to achieve long-term transgene expression *in vitro* and *in vivo* [81,82]. Moreover, they do not elicit immune response [83]. These vectors transduce >95% of cultured human NT2-derived neurons, primary human neurons [84,85] and microglia [86] without detectable toxicity. When it is inoculated stereotaxically into the rat caudate putamen (CP), SV (gp120) caused a lesion in which neuron and other cell apoptosis continue for at least 12 weeks. Human immunodeficiency virus gp120 is expressed throughout this time, and some apoptotic cells are gp120 positive. MDA and HNE assays indicated that there was lipid peroxidation in these lesions. Similarly, protein oxidation was demonstrated by immunostaining for dinitrophenol (DNP) in brain cryosections, 1 week after injection of SV (gp120). Thus, *in vivo* inoculation of SV (gp120) into the rat CP causes ongoing oxidative stress and apoptosis in neurons and may therefore represent a useful animal model for studying the pathogenesis and treatment of HIV-1 envelope-related brain damage.

3.4. Oxidative Stress Associated with Vpr

Some recent studies have demonstrated the role of extracellular Vpr in impairing astrocytic metabolism by affecting the levels of the intracellular pools of both ATP and GSH, the main endogenous antioxidant molecule. Vpr-induced augmented production of ROS was related to an increase in the level of oxidized glutathione (GSSG) and a reduction in the overall GSH/GSSG ratio. This event was almost entirely suppressed by treatment with an anti-Vpr antibody or cotreatment with the antioxidant molecule *N*-acetyl-cysteine (NAC) [87].

4. Animal Models of HAND

There are no perfect models for HAND. Several animal systems have been used to study the pathogenesis of HIV-1-induced neurological disease. Many of them are based on other lentiviruses (*i.e.*, simian immunodeficiency virus infection of macaques, feline immunodeficiency virus infection of cats, Visna-Maedi virus infection in sheep) [88–90]. However, only small percentages of animals develop neurological manifestations in these models and the costs for using these species may be high. Transgenic expression of gp120 in mice has been studied [91], but the gp120 in that model is mainly expressed in astrocytes, whereas in humans HIV-1 chiefly infects microglial cells. Other models based on introduction of HIV-infected macrophages into the brains of SCID mice have been proposed, but they suffer from the fact of human macrophages delivered into a murine brain [92]. Some models of ongoing exposure to Tat have been developed. For example, GFAP-driven, doxycycline-inducible Tat transgenic mice have been useful for mechanistic studies of Tat contribution to HAND. However, the reported data concerning neuronal TUNEL positivity are still debated [93].

We [74,94,95] and others [26,96] have used model systems in which recombinant gp120, or Tat, proteins are directly injected into the striatum. The neurotoxicity of such recombinant proteins is highly reproducible and can be used as an interesting tool for testing novel therapeutic interventions. Administration of recombinant proteins is useful in understanding the effects of HIV-1 gene products, and so their individual contribution to the pathogenesis of HAND. However, HIV-1 infection of the brain is a chronic process, and its study would benefit from a model system allowing longer term exposure to HIV-1 gene product.

This is in part the reason why we developed experimental models of chronic HIV-1 neurotoxicity based on recombinant SV40 (rSV40) vector-modified expression of gp120 [80] or Tat [74] in the brain.

5. Antioxidant Therapeutic Approaches in HAND

As HIV-1 infection of the brain lasts the lifetime of affected individuals, and as eradication of CNS HIV-1 is currently not possible, control of the damage caused by the virus may represent a useful approach to treatment. This could entail limiting oxidative stress-related neurotoxicity.

5.1. Experimental Data

Antioxidant therapeutic options targeting oxidative stress can be artificially divided as targeting upstream and downstream pathways.

5.1.1. Upstream Antioxidant Therapy

Upstream preventive treatment is based on prevention of free radical generation, regulation of neuronal protein interaction with redox metals (*i.e.*, Fe) and maintaining normal cellular metabolism.

Some components have been studied in models of HAND or can be useful in this context. Vitamin E can block the neurotoxicity induced by CSF of patients with HIV dementia [68]. Exposure to the soluble vitamin E analog Trolox prevents against neurodegenerative effects of recombinant HIV-1 Tat [97]. Some natural compounds have been tested in animal models of HAND. *Ginkgo biloba* extract EGb 761, through its antioxidant role, protects against HIV-1 Tat neurotoxicity [98].

Flavinoids are a group of compounds made by plants that have antioxidant and neuroprotective properties. This class of molecules has weak estrogen-receptor-binding properties and thus, do not have the side effects of estradiol. It has been described that diosgenin, a plant-derived estrogen present in yam and fenugreek can prevent neurotoxicity by HIV-1 proteins and by CSF from patients with HIV dementia [68]. Other interesting molecules have not been tested in HAND yet; they include resveratrol, found in grape skins, red wine, and peanuts, as well as genistein and quercetin, found in soybeans. Polyphenols are a group of compounds with antioxidant properties. Among them, curcumin can induce stress response-protective genes, such as heme oxygenase 1 (HO-1), and can protect against heavy-metal insult to the brain [58]. Selenium is a key molecule in GPx1 metabolism. Some HIV-infected patients have low levels of selenium. Because selenium supplementation increases GPx1 activity, it might be beneficial in these patients. *N*-acetyl-L-cysteine (NAC) is a nutritional supplement precursor in the formation of the antioxidant glutathione in the body and its sulfhydryl group confers antioxidant effects and is able to reduce free radicals. NAC injected i.p. into rodents increases glutathione levels in the brain and protects the CNS against the damaging effects of hydroxyl radicals and lipid peroxidation product acrolein [99]. *N*-acetylcysteine amide (NACA), a modified form *N*-acetyl-L-cysteine (NAC), where the carboxyl group has been replaced by an amide group, has been found to be more effective in neurotoxic cases because of its ability to permeate cell membranes and the blood-brain barrier (BBB). Treatment of animals injected intravenously with gp120, Tat and methamphetamine METH by NACA significantly rescued the animals from oxidative stress. Further, NACA-treated animals had significantly less BBB permeability as compared to the group treated with gp120 + Tat + METH alone, indicating that NACA can protect the BBB from oxidative stress-induced damage in gp120, Tat and METH exposed animals [57].

5.1.2. Downstream Antioxidant Therapy

The therapeutic coverage of post oxidative stress events can be done by downstream antioxidant therapy. Non-steroidal anti-inflammatory drugs (NSAIDS) limit the infiltration of macrophages and can reduce the inflammatory cascade induced by oxidative stress. CPI-1189, a nitrone related compound, is supposed to regulate the pro-inflammatory cytokine cascade of genes in primary glial cells [54]. Minocycline is a tetracycline-derived compound that demonstrated neuroprotective profile in several models of neurodegeneration. The molecule has significant anti-inflammatory actions and can easily cross the BBB. *In vitro* data show that minocycline protected mixed neuronal cultures in an oxidative stress assay and has effective antioxidant properties with radical-scavenging potency similar to that of vitamin E [100]. Furthermore, minocycline treatment suppressed viral load in the brain, decreased the expression of CNS inflammatory markers and reduced the severity of encephalitis in a SIV model of HIV dementia [101]. A chemical moiety that resembles vitamin E in its chemical structure is the female sex hormone estrogen (estradiol) that contains a phenolic free radical scavenging site and acts as an antioxidant. It actually has the capability to prevent an upstream neurodegeneration and downstream the oxidative overload [54]. Estrogen replacement may result in improvement of cognitive function in several neurodegenerative disorders and conversely estrogen deficiency has been considered as a risk factor in some of them. Estradiol can protect against the neurotoxic effects of HIV-1 proteins in human neuronal cultures, probably by protecting the neuronal mitochondria in a receptor-independent manner [68]. However, estradiol has well known side effects in women (potential risk of developing breast or uterine cancer), and cannot be used in men or children because of feminizing effects [58]. It has been shown that several novel antioxidants (ebselen, diosgenin) can protect *in vitro* against neurotoxicity induced by CSF from patients with HV dementia [68].

It is likely that neuroprotective therapies should benefit from multiple and combination approaches targeting different aspects and pathways of the oxidative-stress insult. For example, coupling a potent antioxidant with a compound that modifies downstream signaling pathways (*i.e.*, minocycline) could provide a synergistic neuroprotective effects, at lower doses (and thus with less toxicity) that each molecule could achieve alone. The combination of HAART with an antioxidant compound and a molecule involved in downstream antioxidant therapy could be a promising avenue in the treatment of HAND [58]. However, it should be reminded that one of the challenges in designing antioxidants to protect the CNS against ROS is the crossing of the BBB.

5.2. Clinical Trials

A few antioxidants have been tried in small prospective controlled studies in HAND. However, the findings have all been relatively disappointing so far. Selegiline (L-deprenyl), which mechanism of action is speculative, albeit it might decrease the production of ROS and serve as an anti-apoptotic factor, was used in 2 double-blind controlled studies in the pre-HAART era. The first trial involving patients with minor cognitive and motor dysfunction (MCMD) showed improvement in verbal learning and trends for improvement in recall [102,103]. The second study was a smaller study in patients with MCMD and HIV dementia and showed significant improvement in delayed recall. However, other tests were not improved. A slight improvement was noted in patients treated with OPC-14117, a lipophilic compound structurally similar to vitamin E that acts as an antioxidant by scavenging superoxide radicals [104]. CPI-1189, a lipophilic antioxidant that scavenges superoxide anion radicals and block the neurotoxicity of gp120 and TNF-α [105], showed no effect on neurocognition in patients with MCMD and HIV dementia [106].

5.3. Gene Delivery of Antioxidant Enzymes in HAND

5.3.1. Introduction

In order to deliver potent antioxidant compounds to the brain, we used gene transfer of antioxidant enzymes. Gene transfer of antioxidant enzymes has been studied in numerous models of neurological disorders by using diverse viral vectors [107–109]. We used rSV40 vectors to deliver SV (SOD1) or SV (GPx1) carrying the antioxidant enzymes Cu/Zn superoxide dismutase (SOD1) or glutathione peroxidase (GPx1) respectively, into the rat caudate putamen (CP). The safety of SV (SOD1) and

SV (GPx1) delivered intra-CP has been demonstrated in rats and in Rhesus macaques monkeys, and resulting transgene expression is very durable [110]. Transgene expression of antioxidant enzymes can also be achieved through intravenous injection [111].

Mitochondria are a major site of production of superoxide in normal cells and probably contribute to increased oxidative stress in numerous diseases. Overexpression of mitochondrial Mn^{2+}-superoxide dismutase results in moderate reductions in infarction in temporary ischemia. Glutathione, the major water-soluble antioxidant, is localized in both the cytosol and the mitochondria. Mice overexpressing the cytosolic enzyme $Cu^{2+}Zn^{2+}$-superoxide dismutase develop smaller infarcts than wild-type ones, with a decrease in multiple events associated with mitochondrially mediated apoptosis, including the release of cytochrome c [112]. It is thus possible that cytosolic overexpression of antioxidant enzymes delivered by SV40-derived vectors can mitigate the apoptotic events linked to mitochondria.

5.3.2. Effects of Gene Delivery of Antioxidant Enzymes on Oxidative Stress, Apoptosis and Neuronal Loss in Animal Models of HAND

We showed that prior administration of recombinant SV40 vectors carrying antioxidant enzymes SOD1 or GPx1 protected either from Tat-induced oxidative injury (*i.e.*, lipid peroxidation) caused by intra-CP injection of Tat, or against SV (gp120)-induced oxidative injury. This reduction in oxidative stress due to gene transfer of antioxidant enzymes was associated with a protection against gp120- and Tat-elicited apoptosis and neuronal loss. Both striatal (either in acute or chronic models of HAND) and dopaminergic neurons were protected against gp120-induced insult [80,94,95,113,114].

Vector administration into the lateral ventricle (LV) [110] or cisterna magna (CM) [115], particularly if preceded by intraperitoneal mannitol, protects from intra-CP gp120-induced neurotoxicity comparably to intra-CP vector administration.

Caspases are involved in apoptosis linked to HAND. Caspases are implicated in neuronal death in neurodegenerative and other Central Nervous System (CNS) diseases.

Intrinsic apoptosis pathway is required for fetal and postnatal brain development, but is downregulated through the suppression of the expression of one of its key mediator, caspase-3 [114]. During stroke and neurodegenerative diseases, some caspases are upregulated in the brain [113]. Cerebral ischemia triggers both the intrinsic and extrinsic pathways of apoptosis [55,59]. Mounting evidence suggests the involvement of caspases in the disease process associated with neurodegenerative diseases such AD [115] and amyotrophic lateral sclerosis (ALS) [114].

The involvement of caspases in HIV-1 neurotoxicity has been documented *in vitro* and *in vivo*. Higher levels of caspase-3 and caspase-6 have been shown in the brains of patients with HAD [12,116,117]. Both HIV-1 neurotoxins gp120 and Tat significantly increase caspase-3 activation in striatal neurons *in vitro*. However, gp120 acts in large part through the activation of caspase(s), while Tat-induced neurotoxicity is also accompanied by activating an alternative pathway involving endonuclease G [118]. Tat can induce both caspases 3/7 and 9 in hippocampal cell cultures [119]. Increased expression of caspase-3 has been shown in neurons following exposure to Tat [18,21,71,77,118] and to gp120 [120–122]. In HIV-1 transgenic mice, Tat induction increased the percentage of neurons expressing caspase-3 [95]. Caspase-3-positive cells were also observed in a model of protracted exposure to gp120, SV(gp120) [80].

We studied the effect of gp120 on different caspases (3, 6, 8, 9) expression. Caspases production increased in the rat CP 6 h after gp120 injection into the same structure. The expression of caspases peaked by 24 h. Caspases colocalized mainly with neurons. There was a relationship with the concentration of gp120 injected. Both initiator (caspases 8 and 9) and effector/executioner (caspases 3 and 6) were increased after gp120 injection. We showed that about 70% of caspase-8- and 9-positive cells were TUNEL-positive while about 60% of caspase-3- and 6-positive cells were TUNEL-positive one day after intra-CP injection of gp120 [123]. Not all caspases-positive cells undergo apoptosis, at least as assessed by the methods used here and/or at the time points we considered. It is also possible that apoptosis will occur in the remaining caspases-positive cells at later time points. Gp120-induced caspase-3 activity may also be causing nonlethal neuron injury. As previously noted [95], if cell death in response to caspase-3 depends on total enzyme activity within a cell, the caspase-3 activity detected may be below the threshold required to initiate neuron death. This is difficult to determine based on immunocytochemistry. It has also been shown that activated caspase-3 rapidly degrades itself [124].

A link between oxidative stress and activation of some caspases seems highly probable. Prior gene delivery of the antioxidant enzymes SOD1 or GPx1 into the CP before injecting gp120 results in reduced levels of gp120-induced caspases, recapitulating the effect of antioxidant enzymes on gp120-induced apoptosis observed by TUNEL. Thus, HIV-1 gp120 increased caspases expression in the CP. Prior antioxidant enzyme treatment mitigated production of these caspases, probably by reducing ROS levels. While the present study strongly implicates caspases 3, 6, 8 and 9, additional studies are needed to determine the relative contribution of the various caspases to neuronal demise in HAND.

5.3.3. Gp120-Mediated Abnormalities of the Blood-Brain Barrier are Mitigated by Gene Transfer of Antioxidant Enzymes

ROS are important in the pathogenesis of HIV-induced CNS injury [125] and can be induced in brain endothelial cells by HIV-1 gp120 and Tat [126–128]. Although damage to the BBB has been documented in patients with HIV-related encephalopathy [129–131], the exact mechanism by which this injury occurs is still debated [15,132–141]. We used animal models of HAND to characterize abnormalities of the BBB in this context. Exposure to gp120, whether acute (by direct intra-CP injection) or chronic using SV (gp120), an experimental model of ongoing production of gp120 disrupted the BBB, and led to leakage of vascular contents into the area of gp120 exposure. Gp120 was directly toxic to brain endothelial cells and gp120-mediated BBB abnormalities were related to lesions of brain microvessels [142]. Abnormalities of the BBB may reflect the activity of proteolytic enzymes, particularly matrix metalloproteinases (MMPs). MMPs are a family of neutral proteases that are grouped according to their protein structures. MMP-2 and MMP-9 are considered gelatinases [143], and are enzymatically activated by the cleavage of precursor propeptides. These target laminin, a major BBB component, and attack the tight junctions between endothelial cells and BBB basal laminae. MMP-2 and MMP-9 were upregulated following intra-CP gp120-injection. Gp120 greatly diminished total CP content of laminin and tight junction proteins. ROS have been reported to activate MMPs. Injecting gp120 into the CP induced lipid peroxidation, assessed by increased MDA levels. One product of gp120-triggered lipid peroxidation, HNE, was immunolocalized to vascular endothelial cells. Moreover, gene transfer of antioxidant enzymes using recombinant SV (SOD1) and SV (GPx1) protected against gp120-induced BBB abnormalities. BBB injury has also been linked to NMDA, which upregulates the proform of MMP-9 and increases MMP-9 gelatinase activity [144]. Using the NMDA receptor (NMDAR-1) inhibitor, memantine, we observed partial protection from gp120-induced BBB injury [79].

MMPs are upregulated in different neurological diseases and models of CNS injury [145–151]. Various factors, such as ROS, NO, and proteases such as plasmin and stromelysin-1, are involved in MMP activation and upregulation in CNS injury [152–154]. MMPs have been reported in the cerebrospinal fluid of HIV-1 infected patients [155,156] as well as in models of HIV-1 encephalopathy [157–160]. In rapidly progressing simian immunodeficiency virus-infected monkeys, MMP-9 levels correlate with motor and cognitive deficits [161]. Moreover, cerebrospinal fluid levels of the urokinase-type plasminogen activator receptor, which plays an important role in degradation of extracellular matrix, and hence BBB injury, are elevated in patients with HIV dementia [162].

Relatively little is known about the respective roles of ROS and oxidative stress in the balance between MMPs and their endogenous tissue inhibitors (TIMPs). More than 20 MMPs and four TIMPs act together to control tightly temporally restricted, focal proteolysis of extracellular matrix (ECM) [163]. Once activated, MMPs are subject to inhibition by specific TIMPs that bind MMPs non-covalently [163]. Tissue destruction by MMPs is regulated by TIMPs and TIMPs prevent excessive MMP-related degradation of extracellular matrix components. The balance between MMPs and TIMPs is linked to ECM remodeling and imbalance between TIMPs and MMPs can lead to excessive degradation of matrix components as in rheumatoid arthritis. Tumor metastasis and angiogenesis may also reflect such imbalances.

In the myocardium, ROS activate MMPs, decrease TIMPs levels and collagen synthesis [164]. A relationship between oxidative damage, MMP production and BBB disruption has been found in some lesions of the striatum [154]. We studied the effect of gp120 on TIMP1- and TIMP-2 production. TIMP-1 and TIMP-2 levels increased 6 h after gp120 injection into rat CP. TIMP-1 and TIMP-2 colocalized mainly with neurons (92% and 95% respectively). By 24 h, expression of these protease inhibitors diverged, as TIMP-1 levels remained high but TIMP-2 subsided. Gene delivery of the antioxidant enzymes SOD1 or GPx1 into the CP before injecting gp120 there reduced levels of gp120-induced TIMP-1 and TIMP-2, recapitulating the effect of antioxidant enzymes on gp120-induced MMP-2 and MMP-9. A significant correlation was observed between MMP/TIMP upregulation and BBB leakiness. Thus, HIV-1 gp120 upregulated TIMP-1 and TIMP-2 in the CP. Prior antioxidant enzyme treatment mitigated production of these TIMPs, probably by reducing MMP expression. This might be explained by reduced ROS generation, either as effectors of damage or as signaling intermediates, or both, by antioxidant gene transfer with subsequent decrease in MMP expression. Moreover, there was a significant correlation between gp120-related BBB disturbances and MMP/TIMP upregulation. Following prior antioxidant gene delivery, a relationship was also seen between the reduction in Evans Blue (EB) extravasation and MMP-9/TIMP-1 decreased production [165].

Thus, MMPs and their inhibitors, TIMPs, are upregulated in response to oxidative stress produced in a rat model of HIV encephalopathy. In this setting, increase TIMPs may counterbalance the increase in MMPs. The centrality of ROS to this process is demonstrated by the fact that prior gene delivery of antioxidant enzymes mitigates production of TIMPs, possibly by reducing MMP expression. These results suggest that gp120-related oxidative stress induces MMP upregulation, potentially which triggers TIMP production

5.3.4. SV40-Mediated Gene Delivery of Antioxidant Enzymes Reduces gp120-Induced Neuroinflammation

If neuron loss [26,98,113,114] and astrogliosis [26] have been described in animals receiving gp120 directly into their brains, a temporal relationship between neuronal degeneration, astrocytic reaction, proinflammatory cytokine production and microglial proliferation remained to be established. We challenged rat CPs with 100–500 ng HIV-1BaL gp120, with or without prior rSV40-delivered SOD1 or GPx1. CD11b-positive microglia were increased 1 day post-challenge; Iba-1- and ED1-positive cells peaked at 7 days and 14 days respectively. Astrocyte infiltration was maximal at 7–14 days. MIP-1α was produced immediately, mainly by neurons. ED1- and GFAP-positive cells correlated with neuron loss and gp120 dose. We also tested the effect of more chronic gp120 exposure on neuroinflammation using an experimental model of continuing gp120 exposure. SV (gp120), a recombinant SV40-derived gene transfer vector was inoculated into the rat CP, leading to chronic expression of gp120, ongoing apoptosis in microglia and neurons, and oxidative stress. Increase in microglia and astrocytes was seen following intra-CP SV (gp120) injection, suggesting that continuing gp120 production increased neuroinflammation. SV (SOD1) or SV (GPx1) significantly reduced MIP-1α and limited neuroinflammation following gp120 administration into the CP, as well as microglia and astrocytes proliferation after injection of SV (gp120) in the striatum. Thus, gp120-induced CNS injury, neuron loss and inflammation may be mitigated by antioxidant gene delivery [166]. Similar results were observed when we injected Tat in the CP instead of gp120 [73].

Free radical production may be accompanied by elevated expression of MIP-1 alpha contributing to microglial recruitment and delayed neuronal death in several models of CNS injury [153,167–169]. The radical scavengers, like vitamin E analogs may inhibit free radicals and MIP-1α production, and recruitment of microglia in the injured area [169]. Our findings extend the principle of antioxidant protection from neuroinflammation to HIV-related injury, and suggest that rSV40 antioxidant gene delivery may be therapeutically applicable in the case of ongoing injury and neuroinflammation such as HAND.

HIV-1 envelope gp120 induces neuroinflammation when injected in the rat CP. Gp120-induced neuroinflammation correlates with neuron loss. An increase in expression of MIP-1α may play a role in this phenomenon, as well as ROS, as evidenced by the protective effects of rSV40-delivered antioxidant enzymes. The participation of other chemokines/cytokines in gp120-induced lesions *in vivo* remains to be established. The modulation of the interaction between these chemokines/cytokines and their ligands needs to be investigated.

6. Conclusions

HIV-1-associated neurocognitive disorder (HAND) is an increasingly common, progressive disease characterized by neuronal loss and progressively deteriorating CNS function. HIV-1 gene products, particularly gp120 and Tat, elicit ROS that lead to oxidant injury, cause neuron apoptosis, as well as subsequent consequences (e.g., neuroinflammation, abnormalities of the BBB). Understanding of, and developing therapies for, HAND requires accessible models of the disease. We have devised experimental approaches to studying the acute and chronic effects of gp120 and Tat on the CNS. These approaches to gp120 and Tat administration may therefore represent useful animal models for studying the pathogenesis and treatment of HIV-1 gp120- and Tat-related damage. Gene delivery of antioxidant enzymes by recombinant SV40-derived vectors protects against gp120 and Tat-induced oxidative stress and neuronal apoptosis, opening new avenues for potential therapeutics of HAND.

Acknowledgments

This work was supported by NIH grants MH70287, MH69122 and AH48244 to DS.

Conflict of Interest

The authors declare no conflict of interest.

References

1. McArthur, J.C.; Hoover, D.R.; Bacellar, H.; Miller, E.N.; Cohen, B.A.; Becker, J.T.; Graham, N.M.; McArthur, J.H.; Selnes, O.A.; Jacobson, L.P.; *et al*. Dementia in AIDS patients: Incidence and risk factors. Multicenter AIDS Cohort Study. *Neurology* **1993**, *43*, 2245–2252.
2. Major, E.O.; Rausch, D.; Marra, C.; Clifford, D. HIV-associated dementia. *Science* **2000**, *288*, 440–442.
3. Koutsilieri, E.; Sopper, S.; Scheller, C.; ter Meulen, V.; Riederer, P. Parkinsonism in HIV dementia. *J. Neural Transm.* **2002**, *109*, 767–775.
4. Antinori. A.; Arendt, G.; Becker, J.T.; Brew, B.J.; Byrd, D.A.; Cherner, M.; Clifford, D.B.; Cinque, P.; Epstein, L.G.; Gookin, K.; *et al*. Updated research nosology for HIV-associated neurocognitive disorders. *Neurology* **2007**, *69*, 1789–1799.
5. Woods, S.P.; Moore, D.J.; Weber, E.; Grant, I. Cognitive neuropsychology of HIV-associated neurocognitive disorders. *Neuropsychol. Rev.* **2009**, *19*, 152–168.
6. McArthur, J.C.; Brew, B.J.; Nath, A. Neurological complications of HIV infection. *Lancet Neurol.* **2005**, *4*, 543–555.
7. Nath, A.; Sacktor, N. Influence of highly active antiretroviral therapy on persistence of HIV in the central nervous system. *Curr. Opin. Neurol.* **2006**, *19*, 358–361.
8. Ances, B.M.; Ellis, R.J. Dementia and neurocognitive disorders due to HIV-1 infection. *Semin. Neurol.* **2007**, *27*, 86–92.
9. Mattson, M.P.; Haughey, N.J.; Nath, A. Cell death in HIV dementia. *Cell Death Diff.* **2005**, *12*, 893–904.
10. Rumbaugh, J.A.; Nath, A. Developments in HIV neuropathogenesis. *Curr. Pharm. Des.* **2006**, *12*, 1023–1044.
11. Gonzalez-Scarano, F.; Martin-Garcia, J. The neuropathogenesis of AIDS. *Nat. Rev. Immunol.* **2005**, *5*, 69–81.

12. Kaul, M.; Garden, G.A.; Lipton, S.A. Pathways to neuronal injury and apoptosis in HIV-associated dementia. *Nature* **2001**, *410*, 988–994.
13. Van de Bovenkamp, M.; Nottet, H.S.; Pereira, C.F. Interactions of human immunodeficiency virus-1 proteins with neurons: Possible role in the development of human immunodeficiency virus-1 associated dementia. *Eur. J. Clin. Investig.* **2002**, *32*, 619–627.
14. Eugenin, E.A.; D'Aversa, T.G.; Lopez, L.; Calderon, T.M.; Berman, J.W. MCP-1 (CCL2) protects human neurons and astrocytes from NMDA or HIV-tat-induced apoptosis. *J. Neurochem.* **2003**, *85*, 1299–1311.
15. Eugenin, E.A.; Osiecli, K.; Lopez, L.; Goldstein H.; Calderon, T.M.; Berman, J.W. CCL2/monocyte chemoattractant protein-1 mediates enhanced transmigration of human immunodeficiency virus (HIV)-infected leukocytes across the blood-brain barrier: A potential mechanism of HIV-CNS invasion and neuroAIDS. *J. Neurosci.* **2006**, *26*, 1098–1106.
16. Ghezzi, S.; Noolan, D.M.; Aluigi, M.G.; Vallanti, G.; Cota, M.; Benelli, R.; Morini, M.; Reeves, J.D.; Vicenzi, E.; Poli, G.; *et al.* Inhibition of CXCR-3-dependent HIV-1 infection by extracellular HIV-1 Tat. *Biochem. Byophys. Res. Commun.* **2000**, *270*, 992–996.
17. Magnuson, D.S.; Knudsen, B.E.; Geiger, J.D.; Brownstone, R.M.; Nath, A. Human immunodeficiency virus type 1 Tat activates non-*N*-methyl-*o*-aspartate excitatory amino receptors and causes neurotoxicity. *Ann. Neurol.* **1995**, *37*, 373–380.
18. Bonavia, R.; Bajetto, A.; Barbero, S.; Albini, A., Noonan, D.M.; Schettini, G. HIV-1 Tat causes apoptosis death and calcium homeostasis alterations in rat neurons. *Biochem. Biophys. Res. Commun.* **2001**, *288*, 301–308.
19. Haughey, N.J.; Nath, A.; Mattson, M.P. HIV-1 Tat through phosphorylation of NMDA receptors potentiates glutamate excitotoxicity. *J. Neurochem.* **2001**, *78*, 457–467.
20. Norman, J.P.; Perry, S.W.; Reynolds, H.M. HIV-1 Tat activates neuronal ryanodine receptors with rapid induction of the unfolded protein response and mitochondrial hyperpolarization. *PLoS One* **2008**, 3, e3731.
21. Kruman, I.I.; Nath, A.; Mattson, M.P. HIV-1 protein Tat induces apoptosis of hippocampal neurons by a mechanism involving caspase activation, calcium overload, and oxidative stress. *Exp. Neurol.* **1998**, *154*, 276–288.
22. Nath, A.; Haughey, N.J.; Jones, M.; Anderson, C.; Bell, J.E.; Geiger, J.D. Synergistic neurotoxicity by human immunodeficiency virus proteins Tat and gp120: Protection by memantine. *Ann. Neurol.* **2000**, *47*, 186–194.
23. Haughey, N.J.; Cutler, R.G.; Tamara, A.; McArthur, J.C.; Vargas, D.L.; Pardo, C.A.; Turchan, J.; Nath, A.; Mattson, M.P. Perturbation of sphingolipid metabolism and ceramide production in HIV-dementia. *Ann. Neurol.* **2004**, *5*, 257–267.
24. Bonfoco, E.; Krainc, D.; Ankarcrona, M.; Nicotera, P.; Lipton, S.A. Apoptosis and necrosis: Two distinct events induced, respectively, by mild and intense insults with *N*-methyl-D-aspartate or nitric oxide/superoxide in cortical cell cultures. *Proc. Natl. Acad. Sci. USA* **1995**, *92*, 7162–7166.
25. Jones, M.; Olafson, K.; del Bigio, M.R.; Peeling, J.; Nath, A. Intraventricular injection of human immunodeficiency virus type 1 (HIV-1) tat protein causes inflammation, gliosis, apoptosis, and ventricular enlargment. *J. Neuropathol. Exp. Neurol.* **1998**, *57*, 563–570.

26. Bansal, A.K.; Mactutus, C.F.; Nath, A.; Maragos, W.; Hauser, K.F.; Booze, R.M. Neurotoxicity of HIV-1 proteins gp120 and Tat in the rat striatum. *Brain Res.* **2000**, *879*, 42–49.
27. Askenov, M.Y.; Hasselrot, U.; Bansal, A.K.; Wu, G.; Nath, A.; Anderson, C.; Mactutus, C.F.; Booze, R.M. Oxidative damage induced by the injection of HIV-1 Tat protein in the rat striatum. *Neurosci. Lett.* **2001**, *305*, 5–8.
28. Askenov, M.Y.; Hasselrot, U.; Wu, G.; Nath, A.; Anderson, C.; Mactutus, C.F.; Booze, R.M. Temporal relationship between HIV-1 Tat-induced neuronal degeneration, OX-42 immunoreactivity, reactive astrocytosis, and protein oxidation in the rat striatum. *Brain Res.* **2003**, *987*, 1–9.
29. Theodore, S.; Cass, W.A.; Maragos, W.F. Methamphetamine and human immunodeficiency virus protein Tat synergize to destroy dopaminergic terminals in the rat striatum. *Neuroscience* **2006**, *137*, 925–935.
30. Wiley, C.A.; Baldwin, M.; Achim, C.L. Expression of HIV regulatory and structural mRNA in the central nervous system. *AIDS* **1996**, *10*, 843–847.
31. Hudson, L.; Liu, J.; Nath, A.; Jones, M.; Raghavan, R.; Naravan, O.; Male, D.; Everall, I. Detection of the human immunodeficiency virus regulatory protein Tat in CNS tissues. *J. Neurovirol.* **2000**, *6*, 144–155.
32. Garden, G.A.; Guo, W.; Jayadev, S.; Tun, C.; Balcaitis, S.; Choi, J.; Montine, T.J.; Moller, T.; Morrison, R.S. HIV associated neurodegeneration requires p53 in neurons and microglia. *FASEB J.* **2004**, *18*, 1141–1143.
33. Xu, Y.; Kulkosky, J.; Acheampong, E.; Nunnari, G.; Sullivan, J.; Pomerantz, R.J. HIV-1-mediated apoptosis of neuronal cells: Proximal molecular mechanisms of HIV-1-induced encephalopathy. *Proc. Natl. Acad. Sci. USA* **2004**, *101*, 7070–7075.
34. Meucci, O.; Fatatis, A.; Simen, A.A.; Bushell, T.J.; Gray, P.W.; Miller, R.J. Chemokines regulate hippocampal neuronal signalling and gp120 neurotoxicity. *Proc. Natl. Acad. Sci. USA* **1998**, *95*, 14500–14505.
35. Regulier, E.G.; Reiss, K.; Khalili, K.; Amini, S.; Zagury J.F.; Katsikis, P.D.; Rappaport, J. T-cell and neuronal apoptosis in HIV infection: Implications for therapeutic intervention. *Int. Rev. Immunol.* **2004**, *23*, 25–59.
36. Kaul, M.; Lipton, S.A. Chemokines and activated macrophages in HIV gp120-induced neuronal apoptosis. *Proc. Natl. Acad. Sci. USA* **1999**, *96*, 8212–8216.
37. Lipton, S.A.; Choi, Y.B.; Pan, Z.H.; Lei, S.Z.; Chen, H.S.; Sucher, N.J.; Loscalzo, J.; Singel, D.J.; Stamler, J.S. A redox-based mechanism for the neuroprotective and neurodestructive effects of nitric oxide and related nitrosocompounds. *Nature* **1993**, *364*, 626–632.
38. Dreyer, E.B.; Kaiser, P.K.; Offermann, J.T.; Lipton, S.A. HIV-1 coat protein neurotoxicity prevented by calcium channel antagonists. *Science* **1990**, *248*, 364–367.
39. Adamson, D.C.; Wildemann, B.; Sasaki, M.D.; Glass, J.D.; McArthur, J.C.; Christov, V.I.; Dawson, T.M.; Dawson, V.L. Immunologic NO synthase elevation in severe AIDS dementia and induction by HIV-1 gp41. *Science* **1996**, *274*, 1917–1920.
40. Adamson, D.C.; Kopnisky, K.L.; Dawson, T.M.; Dawson, V.L. Mechanisms and structural determinants of HIV-1 coat protein, gp41-induced neurotoxicity. *J. Neurosci.* **1999**, *19*, 64–71.

41. Hoshino, S.; Sun, B.; Konishi, M.; Shimura, M.; Segawa, T.; Hagiwara, Y.; Koyanagi, Y.; Iwamoto, A.; Mimaya, J.; Terunuma, H.; *et al*. Vpr in plasma of HIV type 1-positive patients is correlated with the HIV type 1 RNA titers. *AIDS Res. Hum. Retrovir.* **2007**, *23*, 391–397.
42. Levy, D.N.; Refaeli, Y.; Weiner, D.B. Extracellular Vpr protein increases cellular permissiveness to human immunodeficiency virus replication and reactivates virus from latency. *J. Virol.* **1995**, *69*, 1243–1252.
43. Patel, C.A.; Mukhtar, M.; Pomerantz, R.J. HIV-1 Vpr induces apoptosis in human neuronal cells. *J. Virol.* **2000**, *74*, 9717–9726.
44. Rom, I.; Deshmane, S.L.; Mukerjee, R.; Khalili, K.; Amini, S.; Sawaya, B.E. HIV-1 Vpr deregulates calcium secretion in neural cells. *Brain Res.* **2009**, *1275*, 81–86.
45. Trillo-Pazos, G.; McFarlane-Abdulla, E.; Campbell, I.C.; Pilkington, G.J.; Everall, I.P. Recombinant nef HIV-IIIB protein is toxic to human neurons in culture. *Brain Res.* **2000**, *864*, 315–326.
46. Ranki, A.; Nyberg, M.; Ovod, V.; Haltia, M.; Elovaara, I.; Raininko, R.; Haapasalo, H.; Krohn, K. Abundant expression of HIV Nef and Rev proteins in brain astrocytes *in vivo* is associated with dementia. *AIDS* **1995**, *9*, 1001–1008.
47. Mabrouk, K.; van Rietschoten, J.; Vives, E.; Darbon, H.; Rochat, H.; Sabatier, J.M. Lethal neurotoxicity in mice of the basic domains of HIV and SIV Rev proteins. Study of these regions by circular dichroism. *FEBS Lett.* **1991**, *289*, 13–17.
48. Li, J.; Bentsman, G.; Potash, M.J.; Volsky, D.J. Human immunodeficiency virus type 1 efficiently binds to human fetal astrocytes and induces neuroinflammatory responses independent of infection. *BMC Neurosci.* **2007**, *8*, 31.
49. Gorry, P.R.; Howard, J.L.; Churchill, M.J.; Churchill, M.J.; Anderson, J.L.; Cunningham, A.; Adrian, D.; McPhee, D.A.; Purcell, D.F. Diminished production of human immunodeficiency virus type 1 in astrocytes results from inefficient translation of gag, env, and nef mRNAs despite efficient expression of Tat and Rev. *J. Virol.* **1999**, *73*, 352–361.
50. Giulian, D.; Vaca, K.; Noonan, C.A. Secretion of neurotoxins by mononuclear phagocytes infected with HIV-1. *Science* **1990**, *250*, 1593–1596.
51. Liu, X.; Jana, M.; Dasgupta, S.; Koka, S.; He, J.; Wood, C.; Pahan, K. Human immunodeficiency virus type 1 (HIV-1) Tat induces nitric-oxide synthase in human astroglia. *J. Biol. Chem.* **2002**, *277*, 39312–3919.
52. Conant, K.; Garzino-Demo, A.; Nath, A.; McAthur, J.C.; Halliday, W.; Power, C.; Gallo, R.C.; Major, E.O. Induction of monocyte chemoattractant protein-1 in HIV-1 Tat-stimulated astrocytes and elevation in AIDS dementia. *Proc. Nat. Acad. Sci. USA* **1998**, *95*, 3117–3121.
53. Zhou, B.Y.; Liu, Y.; Kim, B.; Xiao, Y.; He, J.J. Astrocyte activation and dysfunction and neuron death by HIV-1 Tat expression in astrocytes. *Mol. Cell. Neurosci.* **2004**, *27*, 296–305.
54. Uttara, B.; Singh, A.V.; Zamboni, P.; Mahajan, R.T. Oxidative stress and neurodegenerative diseases: A review of upstream and downstream antioxidant therapeutic options. *Curr. Neuropharmacol.* **2009**, *7*, 65–74.
55. Broughton, B.R.S.; Reutens, D.C.; Sobey C.G. Apoptotic mechanisms after cerebral ischemia. *Stroke* **2009**, *40*, e331–e339.

56. Butterfield, D.A.; Castegna, A.; Lauderback, C.M.; Drake, J. Evidence that amyloid β-peptide induced lipid peroxidation and its sequelae in Alzheimer's disease brain contribute to neuronal death. *Neurobiol. Aging* **2002**, 23, 655–664.
57. Banerjee, A.; Zhanq, X.; Manda, K.R.; Banks, W.A.; Ercal, N. HIV proteins (gp120 and Tat) and methamphetamine in oxidative stress-induced damage in the brain: Potential role of the thiol antioxidant *N*-acetylcysteine amide. *Free Rad. Biol. Med.* **2010**, *48*, 1388–1398.
58. Steiner, J.; Haughey, N.; Li, W.; Venkatesan, A.; Anderson, C.; Reid, R.; Malpica, T.; Pocernich, C.; Butterfield, D.A.; Nath, A. Oxidative stress and therapeutic approaches in HIV dementia. *Antioxid. Redox Sign.* **2006**, *8*, 2089–2100.
59. Sims, N.R.; Muyderman, H. Mitochondria, oxidative metabolism and cell death in stroke. *Biochim. Biophysis. Acta* **2010**, *1802*, 80–91.
60. Dexter, D.T.; Carter, C.J.; Wells, F.R.; Javoy-Agid, F.; Agid, Y.; Lees, A.; Jenner, P.; Marsden, C.D. Basal lipid perxidation in substantia nigra is increased in Parkinson's disease. *J. Neurochem.* **1987**, *52*, 381–389.
61. Beal, M.F. Aging, energy, and oxidative stress in neurodegenerative diseases. *Ann. Neurol.* **1995**, *38*, 357–366.
62. Smith, M.A.; Perry, G. Free radical damage, iron, and Alzheimer's disease. *J. Neurol. Sci.* **1995**, *134*, 92–94.
63. Smith, M.A.; Sayre, L.M.; Monnier, V.M.; Perry, G. Radical ageing in Alzheimer's disease. *Trends Neurosci.* **1995**, *18*, 172–176.
64. Cao, W.; Carney, J.M.; Duchon, A.; Floyd, R.A.; Chevion, M. Oxygen free radicals involvement in ischemia and reperfusion of the brain injury to brain. *Neurosci. Lett.* **1998**, *88*, 233–238.
65. Montoliu, C.; Valles, S.; Renau-Piqueras, J.; Guerri, C. Ethanol-induced oxygen radical formation and lipid peroxidation in rat brain: Effect of chronic alcohol consumption. *J. Neurochem.* **1994**, *63*, 1855–1862.
66. Smith, C.D.; Carney, J.M.; Starke-Reed, P.E.; Oliver, C.N.; Stadtman, E.R.; Floyd, R.A.; Markesberry, W.R. Excess brain protein oxidation and enzyme dysfunction in normal aging and in Alzheimer's disease. *Proc. Natl. Acad. Sci. USA* **1991**, *88*, 10540–10543.
67. Mollace, V.; Nottet, H.S.; Clayette, P.; Turco, M.C.; Muscoli, C.; Salvemini, D.; Perno, C.F. Oxidative stress and neuroAIDS: Triggers, modulators and novel antioxidants. *Trends Neurosci.* **2001**, *24*, 411–416.
68. Turchan, J.; Pocernich, C.B.; Gairola, C.; Chauhan, A.; Schifitto, G.; Butterfield, D.A.; Buch, S.; Naravan, O.; Sinai, A.; Geiger, G.; *et al*. Oxidative stress in HIV demented patients and protection *ex vivo* with novel antioxidants. *Neurology* **2003**, *60*, 307–314.
69. Cutler, R.G.; Haughey, N.J.; Tammara, A.; McArthur, J.C.; Nath, A.; Reid, R.; Vargas, D.L.; Pardo, C.A.; Mattson, M.P. Dysregulation of sphingolipids and sterol metabolism by ApoE4 in HIV dementia. *Neurology* **2004**, *63*, 626–630.
70. Agrawal, L.; Louboutin, J.P.; Strayer, D.S. Preventing HIV-1 Tat-induced neuronal apoptosis using antioxidant enzymes: Mechanistic and therapeutic implications. *Virology* **2007**, *363*, 462–472.

71. Kruman, I.I.; Bruce-Keller, A.J.; Bredesen, D.; Waeg, G.; Mattson, M.P. Evidence that 4-hydroxynonenal mediates oxidative stress-induced neuronal apoptosis. *J. Neurosci.* **1997**, *17*, 5089–5100.
72. Bruce-Keller, A.J.; Li, Y.J.; Lovell, M.A.; Kraemer, P.J.; Gary, D.S.; Brown, R.R.; Markesbery, W.R.; Mattson, M.P. 4-Hydroxynonenal, a product of lipid peroxidation, damages cholinergic neurons and impairs visuospatial memory in rats. *J. Neuropathol. Exp. Neurol.* **1998**, *57*, 257–267.
73. Bruce-Keller, A.J.; Barger, S.W.; Moss, N.I.; Pham, J.T.; Keller, J.N.; Nath, A. Proinflammatory and pro-oxidant properties of Tat in a microglial cell line: Attenuation by 17b-estradiol. *J. Neurochem.* **2001**, *78*, 1315–1324.
74. Agrawal, L.; Louboutin, J.P.; Reyes, B.A.S.; van Bockstaele, E.J.; Strayer, D.S. HIV-1 Tat neurotoxicity: A model of acute and chronic exposure, and neuroprotection by gene delivery of antioxidant enzymes. *Neurobiol. Dis.* **2012**, *45*, 657–670.
75. Nath, A.; Conant, K.; Chen, P.; Scott, C.; Major, E.O. Transient exposure to HIV-1 Tat protein results in cytokine production in macrophages and astrocytes: A hit and run phenomenon. *J. Biol. Chem.* **1999**, *274*, 17098–17102.
76. Andersen, J.K. Oxidative stress in neurodegeneration: Cause or consequence? *Nat. Med.* **2004**, *5*, S18–S25.
77. Kruman, I.I.; Mattson, M.P. Pivotal role of mitochondrial calcium uptake in neural cell apoptosis and necrosis. *J. Neurochem.* **1999**, *72*, 529–540.
78. Shah, A.; Kumar, S.; Simon, S.D.; Singh, D.P.; Kumar, A. HIV gp120- and methamphetamine-mediated oxidative stress induces astrocyte apoptosis via cytochrome P4502E1. *Cell Death Dis.* **2013**, *4*, e850.
79. Louboutin, J.P.; Agrawal, L.; Reyes, B.A.S.; van Bockstaele, E.J.; Strayer, D.S. HIV-1 gp120-induced injury to the blood-brain barrier: Role of metalloproteinases 2 and 9 and relationship to oxidative stress. *J. Neuropathol. Exp. Neurol.* **2010**, *69*, 801–816.
80. Louboutin, J.P.; Agrawal, L.; Reyes, B.A.S.; van Bockstaele, E.J.; Strayer, D.S. A rat model of human immunodeficiency virus 1 encephalopathy using envelope glycoprotein gp120 expression delivered by SV40 vectors. *J. Neuropathol. Exp. Neurol.* **2009**, *68*, 456–473.
81. Strayer, D.S. Gene therapy using SV40-derived vectors: What does the future hold? *J. Cell Physiol.* **1999**, *181*, 375–384.
82. Strayer, D.S.; Kondo, R.; Milano, J.; Duan, L.X. Use of SV40-based vectors to transduce foreign genes to normal human peripheral blood mononuclear cells. *Gene Ther.* **1997**, *4*, 219–225.
83. McKee, H.J.; Strayer, D.S. Immune responses against SIV envelope glycoprotein, using recombinant SV40 as a vaccine delivery vector. *Vaccine* **2002**, *20*, 3613–3625.
84. Cordelier, P.; Calarota, S.A.; Pomerantz, R.J.; Xiaoshan, J.; Strayer, D.S. Inhibition of HIV-1 in the central nervous system by IFN-α2 delivered by an SV40 vector. *J. Interferon Cytokine Res.* **2003**, *23*, 477–488.
85. Cordelier, P.; van Bockstaele, E.; Calarota, S.A.; Strayer, D.S. Inhibiting AIDS in the central nervous system: Gene delivery to protect neurons from HIV. *Mol. Ther.* **2003**, *7*, 801–810.
86. Cordelier, P.; Strayer, D.S. Using gene delivery to protect HIV-susceptible CNS cells: Inhibiting HIV replication in microglia. *Virus Res.* **2006**, *118*, 87–97.

87. Ferrucci, R.; Nonnemacher, M.R.; Cohen E.A.; Wigdahl, B. Extracellular human immunodeficiency 1 virus type 1 viral protein R causes reductions in astrocytic ATP and glutathione levels compromising the antioxidant reservoir. *Virus Res.* **2012**, *167*, 358–369.
88. Hurtrel, M.; Ganiere, J.P.; Guelfi, J.F.; Chakrabarti, L.; Maire, M.A.; Gray, F.; Montagnier, L.; Hurtrel, B. Comparison of early and late feline immunodeficiency virus encephalopathies. *AIDS* **1992**, *6*, 399–406.
89. Thormar, H. Maedi-visna virus and its relationship to human deficiency virus. *AIDS Rev.* **2005**, *7*, 233–245.
90. Lackner, A.A.; Veazey, R.S. Current concepts in AIDS pathogenesis: Insights from the SIV/macaque model. *Annu. Rev. Med.* **2007**, *58*, 461–476.
91. Toggas, S.M.; Masliah, E.; Rockenstein, E.M.; Rall, G.F.; Abraham, C.R.; Mucke, L. Central nervous system damage produced by expression of the HIV-1 coat protein gp120 in transgenic mice. *Nature* **1994**, *367*, 188–193.
92. Avgeropoulos, N.; Kelley, B.; Middaugh, L.; Arrigo, S.; Persidsky, Y.; Gendelman, H.E.; Tyor, W.R. SCID mice with HIV encephalitis develop behavioral abnormalities. *J. Acquir. Immune Defic. Syndr.* **1998**, *18*, 13–20.
93. Bruce-Keller, A.J.; Turchan-Cholewo, J.; Smart, E.J.; Geurin, T.; Chauhan, A.; Reid, R.; Xu, R.; Nath, A.; Knapp, P.E.; Hauser, K.F. Morphine causes rapid increases in glial activation and neuronal injury in the striatum of inducible HIV-1 Tat transgenic mice. *Glia* **2008**, *56*, 1414–1427.
94. Agrawal, L.; Louboutin, J.P.; Reyes, B.A.S.; van Bockstaele, E.J.; Strayer, D.S. Antioxidant enzyme gene delivery to protect from HIV-1 gp120-induced neuronal apoptosis. *Gene Ther.* **2006**, *13*, 1645–1656.
95. Louboutin, J.P.; Agrawal, L.; Reyes, B.A.S.; van Bockstaele, E.J.; Strayer, D.S. Protecting neurons from HIV-1 gp120-induced oxidant stress using both localized intracerebral and generalized intraventricular administration of antioxidant enzymes delivered by SV40-derived vectors. *Gene Ther.* **2007**, *14*, 1650–1661.
96. Nosheny, R.L.; Bachis, A.; Acquas, E.; Mocchetti, I. Human immunodeficiency virus type 1 glycoprotein gp120 reduces the levels of brain-derived neurotrophic factor *in vivo*: Potential implication for neuronal cell death. *Eur. J. Neurosci.* **2004**, *20*, 2857–2864.
97. Butler, T.R.; Smith, K.J.; Self, R.L.; Braden, B.B.; Prendergast, M.A. Neurodegenerative effects of recombinant HIV-1 Tat(1–86) are associated with inhibition of microtubule formation and oxidative stress-related reductions in microtubule-associated protein-2(a,b). *Neurochem. Res.* **2011**, *36*, 819–828.
98. Zou, W.; Kim, B.O.; Zhou, B.Y.; Liu, Y.; Messing, A.; He, J. Protection against human immunodeficiency virus type 1 Tat neurotoxicity by Ginkgo biloba extract EGb 761 involving glial fibrillary acidic protein. *Am. J. Pathol.* **2007**, *171*, 1923–1935.
99. Pocernich, C.B.; La Fontaine, M.; Butterfield, D.A. *In-vivo* glutathione elevation protects against hydroxyl free radical-induced protein oxidation in rat brain. *Neurochem. Int.* **2000**, *36*, 185–191.
100. Kraus, R.L.; Pasieczny, R.; Lariosa-Willingham, K.; Turner, M.S.; Jiang, A.; Trauger, J.W. Antioxidant properties of minocycline: Neuroprotection in an oxidative stress assay and direct radical-scavenging activity. *J. Neurochem.* **2005**, *94*, 819–827.

101. Zinc, M.C.; Uhrlaub, J.; DeWitt, J.; Voelker, T.; Bullock, B.; Mankowski, J.; Tarwater, P.; Clements, J.; Barber, S. Neuroprotective anti-human immunodeficiency virus activity of minocycline. *JAMA* **2005**, *293*, 2003–2011.
102. Consortium, D. A randomized, double-blind, placebo-controlled trial of deprenyl and thioctic acid in human immunodeficiency virus-associated cognitive impairment: Dana Consortium on the therapy of HIV dementia and related cognitive disorders. *Neurology* **1998**, *50*, 645–651.
103. Sacktor, N.; Schifitto, G.; McDermott, M.P.; Marder, K.; McArthur, J.C.; Kieburtz, K. Transdermal seleginine in HIV-associated cognitive impairment: Pilot, placebo-controlled study. *Neurology* **2000**, *54*, 233–235.
104. Consortium, D. Safety and tolerability of the antioxidant OPC-14117 in HIV-associated cognitive impairment: The Dana Consortium on the therapy of HIV dementia and related cognitive disorders. *Neurology* **1997**, *49*, 142–146.
105. Pulliam, L.; Irwin, I.; Kusdra, L.; Rempel, H.; Flitter, W.D.; Garland, W.A. CPI-1189 attenuates effects of suspected neurotoxins associated with AIDS dementia: A possible role for ERK activation. *Brain Res.* **2001**, *893*, 95–103.
106. Clifford, D.B.; McArthur, J.C.; Schifitto, G.; Kieburtz, K.; McDermott, M.P.; Letendre, S.; Cohen, B.A.; Marder, K.; Ellis, R.J.; Marra, C.M.; *et al.* A randomized clinical trial of CPI-1189 for HIV-associated cognitive-motor impairment. *Neurology* **2002**, *59*, 1568–1573.
107. Watanabe, Y.; Chu, Y.; Andresen, J.J.; Nakane, H.; Faraci, F.M.; Heistad, D.D. Gene transfer of extracellular superoxide dismutase reduces cerebral vasospasm after subarachnoid hemorrhage. *Stroke* **2003**, *34*, 434–440.
108. Hoehn, B.; Yenari, M.A.; Sapolsky, R.M.; Steinberg, G.K. Glutathione peroxidase overexpression inhibits cytochrome C release and proapoptotic mediators to protect neurons from experimental stroke. *Stroke* **2003**, *34*, 2489–2494.
109. Ridet, J.L.; Bensadoun, J.C.; Deglon, N.; Aebischer, P.; Zurn, A.D. Lentivirus-mediated expression of glutathione peroxidase: Neuroprotection in murine models of Parkinson's disease. *Neurobiol. Dis.* **2006**, *21*, 29–34.
110. Louboutin, J.P.; Marusich, E.; Fisher-Perkins, J.; Dufour, J.P.; Bunnell, B.A.; Strayer, D.S. Gene transfer to the Rhesus monkey brain using SV40-derived vectors is durable and safe. *Gene Ther.* **2011**, *18*, 682–691.
111. Louboutin, J.P.; Chekmasova, A.A.; Marusich, E.; Chowdhury, J.R.; Strayer, D.S. Efficient CNS gene delivery by intravenous injection. *Nature Meth.* **2010**, *7*, 905–907.
112. Agrawal, L.; Louboutin, J.P.; Marusich, E.; Reyes, B.A.S.; van Bockstaele, E.; Strayer, D.S. Dopaminergic neurotoxicity of HIV-1 gp120: Reactive oxygen species as signaling intermediates. *Brain Res.* **2010**, *1306*, 116–130.
113. Louboutin, J.P.; Reyes, B.A.S.; Agrawal, L.; van Bockstaele, E.J.; Strayer, D.S. Strategies for CNS-directed gene delivery: *In vivo* gene transfer to the brain using SV40-derived vectors. *Gene Ther.* **2007**, *14*, 939–949.
114. Louboutin, J.P.; Agrawal, L.; Reyes, B.A.S.; van Bockstaele, E.J.; Strayer, D.S. HIV-1 gp120 neurotoxicity proximally and at a distance from the point of exposure: Protection by rSV40 delivery of antioxidant enzyme. *Neurobiol. Dis.* **2009**, *34*, 462–476.

115. Louboutin, J.P.; Reyes, B.A.S.; Agrawal, L.; van Bockstaele, E.J.; Strayer, D.S. Intracisternal rSV40 administration provides effective pan-CNS transgene expression. *Gene Ther.* **2012**, *19*, 114–118.
116. Petito, C.K.; Roberts, B. Evidence of apoptotic cell death in HIV encephalitis. *Am. J. Pathol.* **1995**, *146*, 1121–1130.
117. Noorbakhsh, F.; Ramachandran, R.; Barsby, N.; Ellestad, K.K.; LeBlanc, A.; Dickie, P.; Baker, G.; Hollenberg, M.D.; Cohen, E.A.; Power, C. MicroRNA profiling reveals new aspects of HIV neurodegeneration: Caspase-6 regulates astrocyte survival. *FASEB J.* **2010**, *24*, 1799–1812.
118. Singh, I.N.; Goody, R.J.; Dean, C.; Ahmad, N.M.; Lutz, S.E.; Knapp, P.E.; Nath, A.; Hauser, K.F. Apoptotic cell death of striatal neurons induced by human immunodeficiency virus-1 Tat and gp120: Differential involvement of caspase-3 and endonuclease G. *J. Neurovirol.* **2004**, *10*, 141–151.
119. Askenov, M.Y.; Askenova, M.V.; Mactutus, C.F.; Booze, R.M. Attenuated neurotoxicity of the transactivation-defective HIV-Tat protein in hippocampal cell cultures. *Exp. Neurol.* **2009**, *219*, 586–590.
120. Nosheny, R.L.; Bachis, A.; Aden, S.A.; de Bernardi, M.A.; Mocchetti, I. Intrastriatal administration of human immunodeficiency virus-1 glycoprotein 120 reduces glial cell-line derived neurotrophic factor levels and causes apoptosis in the substantia nigra. *J. Neurobiol.* **2006**, *66*, 1311–1321.
121. Nosheny, R.L.; Ahmed, F.; Yakovlev, A.; Meyer, E.M.; Ren, K.; Tessarollo, L.; Mocchetti, I. Brain-derived neurotrophic factor prevents the nigrostriatal degeneration induced by human immunodeficiency virus-1 glycoprotein 120 *in vivo*. *Eur. J. Neurosci.* **2007**, *25*, 2275–2284.
122. Bachis, A.; Aden, S.A.; Nosheny, R.L.; Andrews, P.M.; Mocchetti, I. Axonal transport of human immunodeficiency virus type 1 envelope protein glycoprotein 120 is found in association with neuronal apoptosis. *J. Neurosci.* **2006**, *26*, 6771–6780.
123. Louboutin, J.P.; Reyes, B.A.S.; Agrawal, L.; van Bockstaele, E.J.; Strayer, D.S. Gene delivery of antioxidant enzymes inhibits HIV-1 gp120-induced expression of caspases. *Neuroscience* **2012**, *214*, 68–77.
124. Cribbs, D.H.; Poon, W.W.; Rissman, R.A.; Blurton-Jones, M. Caspase-mediated degeneration in Alzheimer's disease. *Am. J. Pathol.* **2004**, *165*, 353–355.
125. Sacktor, N.; Haughey, N.; Cutler, R.; Tamara, A.; Turchan, J.; Pardo, C.; Vargas, D.; Nath, A. Novel markers of oxidative stress in actively progressive HIV dementia. *J. Neuroimmunol.* **2004**, *157*, 176–184.
126. Ullrich, C.K.; Groopman, J.E.; Ganju, R.K. HIV-1 gp120- and gp160-induced apoptosis in cultured endothelial cells is mediated by caspases. *Blood* **2000**, *96*, 1436–1442.
127. Price, T.O.; Ercal, N.; Nakaoke, R.; Banks, W.A. HIV-1 viral proteins gp120 and Tat induce oxidative stress in brain endothelial cells. *Brain Res.* **2005**, *1045*, 57–63.
128. Price, T.O.; Uras, F.; Banks, W.A.; Ercal, N. A novel antioxidant *N*-acetylcysteine amide prevents gp120- and Tat-induced oxidative stress in brain endothelial cells. *Exp. Neurol.* **2006**, *201*,
193–202.

129. Petito, C.K.; Cash, K.S. Blood-brain barrier abnormalities in the acquired immunodeficiency syndrome: Immunohistochemical localization of serum proteins in postmortem brain. *Ann. Neurol.* **1992**, *32*, 658–666.
130. Power, C.; Kong, P.A.; Crawford, T.O.; Wesselingh, S.; Glass, J.D.; McArthur, J.C.; Trapp, B.D. Cerebral white matter changes in acquired immunodeficiency syndrome dementia: Alterations of the blood-brain barrier. *Ann. Neurol.* **1993**, *34*, 339–350.
131. Avison, M.J.; Nath, A.; Greene-Avison, R.; Schmitt, F.A.; Greenberg, R.N.; Berger, J.R. Neuroimaging correlates of HIV-associated BBB compromise. *J. Neuroimmunol.* **2004**, *157*, 140–146.
132. Toneatto, S.; Finco, O.; van der Putten, H.; Abrignani, S.; Annunziata, P. Evidence of blood-brain barrier alteration and activation in HIV-1 gp120 transgenic mice. *AIDS* **1999**, *13*, 2343–2348.
133. Huang, M.B.; Hunter, M.; Bond, V.C. Effect of extracellular human immunodeficiency virus type 1 glycoprotein 120 on primary human vascular endothelium cell cultures. *AIDS Res. Hum. Retrovir.* **1999**, *15*, 1265–1277.
134. Dallasta, L.M.; Pisarov, L.A.; Esplen, J.E.; Werley, J.V.; Moses, A.V.; Nelson, J.A.; Achim, C.L. Blood-brain barrier tight junction disruption in human immunodeficiency virus-1 encephalitis. *Am. J. Pathol.* **1999**, *155*, 1915–1927.
135. Banks, W.A.; Ibrahimi, F.; Farr, S.A.; Flood, J.F.; Morley, J.E. Effects of wheatgerm agglutinin and aging on the regional brain uptake of HIV-1 gp120. *Life Sci.* **1999**, *65*, 81–89.
136. Banks, W.A.; Freed, E.O.; Wolf, K.M.; Robinson, S.M.; Franko, M.; Kumar, V.B. Transport of human immunodeficiency virus type 1 pseudoviruses across the blood-brain barrier: Role of envelope proteins and adsorptive endocytosis. *J. Virol.* **2001**, *75*, 4681–4691.
137. Banks, W.A.; Robinson, S.M.; Nath, A. Permeability of the blood-brain barrier to HIV-1 Tat. *Exp. Neurol.* **2005**, *193*, 218–227.
138. Cioni, C.; Annunziata, P. Circulating gp120 alters the blood-brain barrier permeability in HIV-1 gp120 transgenic mice. *Neurosci. Lett.* **2002**, *330*, 299–301.
139. Annunziata, P. Blood-brain barrier changes during invasion of the central nervous system by HIV-1. Old and new insights into the mechanism. *J. Neurol.* **2003**, *250*, 901–906.
140. Kanmogne, G.D.; Primeaux, C.; Grammas, P. HIV-1 gp120 proteins alter tight junction protein expression and brain endothelial cell permeability: Implications for the pathogenesis of HIV-associated dementia. *J. Neuropath. Exp. Neurol.* **2005**, *64*, 498–505.
141. Kanmogne, G.D.; Schall, K.; Leibhart, J.; Knipe, B.; Gendelman, H.E.; Persidsky, Y. HIV-1 gp120 compromises blood-brain barrier integrity and enhance monocyte migration across blood-brain barrier: Implication for viral neuropathogenesis. *J. Cereb. Blood Flow MeTab.* **2007**, *27*, 123–134.
142. Louboutin, J.P.; Reyes, B.A.S.; Agrawal, L.; Maxwell, C.R.; van Bockstaele, E.J.; Strayer, D.S. Blood-brain barrier abnormalities caused by exposure to HIV-1 gp120—Protection by gene delivery of antioxidant enzymes. *Neurobiol. Dis.* **2010**, *38*, 313–325.
143. Clark, I.M.; Swingler, T.E.; Sampieri, C.L.; Edwards, D.R. The regulation of matrix metalloproteinases and their inhibitors. *Int. J. Biochem. Cell Biol.* **2008**, *40*, 1362–1378.

144. Manabe, S.; Gu, Z.; Lipton, S.A. Activation of matrix metalloproteinase-9 via neuronal nitric oxide synthase contributes to NMDA-induced retinal ganglion cell death. *Investig. Ophtalmol. Vis. Sci.* **2005**, *46*, 4747–4753.
145. Rosenberg, G.A. Matrix metalloproteinases in neuroinflammation. *Glia* **2002**, *39*, 279–291.
146. Gu, Z.; Kaul, M.; Yan, B.; Kridel, S.J.; Cui, J.; Strongin, A.; Smith, J.W.; Liddington, R.C.; Lipton, S.A. *S*-nitrosylation of matrix metalloproteinases: Signaling pathway to neuronal cell death. *Science* **2002**, *297*, 1186–1190.
147. Yong, V.W.; Power, C.; Forsyth, P.; Edwards, D.R. Metalloproteinases in biology and pathology of the central nervous system. *Nat. Rev. Neurosci.* **2001**, *2*, 502–511.
148. Lo, E.H.; Wang, X.; Cuzner, M.I. Extracellular proteolysis in brain injury and inflammation: Role for plasminogen activators and matrix metalloproteinases. *J. Neurosci. Res.* **2002**, *69*, 1–9.
149. Gursoy-Ozdemir, Y.; Qiu, J.; Matsuoka, N.; Bolay, H.; Bermpohl, D.; Jin, H.; Wang, X.; Rosenberg, GA.; Lo, E.H.; Moskowitz, M.A. Cortical spreading depression activates and upregulates MMP-9. *J. Clin. Investig.* **2004**, *113*, 1447–1455.
150. Zozulya, A.L.; Reinke, E.; Baiu, D.C.; Baiu, D.C.; Karman, J.; Sandor, M.; Fabry, Z. Dendritic cell transmigration through brain microvessel endothelium is regulated by MIP-1α chemokine and matrix metalloproteinases. *J. Immunol.* **2007**, *178*, 520–529.
151. Haorah, J.; Schall, K.; Ramirez, S.H.; Persidsky, Y. Activation of protein kinases and matrix metalloproteinases causes blood-brain barrier injury: Novel mechanisms for neurodegeneration associated with alcohol abuse. *Glia* **2008**, *56*, 78–88.
152. Asahi, M.; Asahi, K.; Jung, J.-C.; del Zoppo, G.J.; Fini, M.E.; Lo, E.H. Role for matrix metalloproteinase 9 after focal cerebral ischemia: Effects of gene knockout and enzyme inhibition with BB-94. *J. Cereb. Blood Flow MeTab.* **2000**, *20*, 1681–1689.
153. Gasche, Y.; Copin, J.-C.; Sugawara, T.; Fujimura, M.; Chan, P.H. Matrix metalloproteinases inhibition prevents oxidative stress-associated blood-brain barrier disruption after transient focal cerebral ischemia. *J. Cereb. Blood Flow MeTab.* **2001**, *21*, 1393–1400.
154. Kim, G.W.; Gasche, Y.; Grzeschik, S.; Copin, J.-C.; Maier, C.M.; Chan, P.H. Neurodegeneration in striatum induced by the mitochondrial toxin 3-nitropropionic acid: Role of matrix metalloproteinase-9 in early blood-brain barrier disruption? *J. Neurosci.* **2003**, *23*, 8733–8742.
155. Sporer, B.; Paul, R.; Koedel, U.; Grimm, R.; Wick, M.; Goebel, F.D.; Pfister, H.W. Presence of matrix metalloproteinase-9 activity in the cerebrospinal fluid of human immunodeficiency virus-infected patients. *J. Infect. Dis.* **1998**, *178*, 854–857.
156. Liuzzi, G.M.; Mastroianni, C.M.; Santacroce, M.P.; Fanelli, M.; D'Agostino, C.; Vullo, V.; Riccio, P. Increased activity of matrix metalloproteinases in the cerebrospinal fluid of patients with HIV-associated neurological diseases. *J. Neurovirol.* **2000**, *6*, 156–163.
157. Marshall, D.C.L.; Wyss-Coray, T.W.; Abraham, C.R. Induction of matrix metalloproteinase-2 in human immunodeficiency virus-1 glycoprotein 120 transgenic mouse brains. *Neurosci. Lett.* **1998**, *254*, 97–100.

158. Toschi, E.; Barillari, G.; Sgadari, C.; Bacigalupo, I.; Cereseto, A.; Carlei, D.; Palladino, C.; Zietz, C.; Leone, P.; Sturzl, M.; *et al.* Activation of matrix-metalloproteinase-2 and membrane-type-1-matrix-metalloproteinase in endothelial cells and induction of vascular permeability *in vivo* by human immunodeficiency virus-1 Tat protein and basic Fibroblast Growth Factor. *Mol. Biol. Cell* **2001**, *12*, 2934–2946.
159. Conant, K.; St Hillaire, C.; Anderson, C.; Galey, D.; Wang, J.; Nath, A. Human immunodeficiency virus type 1 Tat and methamphetamine affect the release and activation of matrix-degrading proteinases. *J. Neurovirol.* **2004**, *10*, 21–28.
160. Russo, R.; Siviglia, E.; Gliozzi, M.; Amantea, D.; Paoletti, A.; Berliocchi, L.; Bagetta, G.; Corasaniti, M.T. Evidence implicating matrix metalloproteinases in the mechanism underlying accumulation of IL-1β and neuronal apoptosis in the neocortex of HIV/gp120-exposed rats. *Int. Rev. Neurobiol.* **2007**, *82*, 407–421.
161. Berman, N.E.; Marcario, J.K.; Yong, C.; Raghavan, R.; Raymond, L.A.; Joag, S.V.; Naravan, O.; Cheney, P.D. Microglial activation and neurological symptoms in the SIV model of neuroAIDS: Association with MHC-II and MMP-9 expression with behavioral deficits and evoked potential changes. *Neurobiol. Dis.* **1999**, *6*, 486–498.
162. Cinque, P.; Nebuloni, M.; Santovito, M.L.; Price, R.W.; Gissien, M.; Hagberg, L.; Bestetti, A.; Vago, G.; Lazzarin, A.; Blasi, F.; *et al.* The urokinase receptor is overexpressed in the AIDS dementia complex and other neurological manifestations. *Ann. Neurol.* **2004**, *55*, 687–694.
163. Dzwonek, J.; Rylski, M.; Kaczmarek, L. Matrix metalloproteinases and their endogenous inhibitors in neuronal physiology of the adult brain. *FEBS Lett.* **2004**, *567*, 129–135.
164. Siwik, D.A.; Colucci, W.S. Regulation of matrix metalloproteinases by cytokines and reactive oxygen/nitrogen species in the myocardium. *Heart Fail. Rev.* **2004**, *9*, 43–51.
165. Louboutin, J.P.; Reyes, B.A.S.; Agrawal, L.; van Bockstaele, E.J.; Strayer, D.S. HIV-1 gp120 upregulates matrix metalloproteinases and their inhibitors in a rat model of HIV encephalopathy. *Eur. J. Neurosci.* **2011**, *34*, 2015–2023.
166. Louboutin, J.P.; Reyes, B.A.S.; Agrawal, L.; van Bockstaele, E.J.; Strayer, D.S. HIV-1 gp120 induced neuroinflammation: Relationship to neuron loss and protection by rSV40-delivered antioxidant enzymes. *Exp. Neurol.* **2010**, *221*, 231–245.
167. Chan, P.H.; Schmidley, J.W.; Fishman, R.A.; Longar, S.M. Brain injury, edema, and vascular permeability changes induced by oxygen-derived free radicals. *Neurology* **1984**, *34*, 315–320.
168. Chan, P.H.; Yang, G.Y.; Carlson, E.; Epstein, C.J. Cold-induced brain edema and infarction are reduced in transgenic mice overexpressing CuZn-superoxide dismutase. *Ann. Neurol.* **1991**, *29*, 482–486.
169. Wang, H.K.; Park, U.J.; Kim, S.Y.; Lee, J.H.; Kim, S.U.; Gwaq, B.J.; Lee, Y.B. Free radical production in CA1 neurons induces MIP-1alpha expression, microglial recruitment, and delayed neuronal death after transient forebrain ischemia. *J. Neurosci.* **2008**, *28*, 1721–1727.

10

Antioxidant Potential of Plumieride against CCL_4-Induced Peroxidative Damage in Rats

Dharmendra Singh [1,2], Priya Vrat Arya [2], Ashutosh Sharma [3], Ved Prakash Aggarwal [2], Mahabeer Prasad Dobhal [3] and Radhey Shyam Gupta [1,*]

[1] Centre for Advanced Studies, Department of Zoology, University of Rajasthan, Jaipur 302 055, India; E-Mail: d.singh2009@gmail.com

[2] Department of Zoology, Dyal Singh College, University of Delhi, Lodhi Road, New Delhi 110 003, India; E-Mails: zoology.dsc@gmail.com (P.V.A.); vpa541@gmail.com (V.P.A.)

[3] Department of Chemistry, University of Rajasthan, Jaipur 302 055, India; E-Mails: ashutoshs_912@rediffmail.com (A.S.); mpdobhal@yahoo.com (M.P.D.)

* Author to whom correspondence should be addressed; E-Mail: gupta_rs@hotmail.com

External Editor: Etsuo Niki

Abstract: In search of a new potent as an antioxidant from natural sources, plumieride—an iridoid isolated from the methanol extract of the bark of *Plumeria bicolor* (family Apocynaceae) was evaluated for its antioxidant potential against CCl_4-induced peroxidative damage in liver of rats. The antioxidant potential was evaluated by using hepatic tissue for SOD (superoxide dismutase), CAT (catalase), GSH (reduced glutathione), GPx (glutathione peroxidase), GR (glutathione reductase) and LPO (lipid peroxidation) alongwith the concomitant blood serum for AST & ALT (aspartate and alanine transaminases), GGT (gamma glutamyl transpeptidase), ALP (alkaline phosphatase), total bilirubin and total protein contents. All the biochemical parameters were significantly ($p \leq 0.001$) altered by CCl_4 (0.3 mL/kg body weight/twice a week, intra-peritoneally for 30 days). Simultaneously, oral treatment with plumieride (5, 10 and 20 mg/kg body weight/day for 30 days), restored all the parameters towards a normal level, remarkably. The histological findings of liver sections further corroborated the antioxidant potential of plumieride compared with standard drug-silymarin. In conclusion, plumieride consists of sugar molecules, which have alcoholic groups. Therefore, the alcoholic groups of sugar increase its antioxidant potential through intermolecular hydrogen bonding along with the thiol(SH) group of non-protein thiols and enzymes resulting in the restoration of the antioxidant system. Therefore, it might be considered a natural antioxidant against peroxidative damage in rats.

Keywords: antioxidants; carbon tetrachloride; free radicals; marker enzymes; plumieride

1. Introduction

Free radicals contribute towards tissue injury through covalent binding and lipid peroxidation whereas the compounds that can scavenge free radicals potentially ameliorate the liver injury [1,2]. Natural products and their purified compounds have received much attention as an alternative solution to numerous health problems as antioxidant agents in recent years [3]. Their antioxidant potential inhibits the generation of free radicals and exhibits significance in providing protection against hepatic damage [4].

Antioxidants and radical scavengers have been employed to study the mechanism of carbon tetrachloride (CCl_4) toxicity as well as to protect liver cells from CCl_4-induced damage by breaking the chain reaction of lipid peroxidation [5]. Plumieride (Figure 1) is an iridoid, isolated as a major constituent from the extract of *Plumeria bicolor* stem bark [6,7]. Further, *in vitro* anticancer potential and various pharmacological activities of plumieride have been conducted on mammals [8] whereas its antioxidant potential through possible mechanisms of action remains uninvestigated [9–13]. These medicinal properties and lack of references motivated us to investigate the antioxidant potential of plumieride from *Plumeria bicolor*. Hence, the present study aimed to investigate the natural antioxidant potential of plumieride, using CCl_4-induced peroxidative damage in the liver of rats.

Figure 1. Chemical structure of plumieride.

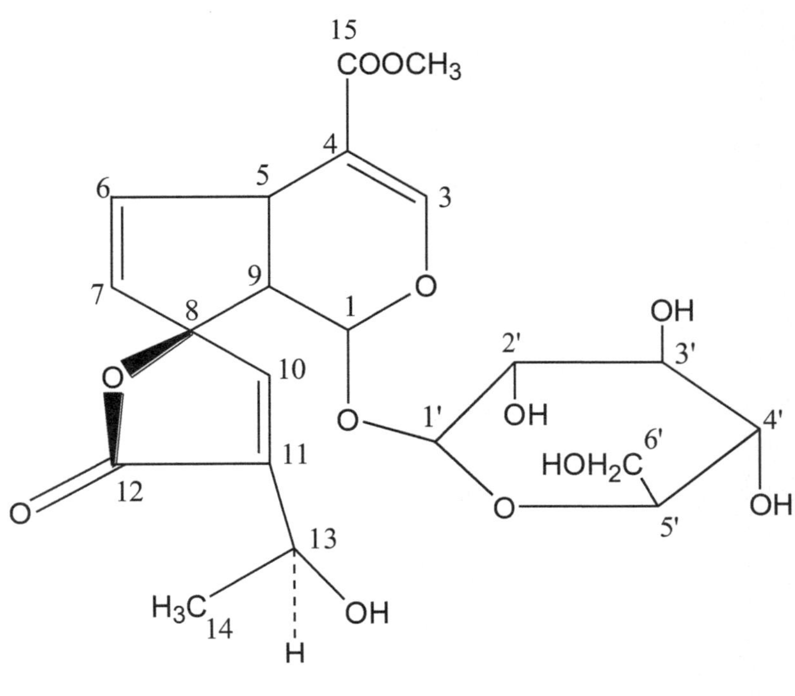

2. Materials and Methods

2.1. Animal Model

Adult, male, wistar albino rats (*Rattus norvegicus*) weighing 150–170 g were used in the present study. The animals were kept in standard laboratory conditions and maintained on rat diet (Lipton India Ltd., Bangalore, India) and tap water *ad libitum* under a natural light-dark cycle.

2.2. Plant Material

The plant material (stem bark of *Plumeria bicolor*) was collected from the campus, University of Rajasthan, Jaipur and authenticated by the Department of Botany, University of Rajasthan, Jaipur, India (Herbarium Sheet No. RUBL-20603).

2.3. Plant Extraction and Isolation of Active Compounds

The bark of the plant was shade dried and grinded to powder. Four kg of powdered bark was extracted with methanol (72 h). The methanol extract was filtered and evaporated to dryness under reduced pressure in a rotary evaporator (Labmate (Asia) Pvt. Ltd., Chennai, India) at <40 °C, which yielded a semi-solid brown mass. The brown mass was treated with acetonitrile for the removal of fats (acetonitrile soluble fraction). Acetonitrile was removed under reduced pressure. Fat free extract was again extracted with benzene. The benzene soluble portion afforded 40 g of crude extract after the removal of solvent. The crude extract so obtained was subjected to column chromatography. For this purpose a column of height 1.2 m with diameter 5 cm filled with 800 g Si-gel G (60–120 mesh) was taken. The column was chromatographed with various solvents. The column was eluted with different solvents using mixtures of benzene-chloroform-methanol in order of increasing polarity. The P_1–P_8 fractions were obtained.

2.4. Purification, Identification and Structure Elucidation of Active Compound

The column was eluted with chloroform and methanol in the ratio of 7:3, the purified compound-A was obtained from fraction P_8 as colourless bright needles, 4.0 g, melting point—227 to 229 °C. The structure of purified compound-A was identified by mass spectrometry (Agilent 1100 Series LC/MSD API-ES spectrometer, Agilent Technologies Inc., Santa Clara, CA, USA), infrared analyses (FTIR-8400S Spectrophotometer, Shimadzu, Japan) and Nuclear Magnetic Resonance (NMR) (JEOL AL-300 MHz Spectrometer, JEOL USA Inc., Peabody, MA, USA.), using ^1H NMR (300.40 MHz) and ^{13}C NMR (75.45 MHz) analyses in pyridine-d_5, respectively.

The mass spectrum of compound-A showed characteristic ion at 471 (M^+H) and the molecular ion peak was considered to be 470 (M^+). On the basis of ^1H NMR spectrum, the number of protons was calculated as 26. The ^{13}C NMR spectrum indicated the presence of 21 carbon atoms. On the basis of these observations, the molecular formula was assigned as $C_{21}H_{26}O_{12}$.

MS m/z: 470 (M^+), 471 (M^+H), 461, 329, 309, 291, 273, 259, 241, 231, 213, 176, 154, 136, 107, *etc.*

In IR spectrum (KBr, cm^{-1}) of the compound-A, the presence of hydroxyl group was confirmed by the absorption at 3350–3200 as a broad band. The presence of α, β unsaturated carbonyl group was indicated at 1750–1742 and the presence of C=C was confirmed at 1655–1640. The absorbance at 1040 was characterized for –C-O stretching.

IR (ν_{max}) cm^{-1} (KBr): 3350, 3200, 1750, 1742, 1655, 1640, 1040.

In the proton NMR spectrum (δ, ppm, pyridine-d_5), a doublet observed at 1.61 (J = 6 Hz) was assigned for three protons of methyl group at C-14. The double doublet observed at 3.06 was assigned for one proton each 9-H. At 5.32 (J = 7 Hz) a doublet was observed for the 1′-H proton and a multiplet at the range of 3.80–4.50 was assigned for the proton present on the β-D-glucopyranose moiety. The two doublets at 5.40 and 6.44 were characteristic to that of protons at C-7 and C-6 of iridoid's skeleton. On the basis of these doublets, compound-A should be a Δ^6 iridoid. Other olefinic proton present at C-10 and C-3 were observed at 7.90 and 7.60, respectively. Absorption signal at 5.32 as a doublet were assigned for proton at C-1′ carbon atom. Thus, the nature and position of all the protons were established.

^{1}H NMR (δ, ppm, pyridine-d_5): 1.61 (3H, *d*, J = 6, 14-CH_3), 3.06 (1H, *dd*, J = 6, 8 Hz, 9-H), 3.63 (3H, *s*, -$COOCH_3$), 3.80–4.50 (~8H, m), 4.76 (1H, *dq*, J = 2, 6 Hz, 13-H), 5.32 (1H, *d*, J = 7 Hz. 1-H), 5.40 (1H, *dd*, J = 2, 6 Hz. 7-H), 5.58 (1H, *d*, J = 6 Hz, 1-H), 6.44 (1H, *dd*, J = 2, 6 Hz, 6-H), 7.60 (1H, *d*, J = 2 Hz., 3-H), 7.90 (1H, *d*, J = 2 Hz., 10-H).

^{13}C NMR (δ, ppm, pyridine-d_5): 23.00 (*q*, C-14), 40.10 (*d*, C-5), 49.90 (*d*, C-9), 51.30 (*q*, -$COOCH_3$), 62.10 (t, C-6′), 62.70 (*d*, C-13), 70.70 (*d*, C-4′), 74.70 (*d*, C-2′), 78.10 (*d*, C-3′), 78.70 (*d*, C-5′), 94.00 (*d*, C-1), 96.40 (*s*, C-8), 100.80 (*d*, C-1′), 109.50 (*s*, C-4), 129.10 (*d*, C-10), 138.70 (*s*, C-11), 140.90 (*d*, C-6), 149.10 (*d*, C-7), 152.00 (*d*, C-3), 166.70 (*s*, C-15), 171.30 (*s*, C-12).

The ^{13}C NMR spectrum (δ, ppm, pyridine-d_5) showing a sharp signal at 166.7 was assigned for C-15. The signals at 23.0, 62.70 and 171.3 were assigned for C-14, C-13 and C-12 carbon atoms, respectively. The C-1 carbon atom to which glucose moiety was attached shows absorbance at 94.0. The presence of six olefinic carbon atoms was confirmed by the absorptions at 152.00 (C-3), 109.50 (C-4), 40.1 (C-5), 140.9 (C-6), 149.10 (C-7), 96.40 (C-8), 49.9 (C-9), 129.1 (C-10) and 138.70 (C-11).

The presence of glucose moiety was confirmed by the characteristic absorption at 100.80 for anomeric carbon (C-1′), 74.70 (C-2′), 78.10 (C-3′), 78.70 (C-4′), 78.70 (C-5′), and 62.10 (C-6′). The remainders of the absorptions were also in good agreement with the reported values for Plumieride [14–16]. Therefore, on the basis of ^{1}HNMR, ^{13}CNMR and mass spectral studies of compound-A from fraction P_8 was characterized as plumieride (Figure 1) with molecular formula $C_{21}H_{26}O_{12}$ and used for the exploration of its antioxidant potential against peroxidative damage in the liver of rats.

2.5. Standard Drug

Silymarin was purchased from MP Biomedicals, Strasbourg, France and it was dissolved in olive oil for oral administration to rats during experimentation at the dose level of 20 mg/kg body weight/day [1].

2.6. Chemicals

All chemicals were analytical grade, and chemicals required for all biochemical assays were obtained from Sigma Chemicals Co., St. Louis, MO, USA.

2.7. Ethical Aspects

The study was approved by the ethical committee (Protocol No: 1678/Go/a/12/CPCSEA/82) of the University Department of Zoology, Jaipur, India. Indian National Science Academy, New Delhi (INSA, 2000) guidelines were followed for maintenance and use of the experimental animals.

2.8. Behavioral and Toxic Effects

The pure compound- Plumieride from *Plumeria bicolor* was administered to all the test groups in graded doses ranging up to 80 mg/kg body weight/day and the rats were observed for any symptoms of mortality and behavioral toxicity for 30 days afterward. The compound was found to be practically non-toxic when given orally to rats and its LD_{50} value was found to be higher than 80 mg/kg body weight [1]. The minimum dose levels *viz.* 5, 10 and 20 mg/kg body weight were used for the oral administration to rats during experimentation [17].

2.9. Experimental Protocol

After acclimatization of 15 days, the animals were divided into the following groups containing six animals in each group:

Group I: Vehicle treated rats were kept on normal diet and served as control for 30 days.

Group II: Rats were intoxicated with carbon tetrachloride at 0.3 mL/kg body weight/twice a week with olive oil (1:1), intra-peritoneally for 30 days.

Group III: Rats orally received plumieride at 5 mg/kg body weight/day with olive oil, and CCl_4 as Group II for 30 days, simultaneously.

Group IV: Rats orally received plumieride at 10 mg/kg body weight/day with olive oil, and CCl_4 as Group II for 30 days, simultaneously.

Group V: Rats orally received plumieride at 20 mg/kg body weight/day with olive oil, and CCl_4 as Group II for 30 days, simultaneously.

Group VI: Rats orally received silymarin at 20 mg/kg body weight/day with olive oil, and CCl_4 as Group II for 30 days, simultaneously.

2.10. Assessment of Liver Function

After 24 h of last dose-delivery, the rats were anaesthetized under mild ether anesthesia. Blood samples were collected by cardiac puncture and allowed to clot at 37 °C. Serum was separated by centrifugation then stored at 4 °C until assayed. The serum-AST, ALT (aspartate and alanine transaminases), GGT (gamma glutamyl transpeptidase), ALP (alkaline phosphatase), total bilirubin and total protein were determined using diagnostic kits. AST (batch No. 61105), ALT (batch No. 60805), GGT (batch No. 34004) kits were purchased from Accurex Biomedical Pvt. Ltd., Mumbai, India, as well as

ALP (lot No. 7093), total bilirubin (lot No. 6801), and total protein (lot No. 6808) kits were purchased from Span Diagnostic Ltd., Surat, India.

After the collection of blood, the liver was immediately excised, washed with cold normal saline, blotted and weighed on an electrical balance. Half of the liver was fixed in Bouin's fixative for histological studies and remaining half was immediately frozen (at −20 °C/−70 °C) for biochemical analysis. After that, a part of it was minced and homogenized in ice-cold 1.15% $^{w}/_{v}$ KCl in a Potter Elvehjem Teflon glass homogenizer for 1 min to make a 10% $^{w}/_{v}$ liver homogenate. The lipid peroxidation (LPO) [18] was measured in the liver homogenate. The activities of hepatic antioxidant enzymes such as SOD (superoxide dismutase) [19], CAT (catalase) [20], GSH (reduced glutathione) [21], GR (glutathione reductase) [22] and GPx (glutathione peroxidase) [23] were also determined, respectively.

2.11. Histopathology

Liver was fixed in Bouin's fixative for 24 h then dehydrated in ethanol series (50%–100%), cleared in xylene, and embedded in paraffin using the standard microtechnique. Sections of the liver (5 μm) were stained with alum haematoxylin and eosin (H & E) for histopathological changes.

2.12. Statistical Process

Statistical analysis was performed using one-way analysis of variance (ANOVA) followed by student *t*-test. The values were mean ± S.E. for six rats in each group. p-value ≤ 0.05 were considered as significant.

3. Results

The results of antioxidant potential of plumieride in CCl_4-intoxicated rats are shown in Tables 1 and 2. CCl_4-intoxication to rats for the period of 30 days resulted in a significant ($p \leq 0.001$) increase in the levels of AST, ALT, GGT, ALP and total bilirubin along with a remarkable reduction ($p \leq 0.001$) in the level of total proteins in serum when compared with normal controls. The effect of plumieride on the serum- AST, ALT, GGT, ALP and total bilirubin in CCl_4-induced rats was found to be dose-dependently significant ($p \leq 0.05$; $p \leq 0.001$) reduction along with the remarkable elevation in the total proteins at all three dose levels (Groups III–V) as compared to CCl_4-treated Group-II. The degree of protection by plumieride (20 mg/kg) was observed statistically similar to the silymarin treated Group VI (Table 1).

Rats treated with CCl_4, caused a significant ($p \leq 0.001$) decline in the hepatic antioxidants such as SOD, CAT, GSH, GPx and GR in comparison to normal controls. Simultaneously, oral treatment with plumieride at all three dose levels (Groups III–V) showed significant ($p \leq 0.05$; $p \leq 0.001$) elevation in the activity of all antioxidant parameters such as SOD, CAT, GSH, GPx and GR. The elimination of hepatic oxidative stress by plumieride (Group V) and silymarin (Group VI) was statistically almost similar in nature (Table 2).

Table 1. Showing antioxidant potential of plumieride and silymarin against CCl_4-induced peroxidative damage in rat liver through serum parameters.

Treatment Design	AST (IU/L)	ALT (IU/L)	GGT (IU/L)	ALP (KAU)	Total Bilirubin (mg/100 mL)	Total Protein (mg/dL)
Control (vehicle treated) Group I	122.27 ± 1.37	104.33 ± 2.45	8.24 ± 0.28	19.37 ± 1.19	0.82 ± 0.05	6.32 ± 0.29
CCl_4 (0.3 mL/kg body weight/twice a week with olive oil, intra-peritoneally, 1:1) Group II	356.45 ± 3.42 ***	330.72 ± 4.57 ***	43.92 ± 2.10 ***	65.33 ± 2.19 ***	2.85 ± 0.14 ***	2.69 ± 0.14 ***
CCl_4 + plumieride (5 mg/kg body weight/day, orally) Group III	275.50 ± 2.66 ^{a}	262.14 ± 2.59 ^{a}	35.10 ± 1.35 ^{b}	56.48 ± 1.59 ^{b}	2.10 ± 0.15 ^{b}	3.12 ± 0.15 ^{ns}
CCl_4 + plumieride (10 mg/kg body weight/day, orally) Group IV	224.26 ± 1.98 ^{a,c}	201.21 ± 1.92 ^{a,c}	28.05 ± 0.72 ^{a,c}	48.10 ± 1.37 ^{a,d}	1.75 ± 0.16 ^{a,ns}	4.56 ± 0.10 ^{a,c}
CCl_4 + plumieride (20 mg/kg body weight/day, orally) Group V	172.24 ± 1.49 ^{a,c,e}	157.20 ± 1.37 ^{a,c,e}	19.10 ± 0.65 ^{a,c,e}	35.15 ± 1.18 ^{a,c,e}	1.27 ± 0.12 ^{a,d,f}	6.42 ± 0.17 ^{a,c,e}
CCl_4 + silymarin (20 mg/kg body weight/day, orally) Group VI	145.18 ± 1.55 ^{a,c,e,g}	128.37 ± 1.92 ^{a,c,e,g}	15.75 ± 1.77 ^{a,c,e,h}	30.47 ± 1.72 ^{a,c,e,i}	1.22 ± 0.08 ^{a,c,f,ns}	6.19 ± 0.18 ^{a,c,e,ns}

Levels of significance; Data are mean ± SEM ($n = 6$); *** $p \leq 0.001$, Group II compared with control (Group I); ^{a} $p \leq 0.001$; ^{b} $p \leq 0.01$; ^{ns} non-significant, Groups III–VI compared with Group II; ^{c} $p \leq 0.001$; ^{d} $p \leq 0.01$; ^{ns} non-significant, Groups IV–VI compared with Group III; ^{e} $p \leq 0.001$; ^{f} $p \leq 0.05$, Groups V & VI compared with Group IV; ^{g} $p \leq 0.001$; ^{h} $p \leq 0.05$; ^{i} $p \leq 0.01$; ^{ns} non-significant, Group VI compared with Group V.

Table 2. Showing antioxidant potential of plumieride and silymarin against CCl_4-induced peroxidative damage in rat liver through tissue parameters.

Treatment Design	LPO (*n* mol TBARS/mg Tissue)	SOD (µmol/mg Protein)	CAT (µmol H_2O_2 Consumed/min/mg Protein)	GSH (*n* mol/g Tissue)	GPx (*n* mol NADPH Consumed/min/mg Protein)	GR (*n* mol NADPH Consumed/min/mg Protein)
Control (vehicle treated) Group I	3.04 ± 0.21	10.24 ± 0.42	62.22 ± 2.33	4.52 ± 0.19	12.18 ± 0.42	18.27 ± 0.62
CCl_4 (0.3 mL/kg b. wt/twice a week with olive oil, intra-peritoneally, 1:1) Group II	11.23 ± 0.89 ***	4.10 ± 0.13 ***	26.21 ± 1.94 ***	1.72 ± 0.09 ***	5.09 ± 0.25 ***	8.82 ± 0.15 ***
CCl_4 + plumieride (5 mg/kg body weight/day, orally) Group III	8.18 ± 0.32 ^{a}	5.32 ± 0.14 ^{a}	32.10 ± 1.52 ^{b}	2.05 ± 0.10 ^{b}	6.62 ± 0.21 ^{a}	10.52 ± 0.17 ^{a}
CCl_4 + plumieride (10 mg/kg body weight/day, orally) Group IV	6.22 ± 0.29 ^{a,c}	6.89 ± 0.16 ^{a,c}	40.21 ± 1.89 ^{a,d}	3.06 ± 0.14 ^{a,c}	ai8.35 ± 0.18 ^{a,c}	12.82 ± 0.22 ^{a,c}
CCl_4 + plumieride (20 mg/kg body weight/day, orally) Group V	3.95 ± 0.35 ^{a,c,e}	7.83 ± 0.18 ^{a,c,f}	48.58 ± 1.23 ^{a,c,f}	3.95 ± 0.13 ^{a,c,e}	10.10 ± 0.15 ^{a,c,e}	16.17 ± 0.21 ^{a,c,e}
CCl_4 + silymarin (20 mg/kg body weight/day, orally) Group VI	3.68 ± 0.42 ^{a,c,e,ns}	8.14 ± 0.33 ^{a,c,f,ns}	51.40 ± 1.67 ^{a,c,f,ns}	3.63 ± 0.12 ^{a,c,e,ns}	10.21 ± 0.24 ^{a,c,e,ns}	15.28 ± 0.33 ^{a,c,e,g}

Levels of significance, Data are mean ± SEM ($n = 6$); *** $p \leq 0.001$, Group II compared with control (Group I); ^{a} $p \leq 0.001$; ^{b} $p \leq 0.05$, Groups III–VI compared with Group II; ^{c} $p \leq 0.001$; ^{d} $p \leq 0.01$, Groups IV–VI compared with Group III; ^{e} $p \leq 0.001$; ^{f} $p \leq 0.01$, Groups V & VI compared with Group IV; ^{g} $p \leq 0.05$; ^{ns} non-significant, Group VI compared with Group V.

Table 2 illustrates a significant ($p \leq 0.001$) increase in the level of hepatic LPO in CCl_4-intoxicated rats as compared to normal control. In contrast, treatment with plumieride at all three dose levels (Groups III–V) showed a significant ($p \leq 0.05$; $p \leq 0.001$) lowering effect on CCl_4-induced elevation of hepatic LPO contents. The lowering effect of LPO by plumieride (Group V) and silymarin (Group VI) was found to be statistically equal against CCl_4-induced lipid peroxidation (Table 2).

The histopathology of CCl_4-induced rats when compared to normal hepatic architecture (Figure 2) showed massive fatty changes, necrosis, ballooning degeneration and the loss of cellular boundaries (Figure 3). The liver sections of plumieride at the dose level of 5 mg/kg body weight plus CCl_4-treated rats (Group III) showed mild prevention of CCl_4-induced degenerative changes with the few pyknotic nuclei and fatty vacuolizations in the cytoplasm (Figure 4). The liver sections of plumieride treated rats at the dose level of 10 mg/kg body weight along with CCl_4 (Group IV) indicated partial amelioration of degenerative effects in hepatocytes but still show cloudy swelling and mild fatty changes (Figure 5). The histomorphological picture of liver sections of plumieride at the dose level of 20 mg/kg body weight along with CCl_4-induction to rats (Group V) showed more or less normal labular patterns devoid of degenerative changes, and cytoplasm was preserved with prominent nucleus without intracellular lipid accumulation (Figure 6) almost comparable to the normal control and silymarin treated Group VI (Figure 7).

Figure 2. Photomicrograph of control rat liver section showing well brought central vein, hepatic cells with preserved cytoplasm and prominent nucleus at H & E × 10.

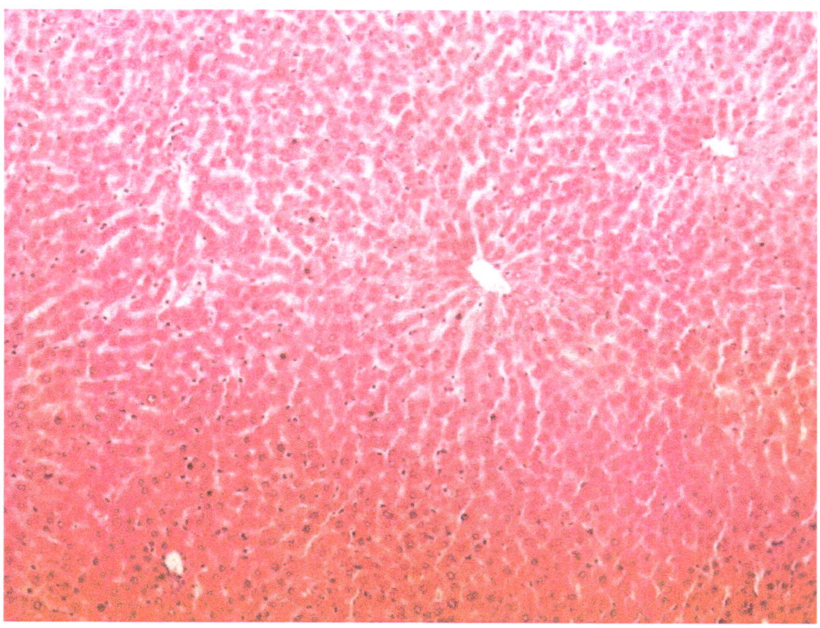

Figure 3. Photomicrograph of rat liver section with CCl_4 treatment showing ballooning degeneration and distended portal vein, mild periportal fibrosis and necrosis at H & E × 100.

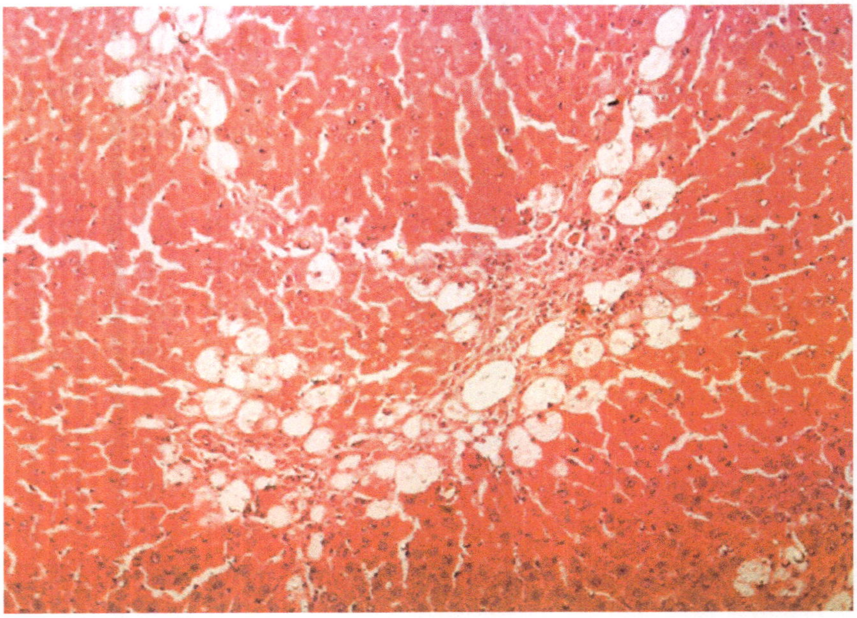

Figure 4. Photomicrograph of rat liver section of CCl_4 + Plumieride (5 mg/kg body weight), showing reasonable reduction in necrosis, fatty changes along with cytoplasmic clearing at H & E × 100.

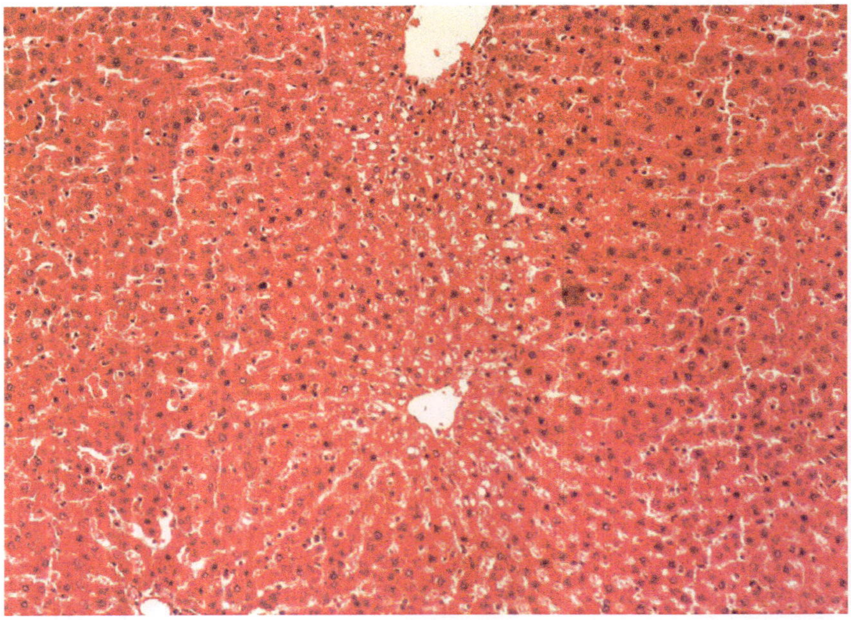

Figure 5. Photomicrograph of rat liver section of CCl_4 + Plumieride (10 mg/kg body weight), reflecting considerable reduction in necrosis, fatty changes and exhibiting cytoplasmic clearing at H & E × 100.

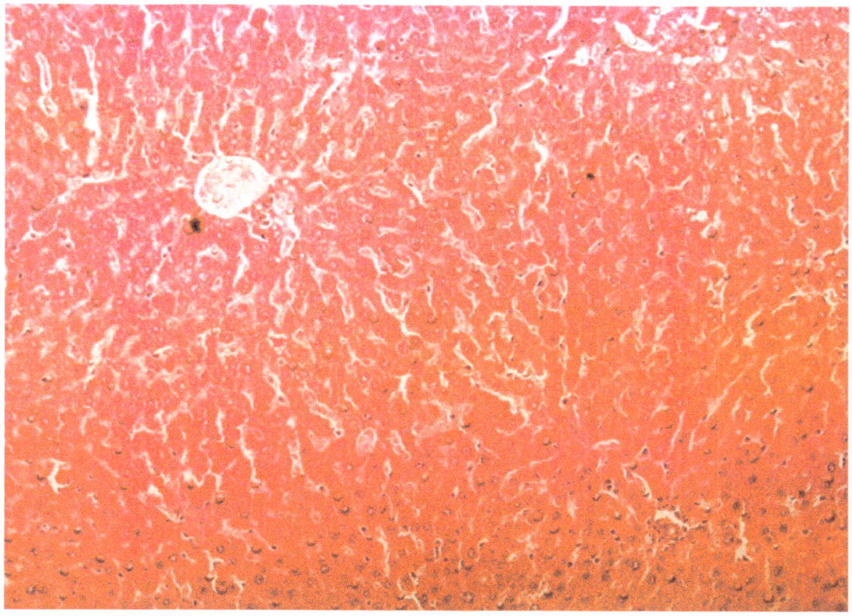

Figure 6. Photomicrograph of rat liver section of CCl_4 + Plumieride (20 mg/kg body weight), showing moderately brought central vein, hepatic cells with preserved cytoplasm and prominent nucleus at H & E × 100.

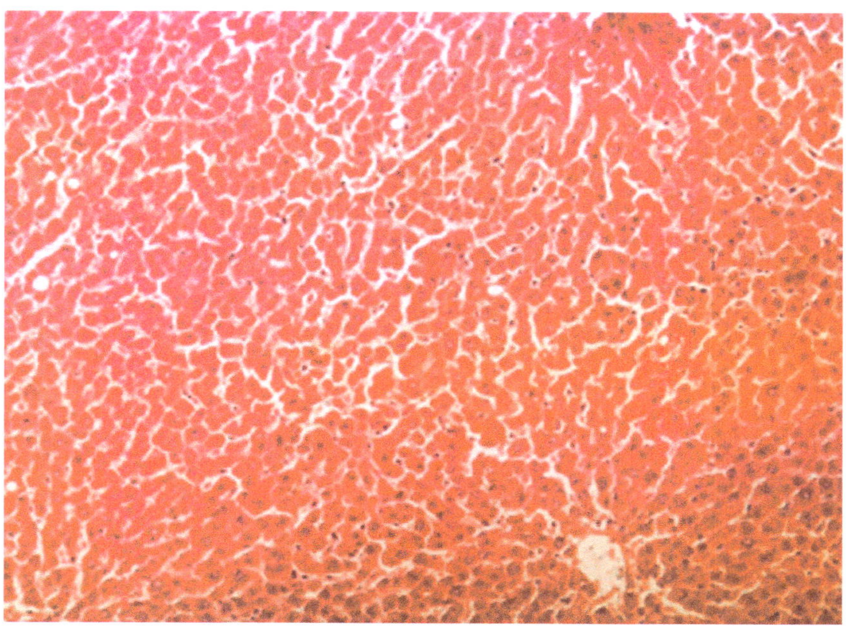

Figure 7. Photomicrograph of rat liver section of CCl_4 + Silymarin (20 mg/kg body weight), showing moderately brought central vein, hepatic cells along with preserved cytoplasm and prominent nucleus at H & E × 100.

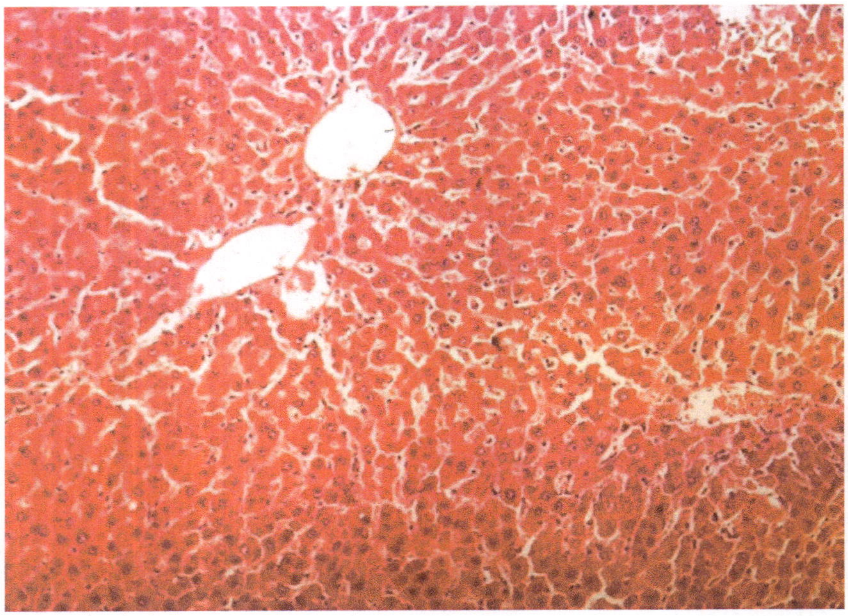

4. Discussion

Reactive oxygen species (ROS) are known for their role in a large number of diseases including hepatic injury because hepatic cells appear to participate in a variety of enzymatic metabolic activities. The natural antioxidant mechanisms of the body can be insufficient and dietary intake of additional antioxidant constituents appear to be necessary [24,25].

CCl_4-induced hypofunctions of the hepatic cell membrane due to hepatic injury are associated with the peroxidation of lipids and reduced antioxidant levels through the production of toxic species—trichloromethyl free radical ($CCl_3^•$) or/and trichloromethyl peroxy radical ($CCl_3OO^•$) which in turn alter the hepatic metabolism via oxidative stress leading to hepatotoxicity [26,27].

The lipid peroxidative degradation of biomembranes is one of the principle causes of hepatotoxicity induced by CCl_4 [4,28]. This is evidenced by the elevation of serum marker enzymes such as AST, ALT, GGT, ALP along with the total bilirubin and reduction in the level of total protein. This is indicative of cellular leakage and loss of functional integrity of cell membrane of the liver tissue [29], concomitantly with the alterations in biliary flow which reflects ALP with the high level of total serum bilirubin contents [30], and finally inhibits the protein synthesis due to trichloromethyl free radical covalent bindings [31]. Reduction in the levels of AST, ALT, GGT and ALP towards the respective normal values by the oral treatment of plumieride and silymarin is an indication of the stabilization of plasma membranes as well as repair of hepatic tissue damage caused by CCl_4 [1,32]. Further, the depletion of raised total bilirubin concentration suggests the possibility of the plumieride being able to stabilize the biliary dysfunctions and improvement of functional status of the liver cells [33]. Additionally, the stabilization of total proteins might be considered as an indicator of the improvement of total protein synthesis in the hepatic cells due to the inhibition of peroxidation of lipids and scavenge the free radicals [34]. This indicates the anti-lipid peroxidation and/or adaptive nature of the systems brought about by plumieride against the damaging effects of free radicals produced by CCl_4.

The LPO is accelerated when free radicals are formed as the result of losing a hydrogen atom from the double bond in the structure of unsaturated fatty acids. Scavenging of free radicals is one of the major antioxidant mechanisms to inhibit the chain reaction of LPO [1,4].

Plumieride restores the antioxidant status by its ability to inhibit the peroxidation of membrane lipids and maintains cell membrane integrity and function. The presence of hydrogen ions in the alcoholic group(s) of plumieride might be responsible for the inhibitory effect, and also the oxygen belonging to the furanic ring might be able to develop a resonance property which is merely a change in the redistribution of electrons, effectively neutralizing them.

SOD and CAT are easily inactivated by lipid peroxides or reactive oxygen species which results in decreased activities of these enzymes in CCl_4 hepatotoxicity [35,36]. The hepatic GSH, GPx and GR play the primary role in protection against trichloromethyl radical-induced liver damage. Kojima *et al.* [37] have also reported that under oxidative stress, GSH is largely consumed by the glutathione-related enzymes thereby resulting in intoxication of toxic metabolites. Therefore, it has been suggested that lipid peroxides generated after CCl_4 exposure is eliminated by GPx and GR in the presence of GSH, resulting in the decreased propagation of lipid peroxidation [5,38]. Administration of plumieride and silymarin showed antioxidant potential by scavenging the endogenous metabolic peroxides generated after CCl_4 induction to rats, which resulted in an increase in the activities of tissue enzymatic antioxidants and glutathione concentration.

Histopathological observations suggested that the ROS and LPO may play an important role in the pathogenesis of hepatocytes as hepatic fibrosis and necrosis with the loss of normal liver architecture. Because of CCl_4 toxicity, a toxic reactive metabolite-trichloromethyl free radical was produced which binds covalently to the macromolecules of the lipid membranes of the adipose tissue and causes peroxidative degradation. As a result, fats from the adipose tissue are translocated and accumulated in the hepatocytes [1,5,39].The degenerative changes showed minimal or absence with plumieride and silymarin treatments. Plumieride, because of low fat accumulation, can scavenge free radicals, interact with oxidative cascade, quench oxygen, chelate metal ions, inhibit oxidative enzymes and LPO; finally, it can restore the antioxidant status of hepatic tissues.

5. Conclusions

Based on our observations, plumieride consists of sugar molecules, which have alcoholic groups. The alcoholic groups of sugar seems to increase its antioxidant potential through intermolecular hydrogen bonding along with the thiol (SH) group of non-protein thiols and enzymes resulting in the restoration of the antioxidant system against peroxidative damage. It may also stimulate hepatic regeneration through an improved synthesis of proteins, or due to its ability to block the bioactivation of CCl_4, by inhibiting the P450 2E1 activity and/or its accelerated detoxification, as well as having the potential to minimize the deleterious effects of free radicals including the peroxy radicals and its antioxidant activity in combination with inhibition of LPO. In summary, plumieride might be considered a natural antioxidant agent against peroxidative damage in mammalian liver tissue.

Acknowledgments

The authors are thankful to the respective authorities for providing the necessary facilities and support.

Author Contributions

Dharmendra Singh, Ashutosh Sharma, Mahabeer Prasad Dobhal and Radhey Shyam Gupta contributed for the experimental design and data analysis. Dharmendra Singh, Priya Vrat Arya, Ved Prakash Aggarwal and Radhey Shyam Gupta have completed the manuscript preparation and data interpretations. All authors read and approved the final manuscript.

Conflicts of Interest

The authors have confirmed that there is no conflict of interest.

References

1. Singh, D.; Singh, R.; Singh, P.; Gupta, R.S. Effects of embelin on lipid peroxidation and free radical scavenging activity against liver damage in rats. *Basic Clin. Pharmacol. Toxicol.* **2009**, *105*, 243–248.
2. Ahn, M.; Park, J.S.; Chae, S.; Kim, S.; Moon, C.; Hyun, J.W.; Shin, T. Hepatoprotective effects of *Lycium chinense* Miller fruit and its constituent betaine in CCl_4-induced hepatic damage in rats. *Acta Histochem.* **2014**, *116*, 1104–1112.
3. Matés, J.M.; Segura, J.A.; Alonso, F.J.; Márquez, J. Natural antioxidants: Therapeutic prospects for cancer and neurological diseases. *Mini Rev. Med. Chem.* **2009**, *9*, 1202–1214.
4. Manubolu, M.; Goodla, L.; Ravilla, S.; Thanasekaran, J.; Dutta, P.; Malmlöf, K.; Obulum, V.R. Protective effect of *Actiniopteris radiata* (Sw.) Link. against CCl_4 induced oxidative stress in albino rats. *J. Ethnopharmacol.* **2014**, *153*, 744–752.
5. Huo, H.Z.; Wang, B.; Liang, Y.K.; Bao, Y.Y.; Gu, Y. Hepatoprotective and antioxidant effects of licorice extract against CCl_4-induced oxidative damage in rats. *Int. J. Mol. Sci.* **2011**, *12*, 6529–6543.
6. Boonclarm, D.; Sornwatana, T.; Arthan, D.; Kongsaeree, P.; Svasti, J. β-Glucosidase catalyzing specific hydrolysis of an iridoid β-glucoside from *Plumeria obtusa*. *Acta Biochim. Biophys. Sin.* **2006**, *38*, 563–570.
7. Saleem, M.; Akhtar, N.; Riaz, N.; Ali, M.S.; Jabbar, A. Isolation and characterization of secondary metabolites from *Plumeria obtusa*. *J. Asian Nat. Prod. Res.* **2011**, *13*, 1122–1127.
8. Dobhal, M.P.; Li, G.; Gryshuk, A.; Graham, A.; Bhatanager, A.K.; Khaja, S.D.; Joshi, Y.C.; Sharma, M.C.; Oseroff, A.; Pandey, P.K.; *et al.* Structural modification of plumieride isolated from *Plumeria bicolor* and the effect of these modification on *in vitro* anticancer activity. *J. Org. Chem.* **2004**, *69*, 6165–6172.
9. Kuigoua, G.M.; Kouam, S.F.; Ngadjui, B.T.; Schulz, B.; Green, I.R.; Choudhary, M.I.; Krohn, K. Minor secondary metabolic products from the stem bark of *Plumeria rubra* Linn. displaying antimicrobial activities. *Planta Med.* **2010**, *76*, 620–625.

10. Singh, D.; Sharma, U.; Kumar, P.; Gupta, Y.K.; Dobhal, M.P.; Singh, S. Antifungal activity of plumericin and isoplumericin. *Nat. Prod. Commun.* **2011**, *6*, 1567–1568.
11. Sharma, U.; Singh, D.; Kumar, P.; Dobhal, M.P.; Singh, S. Antiparasitic activity of plumericin and isoplumericin isolated from *Plumeria bicolor* against *Leishmania donovani*. *Indian J. Med. Res.* **2011**,*134*, 709–716.
12. Kumar, P.; Singh, A.; Sharma, U.; Singh, D.; Dobhal, M.P.; Singh, S. Anti-mycobacterial activity of plumericin and isoplumericin against MDR *Mycobacterium tuberculosis*. *Pulm. Pharmacol. Ther.* **2013**, *26*, 332–325.
13. Rebouças Sde, O.; da Silva, J.; Bertoni, R.S.; Decker, N.; Santos, M.S.; Rossatto, R.R.; Corrêa, D.S.; Ferraz, A.B. Assessment of the genotoxic and mutagenic properties of *Himatanthus articulatus* bark extracts used as phytotherapeutic drug in the Amazon. *J. Ethnopharmacol.* **2013**, *147*, 474–480.
14. Chaudhuri, R.K.; Afifi-Yazar, F.U.; Sticher, O.; Winkler, T. ^{13}C NMR spectroscopy of naturally occurring iridoid glucosides and their acylated derivatives. *Tetrahedron* **1980**, *36*, 2317–2326.
15. Yamauchi, T.; Abe, F.; Taki, M. Protoplumericin, an iridoid bis-glucoside in *Allamanda neriifolia*. *Chem. Pharm. Bull.* **1981**, *29*, 3051–3055.
16. Abe, F.; Mori, T.; Yamauchi, T. Iridoids of Apocynaceae. III. Minor iridoids from *Allamanda neriifolia*. *Chem. Pharm. Bull.* **1984**, *32*, 2947–2956.
17. Porchezhian, E.; Ansari, S.H. Hepatoprotective activity of *Abutilon indicum* on experimental liver damage in rats. *Phytomedicine* **2005**, *12*, 62–64.
18. Ohkawa, H.; Ohishi, N.; Yagi, K. Assay for lipid peroxidation in animal tissue by thiobarbituric acid reaction. *Anal. Biochem.* **1979**, *95*, 351–358.
19. Marklund, S.; Marklund, G. Involvement of superoxide anion radical in auto-oxidation of pyrogallol and a convenient assay for superoxide dismutase. *Eur. J. Biochem.* **1974**, *47*, 469–474.
20. Aebi, H. Catalase *in vitro*. In *Methods in Enzymology*; Colowick, S.P., Kaplan, N.O., Eds.; Academic Press: New York, NY, USA, 1984; Volume 105, pp. 121–126.
21. Moron, M.S.; Dipierre, J.W.; Mannervick, B. Levels of glutathione, glutathione reductase and glutathione-*s*-transferase activities in rat lung and liver. *Biochem. Biophys. Acta* **1979**, *582*, 67–78.
22. Carlberg, I.; Mennervick, B. Glutathione reductase. In *Methods in Enzymology*; Academic Press: New York, NY, USA, 1985; Volume 113, pp. 484–490.
23. Paglia, D.E.; Velentine, W.M. Studies on the quantitative and qualitative characterization of erythrocyte glutathione peroxidase. *J. Lab. Clin. Med.* **1967**, *70*, 158–169.
24. Pradeep, K.; Rajmohan, C.V.; Anand, K.G.; Karthikayan, S. Effect of pretreatment of *Cassia fistula* Linn. leaf extract against subacute CCl_4 induced hepatotoxicity in rats. *Indian J. Exp. Biol.* **2005**, *43*, 526–530.
25. Saikia, L.R.; Upadhyaya, S. Antioxidant activity, phenol and flavonoid content of some less known medicinal plants of Assam. *Int. J. Pharm. Bio. Sci.* **2011**, *2*, 383–388.
26. Basu S. Carbon tetrachloride-induced lipid peroxidation: Eicosanoid formation and their regulation by antioxidant nutrients. *Toxicology* **2003**, *189*, 113–117.
27. Zeashan, H.; Amresh, G.; Singh, S.; Rao, C.V. Hepatoprotective activity of *Amaranthus spinosus* in experimental animals. *J. Food Chem. Toxicol.* **2008**, *46*, 3417–3421.

28. Kaplowitz, N.; Aw, T.Y.; Simon, F.R.; Stolz, A. Drug induced hepatotoxicity. *Ann. Intern. Med.* **1986**, *104*, 826–839.
29. Kalegari, M.; Gemin, C.A.; Araújo-Silva, G.; Brito, N.J.; López, J.A.; Oliveira Tozetto, S.D.; das Graças Almeida, M.; Miguel, M.D.; Stien, D.; Miguel, O.G.; *et al.* Chemical composition, antioxidant activity and hepatoprotective potential of *Rourea induta* Planch. (Connaraceae) against CCl_4-induced liver injury in female rats. *Nutrition* **2014**, *6*, 713–718.
30. Bhakta, T.; Mukherjee, P.K.; Mukherjee, K.; Banerjee, S.; Mandal, S.C.; Maity, T.K.; Pal, M.; Saha, B.P. Evaluation of hepatoprotective activity of *Cassia fistula* leaf extract. *J. Ethnopharmacol.* **1999**, *66*, 277–282.
31. Lee, K.J.; Woo, E.; Choi, C.Y.; Shin, D.W.; Lee, D.G.; You, H.J.; Jeong, H.G. Protective effect of acteoside on carbon tetrachloride-induced hepatotoxicity. *Life Sci.* **2004**, *74*, 1051–1064.
32. Shah, N.A.; Khan, M.R.; Ahmad, B.; Noureen, F.; Rashid, U.; Khan, R.A. Investigation on flavonoid composition and anti-free radical potential of *Sida cordata. BMC Complement. Altern. Med.* **2013**, *13*, 276–288.
33. Kumar, G.; Banu, G.S.; Kannan, V.; Pandian, M.R. Antihepatotoxic effect of β-carotene on paracetamol induced hepatic damage in rats. *Indian J. Exp. Biol.* **2005**, *43*, 351–355.
34. Mandal, P.K.; Bishayee, A.; Chatterjee, M. Stimulation of tissue repair by *Mikania cordata* root extract in carbon tetrachloride-induced liver injury in mice. *Phytother. Res.* **1993**, *7*, 103–105.
35. Salvi, M.; Battaglia, V.; Brunati, A.M.; LaRocca, N.; Tibaldi, E.; Pietrangeli, P.; Marcocci, L.; Mondovi, B.; Rossi, C.A.; Toninello, A.; *et al.* Catalase takes part in rat liver mitochondria oxidative stress defense. *J. Biol. Chem.* **2007**, *282*, 24407–24415.
36. Parimoo, H.A.; Sharma, R.; Patil, R.D.; Sharma, O.P.; Kumar, P.; Kumar, N. Hepatoprotective effect of *Ginkgo biloba* leaf extract on lantadenes-induced hepatotoxicity in guinea pigs. *Toxicon* **2014**, *81*, 1–12.
37. Kojima, S.; Matsuki, O.; Nomura, T.; Kubodera, A.; Yamaoka, K. Elevation of mouse liver glutathione level by low-dose gamma ray irradiation and its effect on CCl_4-induced liver damage. *Anticancer Res.* **1998**, *18*, 2471–2476.
38. Meister, A. Glutathione. In *The Liver, Biology and Pathobiology*; Arias, I.M., Boyer, J.L., Jakoby, W.B., Fausto, D., Schacter, D., Shafritz, D.A., Eds.; Ravan Press: New York, NY, USA, 1994; pp. 401–417.
39. Okuno, H.; Hazama, H.; Mutazo, T.; Shiozaki, Y.; Somoshima, Y.T. Drug metabolizing activity in rats with chronic liver injury, induced by carbon tetrachloride relationship with the hydroxyproline content in liver. *Jpn. J. Pharmacol.* **1998**, *41*, 363–369.

A Cystine-Rich Whey Supplement (Immunocal®) Delays Disease Onset and Prevents Spinal Cord Glutathione Depletion in the hSOD1^{G93A} Mouse Model of Amyotrophic Lateral Sclerosis

Erika K. Ross [1], Aimee N. Winter [1], Heather M. Wilkins [1], Whitney A. Sumner [1], Nathan Duval [1], David Patterson [1] and Daniel A. Linseman [1,2,3,*]

[1] Department of Biological Sciences and Eleanor Roosevelt Institute, University of Denver, 2199 S. University Blvd., Denver, CO 80208, USA; E-Mails: Ross.Erika@mayo.edu (E.K.R.); Aimee.Winter@du.edu (A.N.W.); hwilkins@kumc.edu (H.M.W.); wsumner714@gmail.com (W.A.S.); nathan.duval@du.edu (N.D.); dpatter2@du.edu (D.P.)

[2] Research Service, Veterans Affairs Medical Center, 1055 Clermont St., Denver, CO 80220, USA

[3] Division of Clinical Pharmacology and Toxicology, Department of Medicine and Neuroscience Program, University of Colorado Denver, 12700 E 19th Ave., Aurora, CO 80045, USA

* Author to whom correspondence should be addressed; E-Mail: Daniel.Linseman@du.edu

External Editor: Wenlan Liu

Abstract: Depletion of the endogenous antioxidant, glutathione (GSH), underlies progression of the devastating neurodegenerative disease, amyotrophic lateral sclerosis (ALS). Thus, strategies aimed at elevating GSH may yield new therapeutics for ALS. Here, we investigated the effects of a unique non-denatured whey protein supplement, Immunocal®, in the transgenic Gly position 93 to Ala (G93A) mutant hSOD1 (hSOD1^{G93A}) mouse model of ALS. Immunocal® is rich in the GSH precursor, cystine, and is therefore capable of bolstering GSH content. Transgenic hSOD1^{G93A} mice receiving Immunocal® displayed a significant delay in disease onset compared to untreated hSOD1^{G93A} controls. Additionally, Immunocal® treatment significantly decreased the rate of decline in grip strength and prevented disease-associated reductions in whole blood and spinal cord tissue GSH levels in end-stage hSOD1^{G93A} mice. However, Immunocal® did not extend survival, likely due to its inability to preserve the mitochondrial GSH pool in spinal cord. Combination treatment with Immunocal® and the anti-glutamatergic compound, riluzole, delayed disease onset and extended survival in hSOD1^{G93A} mice. These findings demonstrate that sustaining tissue GSH with Immunocal® only modestly delays disease onset and slows the loss of skeletal muscle strength in hSOD1^{G93A} mice. Moreover, the inability of Immunocal® to rescue mitochondrial GSH in spinal cord provides a possible mechanism for its lack of effect on survival and is a limiting factor in the potential utility of this supplement as a therapeutic for ALS.

Keywords: Immunocal®; whey protein; oxidative stress; glutathione; cysteine; amyotrophic lateral sclerosis

1. Introduction

Amyotrophic lateral sclerosis (ALS) is the most common adult-onset motor neuron disease. It is characterized clinically by progressive skeletal muscle weakness, atrophy and paralysis, ultimately leading to respiratory failure and death within two to five years of diagnosis. ALS is characterized pathologically by a progressive loss of motor neurons in the cortex, brainstem and spinal cord [1]. Though its underlying cause remains elusive, oxidative damage due to aberrant production of reactive oxygen species (ROS) and associated mitochondrial dysfunction play key roles in motor neuron death [2–4]. Only approximately 10% of ALS cases are considered familial, with the remaining 90% characterized as sporadic with no known cause. Mutations in Cu/Zn-superoxide dismutase (SOD1) are one of the most common causes of familial ALS. Nearly 150 mutant forms of SOD1 have been identified in ALS patients, and these are collectively responsible for approximately 20% of all cases of familial disease [5].

Mutant forms of SOD1 have been implicated in the aberrant generation of ROS at the mitochondria and subsequent mitochondrial dysfunction, which underlie ALS disease pathology. The mutant form of SOD1 harboring a glycine to alanine mutation at position 93 (SOD1^{G93A}) in particular, displays a gain of toxic function that is characterized by an increased generation of mitochondrial ROS [6]. Mutant SOD1 also accumulates at mitochondria and triggers a shift in the redox state of these organelles [7]. Moreover, crossing of transgenic hSOD1^{G93A} mutant mice with mice heterozygous for the deletion of the mitochondrial-specific SOD2 gene significantly exacerbates motor neuron pathology and reduces lifespan in this model of familial ALS, further indicating a central role for mitochondrial oxidative stress (MOS) in disease pathogenesis [8].

Glutathione (GSH) is an endogenous tri-peptide antioxidant that plays a critical role in detoxifying ROS generated within cells, particularly at mitochondria [9]. Mitochondria possess a discrete pool of GSH, which is critical for the prevention of intrinsic apoptosis and other cell death pathways [10,11]. Decreased levels of GSH have been observed in erythrocytes of patients with sporadic ALS and are correlated with disease progression, indicating that depletion of this key antioxidant is likely one underlying factor in disease progression [12]. Moreover, GSH depletion has been observed *in vivo* in whole spinal cord of end-stage hSOD1^{G93A} mice, and more specifically, the ratio of reduced GSH-to-oxidized glutathione disulfide (GSSG) in spinal cord mitochondria of mutant SOD1 mice is significantly diminished, indicative of MOS and concurrent GSH depletion [13,14].

Because GSH depletion has been implicated in the pathogenesis of both sporadic and familial forms of ALS, treatments aimed at preserving GSH levels may lead to new potential therapeutic options for ALS patients. Treatment with agents, such as *N*-acetylcysteine (NAC) and GSH-monoethyl ester (GSH-MEE), has shown some promise in pre-clinical ALS mouse models; however, the relatively low bioavailability of these agents, and in the case of GSH-MEE, the necessity for central delivery of the drug, limit the utility of these agents for treatment of human patients [15,16]. Similarly, NAC, though it can be orally administered, has very low bioavailability and often requires intravenous administration to increase circulating levels of this compound [15]. Immunocal® (Immunotec Inc., Vaudreuil-Dorion, Quebec, Canada) is a whey protein supplement that contains abundant amounts of cystine, a cysteine precursor, due to its unique non-denaturing preparation. As cysteine is required for the rate limiting step of GSH synthesis, supplementation with cystine-rich compounds is an effective way to enhance de novo tissue GSH synthesis. Cysteine itself is rapidly catabolized in the GI tract and is capable of producing toxicity when administered in a pure form [17]. On the other hand, cystine acts as a cysteine delivery system, which is rapidly reduced into two cysteine molecules upon uptake by target cells, significantly limiting toxicity. Furthermore, Immunocal® displays significantly higher bioavailability than NAC when administered orally [18,19].

Immunocal® was initially developed as a nutritional supplement to increase immune system function, and it is one of only a handful of nutritional supplements that are included in the Physician's Desk Reference (see Table 1 for composition) [20]. This supplement was found to have beneficial effects in clinical disorders for which oxidative stress is a significant underlying factor, including HIV infection and cystic fibrosis [21,22]. Based on these studies, Immunocal® holds significant potential as an agent to bolster GSH levels and, thus, may provide a novel therapeutic approach for the treatment of neurodegenerative diseases for which the underlying pathology involves significant oxidative stress. Here, we sought to determine its effects in the $hSOD1^{G93A}$ mutant mouse model of familial ALS.

Table 1. Immunocal® constituents by mass per one packet of supplement [a,b].

Component	Supplement Content	% of Total Supplement
Whey proteins (serum albumin, α lactalbumin and lactoferrin)	8.8–9.2 g	88%–92%
Fat	~0.05 g	<0.5%
Lactose	~0.15 g	<1.5%
Minerals (Ca, Na)	~0.30 g	<3.0%
Moisture	0.5 g	~5%

[a] One packet of Immunocal® contains approximately 10 g of protein supplement (one serving) in fine powder form and 40 calories per serving. [b] Constituents appear as determined by [22].

2. Experimental Section

2.1. Mouse Model of ALS

All animal procedures were performed according to a protocol approved by the University of Denver Institutional Animal Care and Use Committee. FVB-Tg (SOD1-G93A) mice with the toxic gain of function SOD1 Gly position 93 to Ala mutation (G93A) were obtained from The Jackson Laboratory (Bar Harbor, ME, USA). The colony was maintained and bred in the animal facility at the University of

Denver. Animal genotyping was done by the third party company, Transnetyx (Cordova, TN, USA). Littermates of both sexes (approximately equal numbers of males and females) were included in each group, with an age- and sex-matched non-transgenic (NonTG) mouse as the control, with the exception of the treatment groups containing mice receiving Immunocal® supplement alone. These groups were predominately composed of male hSOD^{G93A} mice, which typically show a slightly shorter life span than their female counterparts (Tables 2 and 3). No significant gender differences in the age of disease onset were observed in our colony (Table 2). For experiments assessing the effects of Immunocal® alone, animals receiving supplementation had ad libitum access to a 3.3% solution of Immunocal® in drinking water beginning at 60 days of age. For experiments utilizing Immunocal® in conjunction with the anti-glutamatergic drug, riluzole, animals receiving Immunocal® supplementation were dosed twice daily, five days a week, with 0.25 mL of a solution containing 3.3% Immunocal® in sterile drinking water via oral gavage, which corresponds to a dose of approximately 660 mg/kg/day (based on a 25-g mouse). The typical daily dose of Immunocal® when taken as a nutritional supplement is two 10-g packets per day or approximately 285 mg/kg/day (based on a 70-kg person). Riluzole was administered ad libitum in drinking water at a dose of 100 μg/mL of water.

Table 2. Gender effects on disease onset and survival in amyotrophic lateral sclerosis (ALS) mice.

G93A SOD1 Transgenic	Males (n = 11)	Females (n = 12)
Onset (days ± SEM)	90 ± 1.0	92.8 ± 1.4
Survival (days ± SEM)	123.3 ± 2.2	128.6 ± 3.1

G93A, Gly position 93 to Ala; SOD1, Cu/Zn-superoxide dismutase.

Table 3. Gender distribution of treatment groups and statistical analysis of disease onset.

Group Number(s)	Treatment	Females	Males	Total N	Mean Onset (days)	SEM
1	NonTG	11	13	24		
2	G93A SOD1 Control	12	11	23	91	1
3	ICAL (ad libitum)	5	8	13	99 **	1
4	ICAL (oral gavage)	1	4	5	98 *	3
5	ICAL (oral gavage) + riluzole	5	5	10	101 ***	2

NonTG, Non-transgenic; ICAL, Immunocal®. * $p < 0.05$, ** $p < 0.01$, *** $p < 0.001$ *vs.* G93A SOD1 control (Student's t-test).

The decision to start Immunocal® supplementation at 60 days of age was based upon accepted practices for designing studies using ALS mouse models as recommended by the Jackson Laboratory [23]. Briefly, when working with mouse models of ALS, preclinical studies are conducted by first treating mice with a potential therapeutic agent between 50 and 70 days of age. If this pre-symptomatic treatment yields a robust therapeutic effect, a second study can be conducted to analyze the efficacy of administering the agent at or after disease onset. Seeing that Immunocal® administration produced a very modest positive effect when given pre-symptomatically, we did assess its applicability at disease onset (approximately 90 days of age) in a small number of mice. However, Immunocal® administration beginning at this stage of the disease did not appear to affect either disease progression or survival (data not shown).

2.2. Clinical Tests

Paw grip endurance (PaGE) testing was performed, and scores were determined by the latency of the animal's hind limbs to detach from a conventional housing wire cage lid after inversion. Briefly, mice were placed on top of the wire cage lid and given a few seconds to acclimate before the cage lid was gently inverted in one smooth motion, prompting the mouse to grip the wire. Care was taken to ensure that no jostling occurred during inversion, which might have caused the mouse to fall. The lid was held still and suspended while the mouse gripped the wire lid, and a stop watch was used to determine the point at which the mouse's hind limbs detached from the wire lid. Time was stopped the moment the mouse's hind limbs detached from the cage lid or after 30 s with no detachment, and the score was recorded as the latency to fall. Mice were given three scored attempts. Final scores were recorded as the average of these three trials for each time point, with a maximum possible score of 30 s. The PaGE test was carried out twice weekly [24]. Scores are reported as the average of all animals' final scores ± SEM for each time point. Time points correspond to the age of the animal at the time of testing and are represented as a span of 5 days due to the fact that multiple groups of animals having slightly different ages were tested concomitantly during the twice-weekly testing regimen. Animals were weighed every other day starting on Day 30. Disease onset was determined by the appearance of hind limb trembling, inability to splay the hind legs or failure of the mouse to extend either hind leg when suspended by its tail, which would indicate the first appearance of muscle weakness or paralysis. Though onset was not determined in a blinded fashion, at least two investigators confirmed the appearance of neurological symptoms of the disease in an effort to lessen subjectivity when determining disease onset. We assessed disease onset in the manner described above daily beginning at 60 days of age. Determination of disease onset by monitoring mice harboring ALS causing mutations for neurological deficits, such as the inability to splay hind limbs when suspended by the tail, is a well-accepted and common way to determine disease onset [23,25]. Animals were euthanized at the end-stage of disease, which is defined as the point at which the mouse is no longer capable of righting itself or performing regular motor tasks that would be required to reach food and water. This occurs due to extensive paralysis of the hind limbs and weakness in the upper extremities as a result of disease progression. The end-stage of the disease was determined by a failure of the animal to right itself to sternum within 20 s upon being placed on its side.

2.3. Tissue Processing

Tissues, including cerebral cortex, lumbar spinal cord and trunk blood, were harvested from end-stage hSOD1^{G93A} or age and sex-matched NonTG mice post-isoflurane overdose and were immediately frozen in liquid nitrogen (−196 °C). For HPLC-EC analysis, frozen trunk blood was weighed and 300 μL of HCL was added to the sample and vortexed rapidly. It was next centrifuged at 10,000× *g* for 20 min at 4 °C. The supernatant was removed and added to a new tube containing 10% perchloric acid (PCA), which was centrifuged for 10 min at 10,000× *g* at 4 °C. A clear supernatant was removed and filtered. Frozen lumbar spinal cord was weighed and added to 1 mL of 10% PCA before vortexing 3 times for 15 s each time. The supernatant was removed and filtered. Spinal cord GSH values were normalized to protein concentrations, which were determined by a commercially-available protein assay kit (BCA, Thermo Scientific, Rockford, IL, USA). Samples were analyzed in triplicate, and an additional sample was spiked with reduced GSH and glutathione disulfide (GSSG) to verify peak identification.

2.4. High Performance Liquid Chromatography with Electrochemical Detection

GSH and GSSG in samples and known standards were separated by reverse phase HPLC on a C18 bonded silica column at 35 °C (3 μm, 3 × 150 mm for whole blood, 3 μm, 3 × 250 mm for lumbar spinal cord) from Dionex Inc. (Sunnyvale, CA, USA). Analytes were detected using a CoulArray® detector (model 5600A, ESA; ESA Inc., Chelmsford, MA, USA) on three coulometric detector modules. Each electrochemical cell contains four coulometric detectors in series set to a range of potentials from 0 to 900 mV at increments of 100 mV. The mobile phase consisted of 125 mmol/L sodium phosphate and 1% HPLC grade methanol (Fisher Scientific, Pittsburg, PA, USA) in water, pH 2.8 [26]. The flow rate was set to 0.4 mL/min for all samples. CoulArray software was used for baseline correction and analysis.

2.5. Isolation of Mitochondria from Lumbar Spinal Cord

Mitochondria were isolated as previously described by Liang and Patel [27]. Briefly, lumbar spinal cord for each individual animal was dounce homogenized in 2 mL of mitochondrial isolation buffer (0.064 M sucrose, 2 mM EDTA, 20 mM Tris-HCl, pH 7.4). Samples were placed in an equal volume of 24% Percoll gradient and centrifuged at 4 °C for 5 min, 16,000 rpm to make a 12% Percoll gradient. Two milliliters of supernatant were then added to a Percoll gradient containing a bottom layer of 2 mL 40% Percoll and a top layer of 2 mL 19% Percoll. Samples were spun at 4 °C for 10 min, 16,000 rpm. The mitochondrial layer was removed (2 mL of the layer between the 19% and 40% gradients, respectively), washed with mitochondrial buffer at a dilution of 4:1 and spun at 4 °C for 10 min at 11,820 rpm. The supernatant was discarded, and the pellets were washed a second time with 4.5 mL of mitochondrial isolation buffer and 0.5 mL of mitochondrial isolation buffer containing 5 mg/mL BSA, then spun at 4 °C for 10 min at 7500 rpm. Mitochondrial pellets were then re-suspended in 100 μL of a mitochondrial buffer containing 130 mM KCl, 4 mM Tris-HCl, 5 mM sodium pyruvate, 5 mM sodium succinate and 1 mM EGTA, pH 7.4.

2.6. Mitochondrial GSH Loading and Measurement of GSH Levels in Isolated Mitochondria

For loading experiments, isolated mitochondria from either NonTG or hSOD1^{G93A} mice were incubated with 2 mM GSH at 37 °C, 300 rpm for 4 h after which mitochondria were washed three times, and total GSH was measured. A sample of unloaded mitochondria was frozen immediately after isolation to serve as an unloaded control. Values for this sample were subtracted from total GSH following loading to determine the amount of GSH loaded per hour. Total mitochondrial glutathione (both GSH and GSSG) for all experiments using isolated mitochondria was measured using a colorimetric kinetic assay kit from Oxford Biomedical (Rochester Hills, MI, USA) and was performed per the manufacturer's instructions. All GSH measurements were normalized to protein concentration.

2.7. Statistical Analysis

Measurements of GSH were performed in duplicate and repeated a minimum of three times. Data are reported as the mean ± SEM. Statistical significance was analyzed with one-way analysis of variance (ANOVA) followed by a post hoc Tukey's test, or using a paired Student's *t*-test when two matched sets of data were compared. PaGE measurements of grip strength data were compared between groups at each time point using one-way ANOVA and a post hoc Tukey's test. Survival and onset data were analyzed with Kaplan-Meier curves and a log rank test.

3. Results

3.1. Immunocal® Delays Disease Onset, but Does Not Extend Lifespan in the hSOD1^{G93A} Mouse Model of ALS

Here, we investigated the effects of Immunocal® supplementation in the hSOD1^{G93A} mouse model of ALS. Beginning at 60 days-of-age, mice received Immunocal® ad libitum in drinking water. Those mice receiving Immunocal® displayed a significant delay in clinical onset of disease of approximately seven days (7.0 ± 1.1 days) with onset occurring on average at 98.5 ± 1.1 days of age in comparison to untreated hSOD1^{G93A} mice, which had an average disease onset of 91.6 ± 0.9 days of age (Figure 1A). However, treatment with Immunocal® did not produce any measurable difference in lifespan. Mice receiving Immunocal® displayed an average age of 125.2 ± 2.4 days at the end-stage in comparison to untreated hSOD1^{G93A} mice, which reached the end-stage at 124.1 ± 1.5 days of age (Figure 1B).

Figure 1. Immunocal® delays clinical onset in hSOD1^{G93A} mice. (**A**) hSOD1^{G93A} mice receiving Immunocal® ad libitum beginning at 60 days of age (pre-symptomatically) displayed a delay in disease onset and clinical decline compared to untreated mutant mice ($n = 13$). Onset curves are significantly different ($p < 0.001$) as determined by the Gehan–Breslow–Wilcoxon test. (**B**) Median survival is not significantly different between hSOD1^{G93A} mice receiving Immunocal® ad libitum and untreated mutant mice ($n = 13$).

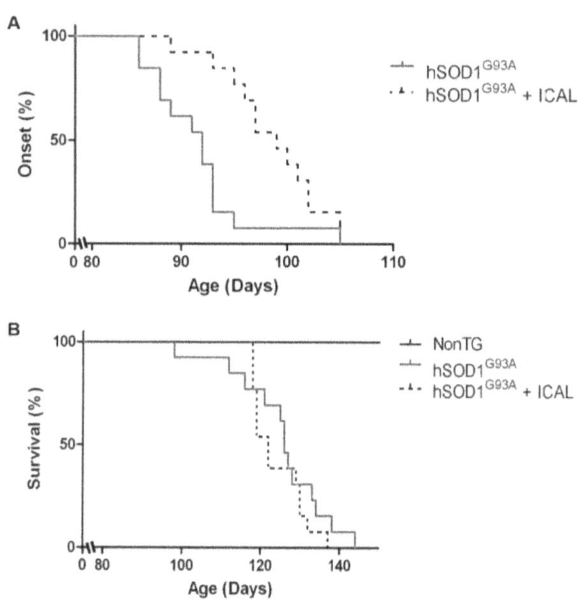

Mice were visually assessed for deficits in motor function and coordination daily and by the PaGE hanging wire grip test twice weekly. PaGE testing revealed a statistically significant decrease in the rate of decline in grip strength between 100 days and 120 days of age when Immunocal®-treated mice were compared to hSOD1^{G93A} mice that did not receive supplementation (Figure 2A). Despite retaining muscle strength, Immunocal® did not show any ability to preserve body weight in transgenic mice receiving the supplement (Figure 2B). Thus, oral treatment with Immunocal® preserved grip strength and modestly delayed the onset of motor dysfunction in this mouse model of familial ALS.

Figure 2. Immunocal® diminishes the rate of decline in grip strength in hSOD1^{G93A} mice. (**A**) The paw grip endurance (PaGE) hanging wire test expressed as latency to fall at indicated ages ($n = 13$); (**B**) body weight of wild-type and hSOD1^{G93A} mice expressed as the percent of peak body weight. All data are represented as the mean ± SEM. *** indicates $p < 0.001$ compared to non-transgenic (NonTG) mice; ** indicates $p < 0.01$ compared to NonTG; † indicates $p < 0.05$ compared to untreated hSOD1^{G93A} mice (one-way ANOVA with a post hoc Tukey's test conducted for each time point).

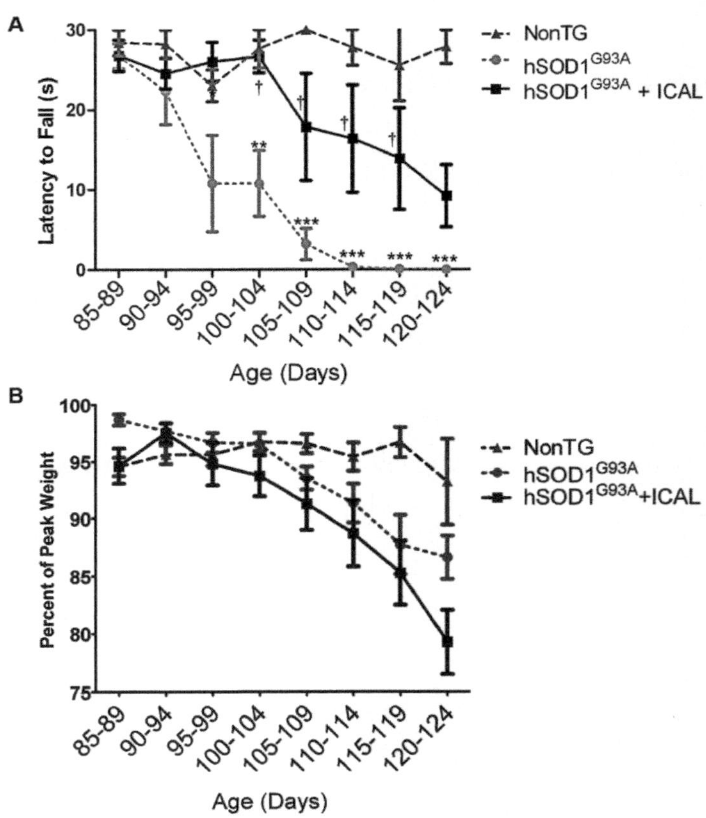

3.2. *Immunocal® Prevents GSH Depletion in Whole Blood and Lumbar Spinal Cord Tissue of hSOD1^{G93A} Mice*

The neuroprotective effects of Immunocal® observed *in vitro* are largely due to its capacity to enhance GSH synthesis by providing the key precursors, cystine and cysteine. To investigate this potential mechanism of action *in vivo*, whole blood and lumbar spinal cord tissue were collected from end-stage hSOD1^{G93A} mice and analyzed for reduced GSH and oxidized GSSG using HPLC-EC. We found that hSOD1^{G93A} mice that did not receive supplementation displayed a significant decrease in whole blood GSH when compared to NonTG littermate controls. Levels of GSSG in whole blood did not significantly change; however, the ratio of GSH-to-GSSG in whole blood was significantly decreased in hSOD1^{G93A} mice compared to NonTG controls. Both the decreases in GSH and the reduction in the GSH/GSSG ratio were prevented in hSOD1^{G93A} mice receiving Immunocal® (Figure 3A). Representative HPLC chromatograms from these animals are shown in Figure 3B.

Figure 3. HPLC-EC detection reveals whole blood GSH is preserved in hSOD1^{G93A} mice receiving Immunocal®. (**A**) Mean GSH and glutathione disulfide (GSSG) concentrations and GSH/GSSG ratios from the whole blood of end-stage trial animals determined using HPLC-EC detection, $n = 13$. ** indicates $p < 0.01$; * indicates $p < 0.05$; ns indicates no significant difference. (**B**) Representative HPLC-EC chromatograms from the whole blood of end-stage animals; labeled peaks indicate GSH oxidizing at 600 and 800 mV.

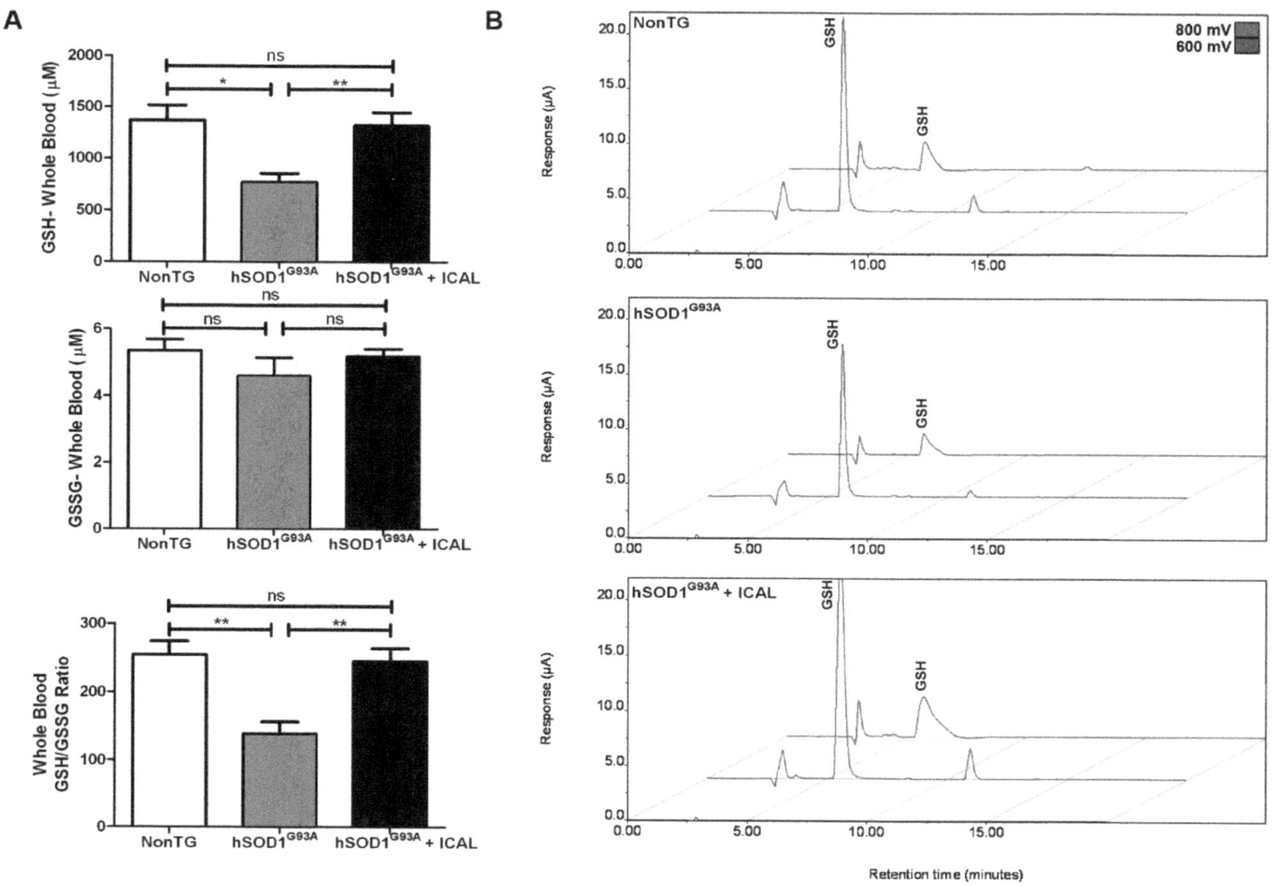

Interestingly, we found that a similar pattern also existed for GSH levels in the lumbar spinal cord tissue of study animals. Spinal cord tissue GSH levels were decreased by approximately 50%; GSSG levels were elevated two-fold; and the ratio of GSH-to-GSSG was significantly decreased in hSOD1^{G93A} mice compared to NonTG controls. Immunocal® treatment prevented these changes in GSH and GSSG and maintained the GSH/GSSG ratio at a level that was indistinguishable from NonTG controls (Figure 4A). Representative chromatograms from these animals are displayed in Figure 4B. These results indicate that the preservation of whole blood and spinal cord tissue GSH levels positively correlates with the beneficial effects of Immunocal® supplementation in the mutant hSOD1^{G93A} mouse model of ALS.

Figure 4. HPLC-EC detection reveals lumbar spinal cord GSH is maintained in hSOD1^{G93A} mice receiving Immunocal®. (**A**) Mean GSH and GSSG concentrations and GSH/GSSG ratios from the lumbar spinal cord of end-stage trial animals determined using HPLC-EC detection, $n = 17$. * indicates $p < 0.05$; ns indicates no significant difference. (**B**) Representative HPLC-EC chromatograms from the lumbar spinal cord of end-stage animals; labeled peaks indicate GSH and GSSG oxidizing at 600 mV.

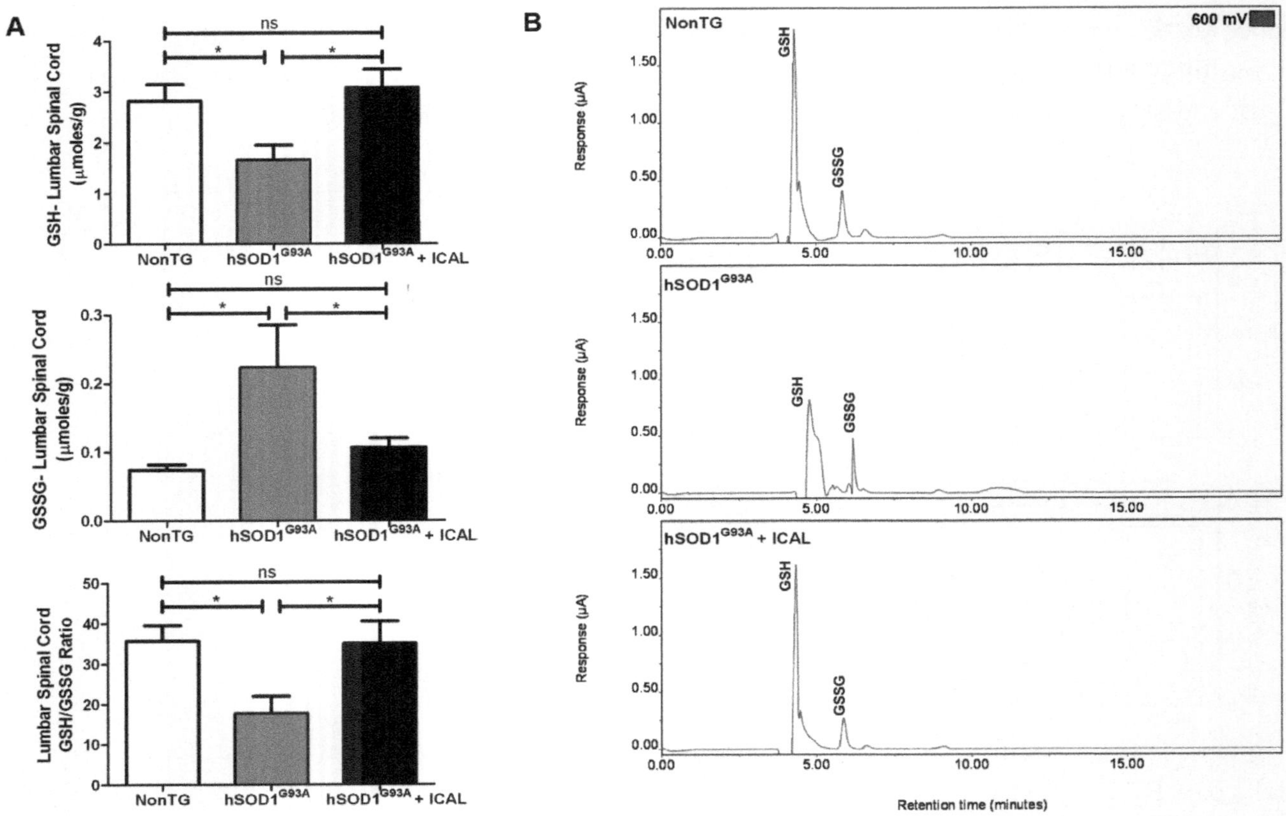

3.3. *Immunocal® Does Not Prevent Depletion of Mitochondrial GSH in Lumbar Spinal Cord of hSOD1^{G93A} Mice*

Although the ability of Immunocal® to preserve total GSH levels in whole blood and lumbar spinal cord tissue of hSOD1^{G93A} mutant mice correlates with preserved grip strength and delayed disease onset, the underlying reason for the lack of effect on survival with Immunocal® supplementation remained unclear. We have previously shown that specific deficits in mitochondrial GSH levels significantly sensitize neurons to oxidative insult [28]. Furthermore, recent evidence demonstrates that the GSH-to-GSSG ratio is significantly reduced in spinal cord mitochondria of mutant SOD1 mice, indicative of MOS and mitochondrial GSH depletion [14]. As MOS is a key feature of ALS disease pathology, we hypothesized that although Immunocal® was able to bolster spinal cord tissue GSH, it may not have sustained mitochondrial GSH levels and, thus, would be unable to prevent MOS.

To test this hypothesis, mitochondria were isolated from the cortex and lumbar spinal cord of hSOD1^{G93A} mice at the end-stage of disease, and total mitochondrial GSH levels were assessed. In comparison to their NonTG counterparts, hSOD1^{G93A} mice displayed a significant decrease in total mitochondrial GSH in lumbar spinal cord at the end-stage of disease (Figure 5A), consistent with prior reports of a reduced GSH to GSSG ratio; however, no deficit was observed at disease onset [14]. A similar trend was observed for mitochondria isolated from the cortex of mutant animals, but did not reach statistical significance. This observation encouraged further investigation into the mechanism by which mitochondrial GSH is depleted in hSOD1^{G93A} mice. Because mitochondria lack the enzymes necessary to synthesize GSH on their own, de novo synthesis takes place in the cytosol, and GSH is subsequently transported into the mitochondria [10]. Thus, we analyzed the ability of mitochondria isolated from the spinal cord and cortex of end-stage mutant mice and their NonTG littermates to take up GSH *in vitro* over time. Intriguingly, mitochondria isolated from hSOD1^{G93A} mutant spinal cord showed a marked decrease in GSH loading efficiency in comparison to NonTG controls (Figure 5B). This effect was not observed in mitochondria isolated from cortex (Figure 5B). We next examined the total GSH content of spinal cord mitochondria isolated from hSOD1^{G93A} mutant mice that had been treated with Immunocal® in comparison to mutant mice receiving no supplement, as well as NonTG controls. Mutant mice that did not receive Immunocal® showed marked depletion of mitochondrial GSH levels in comparison to NonTG controls (Figure 5C). Notably, supplementation with Immunocal® did not rescue this effect, indicating that Immunocal® was unable to preserve mitochondrial GSH levels in the spinal cord of hSOD1^{G93A} mice (Figure 5C).

3.4. Combination Treatment with Immunocal® and Riluzole Shows Complementary Effects on Disease Onset and Survival in hSOD1^{G93A} Mice

The only current FDA approved treatment for ALS is the anti-glutamatergic drug, riluzole. This compound modestly increases the lifespan of hSOD1^{G93A} mice by approximately 7–10 days, which translates to an increase in the life expectancy of ~2–3 months in human patients [29]. However, despite its effect on lifespan, riluzole has no discernible effect on disease onset in the hSOD1^{G93A} mouse model [30]. Because Immunocal® delayed disease onset, but had no effect on survival, we treated hSOD1^{G93A} mice with a combination of Immunocal® and riluzole to determine if these agents had either complementary or synergistic effects on disease onset and survival when given together.

Mutant mice receiving riluzole alone did not display a significant difference in disease onset compared to untreated controls (average disease onset occurred at 94.5 ± 1.3 and 91.2 ± 1.2 days of age, respectively); however, mice receiving both Immunocal® and riluzole in combination demonstrated a delay in disease onset of approximately 10 days (average disease onset occurred at 102.1 ± 2.2 days of age; Figure 6A). This delay in disease onset is comparable to that observed in mice treated with Immunocal® alone. Conversely, hSOD1^{G93A} mice treated with riluzole alone showed a modest, but significant increase in survival of approximately seven days with the end-stage occurring at 131.6 ± 2.6 days of age in comparison to untreated mice, which reached the end-stage at 124.9 ± 1.4 days of age (Figure 6B). This modest increase in lifespan is consistent with previous reports using riluzole in the hSOD1^{G93A} mouse model [30]. Mice receiving both riluzole and Immunocal® displayed a similar extension of lifespan, reaching the end-stage at 130.0 ± 3.0 days of age (Figure 6B).

Figure 5. Spinal cord mitochondrial GSH levels and mitochondrial GSH transport are significantly diminished in hSOD1^{G93A} mice. (**A**) Mitochondria were isolated from NonTG and hSOD1^{G93A} mice at onset (~90 days old) and end-stage (~120 days old) from lumbar spinal cord and whole cortex, and total GSH was measured. All measurements were normalized to protein and represented as a percent of NonTG. *** indicates $p < 0.001$; NS indicates no significant difference, as determined by an unpaired Student's *t*-test, $n = 4$. Error bars indicate SEM. (**B**) Mitochondria were isolated from lumbar spinal cord and cortex of end-stage (~120 days old) hSOD1^{G93A} and age-matched NonTG mice, as described in (**A**). Isolated mitochondria were incubated with 2 mM GSH at 37 °C, 300 rpm for 4 h, after which mitochondria were washed 3× and total GSH was measured. All measurements were normalized to protein and represented as µmoles GSH/mg of mitochondrial protein loaded per hour. * indicates $p < 0.05$; NS indicates no significant difference, as determined by a paired Student's *t*-test, $n = 7$. Error bars indicated SEM. (**C**) Mitochondria were isolated from lumbar spinal cord as described in (**A**) from untreated end-stage (~120 days old) hSOD1^{G93A} mice, hSOD1^{G93A} mice treated with Immunocal® (hSOD1^{G93A} + ICAL) and age-matched NonTG mice. Total GSH was measured. All measurements of total GSH are normalized to protein and represented as nmols/mg of protein. ** indicates $p < 0.01$; NS indicates no significant difference, as determined using a one-way ANOVA with a post hoc Tukey's test, $n = 4$. Error bars indicate SEM.

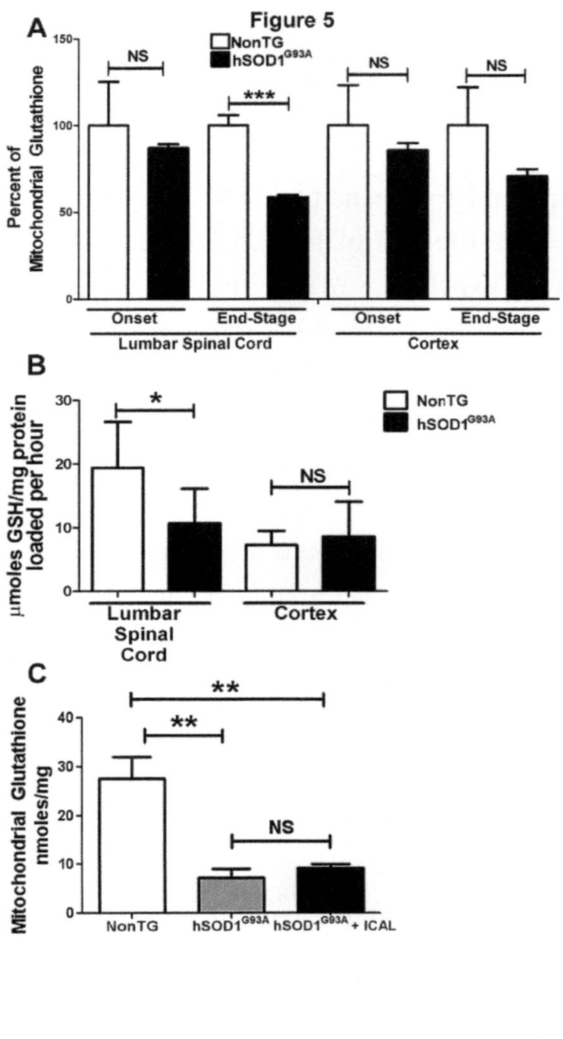

Figure 6. Treatment with Immunocal® an riluzole significantly delays disease onset and extends survival in hSOD1^{G93A} mice. (**A**) hSOD1^{G93A} mice receiving riluzole beginning at 60 days of age (pre-symptomatically) show no delay in disease onset and clinical decline compared to untreated mutant mice ($n = 8$). hSOD1^{G93A} mice receiving riluzole in addition to Immunocal® showed a significant delay in disease onset and clinical decline compared to untreated mutant mice ($p < 0.001$; $n = 10$). Onset curves were compared pair-wise using the Gehan–Breslow–Wilcoxon test. (**B**) hSOD1^{G93A} mice receiving riluzole beginning at 60 days of age (pre-symptomatically) showed a significant extension in survival compared to untreated mutant mice ($n = 7$; $p < 0.05$). Similarly, hSOD1^{G93A} mice receiving riluzole in addition to Immunocal® showed a significant extension in survival compared to untreated mutant mice ($p < 0.05$; $n = 8$). Survival curves were compared pair-wise using the Gehan–Breslow–Wilcoxon test.

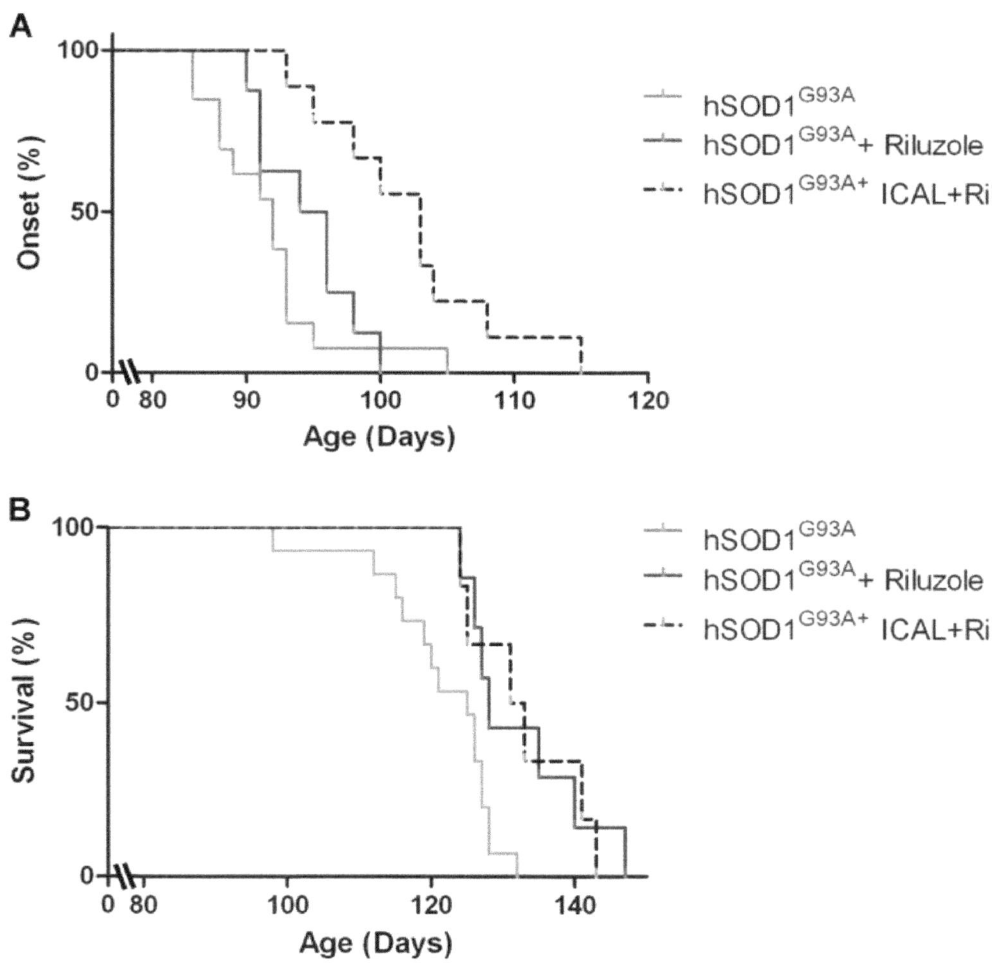

Moreover, PaGE testing indicated that hSOD1^{G93A} mice that received riluzole in their water displayed a minimal enhancement in grip strength as compared to their untreated counterparts (Figure 7A). However, this effect was accentuated in mice that were supplemented with both Immunocal® and riluzole (Figure 7A). Despite these improvements, however, neither mice receiving riluzole alone nor mice treated with the combination of Immunocal® and riluzole showed any significant change in weight loss compared to untreated mutant controls (Figure 7B). Collectively, these data indicate that mice treated with a combination of riluzole and Immunocal® receive modest benefits of both agents, displaying both a delay in disease onset and increased survival, with preserved grip strength and no overt loss of effect from either agent due to combined administration. While the effects of Immunocal® and riluzole appear to be complementary in this sense, no synergism was observed with combined administration.

Figure 7. Treatment with Immunocal® and riluzole diminishes the decline in grip strength in hSOD1^{G93A} mice. (**A**) The PaGE hanging wire test expressed as latency to fall at indicated ages (n = 8); (**B**) body weight of wild-type and hSOD1^{G93A} mice expressed as percent of peak body weight. All data are represented as the mean ± SEM. *** indicates $p < 0.001$ compared to NonTG; ** indicates $p < 0.01$ compared to NonTG; * indicates $p < 0.05$ compared to NonTG; †† indicates $p < 0.01$ compared to untreated hSOD1^{G93A} mice; and † indicates $p < 0.05$ compared to untreated hSOD1^{G93A} mice (one-way ANOVA with a post hoc Tukey's test conducted for each time point).

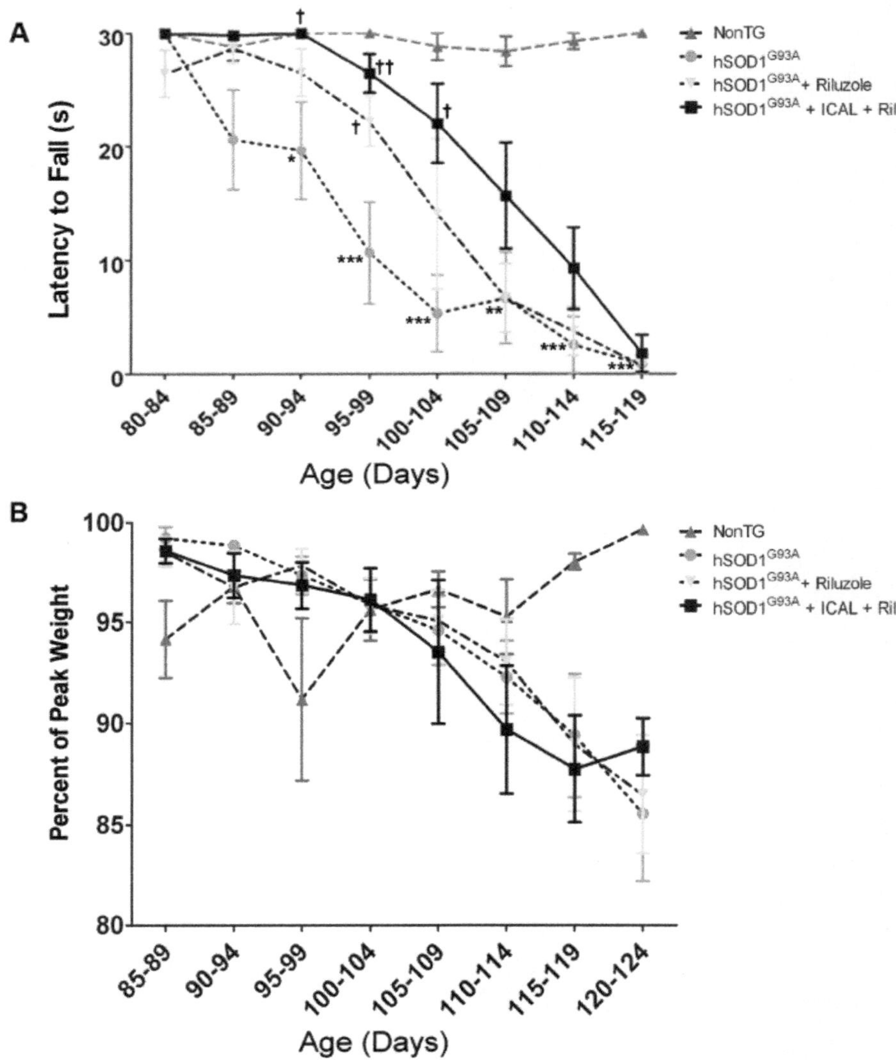

4. Discussion

GSH depletion occurs in many neurodegenerative diseases, including Alzheimer's disease and Parkinson's disease, as well as ALS [13,31,32]. GSH depletion and a decline in antioxidant enzyme activity have been observed in the erythrocytes of sporadic ALS patients with active disease, and interestingly, characteristic pathological changes observed in sporadic disease may be induced by intracellular GSH depletion [12]. For instance, TAR DNA-binding protein-43 (TDP-43) forms cytoplasmic inclusions, which are a hallmark pathology observed in sporadic ALS patients. These inclusions can be recapitulated in cultured neurons subjected to GSH depletion [33]. Moreover, crossing of hSOD1^{G93A} mice with mice lacking the γ-glutamylcysteine ligase regulatory subunit resulted in a significant acceleration of motor neuron disease, a result consistent with GSH depletion being a significant modifier of ALS susceptibility [34]. These cumulative findings suggest a prominent role for GSH depletion in ALS pathogenesis, prompting interest in therapeutically targeting this aspect of the disease.

Here, we investigated the therapeutic potential of Immunocal®, a cystine-rich whey protein supplement, in a mouse model of familial ALS. This supplement has been investigated previously as a means to bolster GSH in diseases for which oxidative stress is a significant underlying factor. For instance, oxidative stress is a known activator of human immunodeficiency virus replication, and based on this, Immunocal® was tested as an approach to attenuate this stress and combat infection by increasing intracellular GSH levels [21]. Oxidative stress also plays a significant role in muscle weakness. Oral Immunocal® administration to normal healthy subjects for three months significantly increased muscle power and work capacity in comparison to individuals that received placebo treatment [35]. Immunocal® supplementation also significantly increased lymphocyte GSH levels in these healthy subjects compared to placebo (36% ± 11% increase). Finally, oxidative stress is also believed to play a significant role in the pathogenesis of cystic fibrosis. In cystic fibrosis patients receiving oral Immunocal® for three months, there was an approximately 47% increase in lymphocyte GSH levels compared to individuals receiving a placebo [22]. These studies demonstrate that Immunocal® is capable of bolstering GSH *in vivo*, although its potential to do so in the central nervous system has not previously been addressed.

Building upon these earlier studies, we have recently found that Immunocal® displays robust neuroprotective activity *in vitro* against a variety of insults that contribute significantly to oxidative damage within the cell and which are directly relevant to the pathogenesis of multiple neurodegenerative diseases [36]. Moreover, the neuroprotective effects of Immunocal® *in vitro* are blocked by inhibiting GSH synthesis, demonstrating the dependence on enhanced GSH. Consistent with these *in vitro* findings and those previous observations in various human diseases, we demonstrate here that oral administration of Immunocal® preserved whole blood and spinal cord tissue GSH levels in end-stage hSOD1^{G93A} mice. Transgenic hSOD1^{G93A} mice that did not receive Immunocal® supplementation displayed a marked decrease in the amount of reduced GSH in both whole blood and lumbar spinal cord tissue, when compared to age-matched NonTG control mice. However, transgenic mice administered Immunocal® displayed GSH levels, which were essentially equal to NonTG controls. This preservation of whole blood and spinal cord tissue GSH correlated with a significant delay in the clinical onset of disease and preservation of paw grip strength in this mouse model of familial ALS. Importantly, the ability of Immunocal® to preserve GSH levels in spinal cord indicates that this supplement is capable of acting on the central nervous system without the need for invasive delivery systems, a feature that is highly desirable for potential therapeutic agents in ALS. Since decreases in GSH have been correlated with the rate of disease progression, we conclude that preservation of blood and spinal cord tissue GSH levels with Immunocal® is likely responsible for the observed delay in disease onset [37]. Furthermore, Immunocal® has been shown specifically to attenuate muscle weakness and increase skeletal muscle work power, which may partially account for its ability to maintain paw grip strength in hSOD1^{G93A} mice [35].

Somewhat surprisingly, despite these positive, albeit modest, findings, Immunocal® did not significantly extend survival in hSOD1^{G93A} mice. This result is particularly unexpected given the recent study by Johnson and colleagues, which demonstrated that crossing of hSOD1^{G93A} mice with mice lacking the γ-glutamylcysteine ligase modifier subunit, involved in the rate limiting step of GSH synthesis, significantly accelerated disease progression [34]. Taking these two results together, it seems reasonable to conclude that reducing GSH synthesis is capable of enhancing neuromuscular disease progression; however, preserving whole blood and spinal cord tissue GSH is not sufficient to significantly extend the survival of ALS mice. There is a possibility that the unequal distribution of males to females in the treatment group receiving ad libitum Immunocal® supplementation may have caused the values for survival to be artificially low; however, this is unlikely, as analysis of Immunocal® treated animals in comparison to untreated mutant controls, when separated by gender, revealed that neither males nor females showed a significant extension in survival (end-stage occurred at 122.3 ± 3.0 and 131.0 ± 3.3 days of age for males and females treated with Immunocal®, respectively; see Table 2 for values of untreated hSOD1^{G93A} controls). The lack of effect on survival could also be attributed to the multifaceted nature of ALS disease pathology. However, here, we present evidence that the lack of effect on survival may be due more specifically to the inability of Immunocal® to rescue mitochondrial GSH levels in the lumbar spinal cord of ALS mice.

A number of *in vitro* studies suggest that mutant SOD1 significantly influences mitochondrial GSH and, as a result, susceptibility of motor neuronal cells to MOS. For instance, an *in vitro* study using NSC34 motor neuron-like cells stably transfected with hSOD1^{G93A} demonstrated that cells expressing this mutant form of SOD1 showed markedly and selectively decreased levels of mitochondrial GSH in comparison to parental cells [38]. Similarly, infection of NSC34 cells with adenoviral hSOD1^{G93A} induces oxidative stress, mitochondrial dysfunction and intrinsic apoptosis, which are significantly alleviated by co-expression of the mitochondrial antioxidant enzymes, SOD2 and GSH peroxidase-4 [39]. Finally, NSC34 cells expressing hSOD1^{G93A}, but not wild-type (WT) SOD1, show marked morphological and functional alterations in mitochondria and exhibit a significant decrease in the reduced GSH-to-oxidized GSSG ratio in mitochondria following exposure to the inflammatory cytokines, tumor necrosis factor α and interferon γ [40]. Thus, hSOD1^{G93A} appears to sensitize motor neuronal cells *in vitro* to MOS and apoptosis by specifically diminishing the mitochondrial GSH pool.

Moreover, mitochondria lack the enzymes necessary to synthesize and thereby maintain the mitochondrial pool of GSH and rely instead on transporters to import GSH from the cytosol [10,11]. Maintenance of mitochondrial GSH levels by these transporters is critical for cellular survival, as selective depletion of this antioxidant pool by inhibiting GSH transport sensitizes primary neuronal cells to oxidative challenge and subsequent apoptosis [28]. We have previously shown that Bcl-2 is a key regulator of the mitochondrial GSH transport process, and inhibition of Bcl-2 *in vitro* induces significant GSH depletion at the mitochondria [41]. As Bcl-2 expression is reduced in ALS, mitochondria may experience deficits in GSH transport during disease progression, which may, in turn, exacerbate mitochondrial GSH depletion by hSOD1^{G93A} [42]. Furthermore, mutant SOD1 has been shown to accumulate at mitochondria and form aggregates with Bcl-2, which may further interfere with the ability of Bcl-2 to regulate GSH transport into mitochondria [43]. Consistent with this hypothesis, we demonstrate that mitochondria isolated from the lumbar spinal cord of end-stage hSOD1^{G93A} mutant mice show both a marked decrease in mitochondrial GSH levels and deficits in GSH uptake *in vitro* in comparison to spinal cord mitochondria isolated from NonTG controls. However, while there is evidence to suggest that the ratio of GSH-to-GSSG is reduced at disease onset due to enhanced oxidative stress conditions, which deplete the reduced form of GSH, no statistically significant depletion of total mitochondrial GSH and GSSG was observed at disease onset, suggesting that deficits in transport may not yet be evident at early stages of the disease [14]. Most significantly, hSOD1^{G93A} mice treated with Immunocal® showed no rescue of lumbar spinal cord mitochondrial GSH levels when compared to untreated transgenic mice at end-stage. Thus, while Immunocal® supplementation is sufficient to preserve tissue GSH levels in the spinal cord of ALS mice, this GSH appears unable to enter the mitochondria, where it would normally act to mitigate organelle damage caused by aberrant ROS generation. We propose this scenario as a plausible reason for the lack of extension in the survival of mutant hSOD1^{G93A} mice administered Immunocal® for two reasons.

Firstly, decreased the levels of Bcl-2, and inhibitory interactions between Bcl-2 and mutant SOD1 may explain some deficits in GSH transport into mitochondria due to impaired regulation of this process. However, there are also other possibilities to consider, which have not been previously explored in the context of ALS. For example, decreases in GSH transport from the cytosol to the mitochondria could be compromised at the level of the mitochondrial GSH transporters themselves. This may occur if proteins, such as the dicarboxylate carrier or the 2-oxyglutarate carrier, both of which play a major role in maintaining mitochondrial GSH levels in brain tissue, are damaged or modified by oxidative species generated within the mitochondria [11,28,41]. Indeed, disruption of the overall architecture of key GSH transport machinery under conditions of mitochondrial oxidative stress could interfere with or abrogate their ability to move GSH from the cytosol to the mitochondria by abolishing the transport function of these proteins or preventing their interaction with key regulators, such as Bcl-2. The 2-oxyglutarate carrier, for example, possesses three critical cysteine residues that are vital for its transport function and could be sensitive to oxidative modification [44]. Therefore, even in conditions where GSH production is enhanced and cytosolic levels of GSH are elevated, such as with Immunocal®, the rescue of the mitochondrial GSH pool may not be possible without first correcting impairments in the mitochondrial glutathione transport machinery.

Secondly, deficits in glutathione transport into the mitochondria could contribute to the adoption of an inflammatory phenotype by surrounding glial cells. Neuroinflammation is a contributing factor to many neurodegenerative disorders and is known to play a significant role in the pathology and progression of ALS [45,46]. Interestingly, GSH depletion results in activation of both astrocytes and microglia due to increased levels of oxidative stress within these cell types and results in secretion of a number of pro-inflammatory and neurotoxic factors [47,48]. The reverse is also true: transition to an inflammatory phenotype through stimulation by agents, such as lipopolysaccharide, also results in GSH depletion and induction of MOS [49]. Moreover, GSH depletion in glial cells causes upregulation of the xc^- Sxc^- transporter, which is responsible for antiporting glutamate for cystine to stimulate GSH production [50,51]. Increased secretion of glutamate can then contribute to excitotoxicity and neuronal death. Inflammation in both astrocytes and microglia can be mitigated by supplementation with GSH, GSH precursors or protection of the critical mitochondrial GSH pool, which reduce oxidative stress within these cells and promote the maintenance of a neuroprotective phenotype [48,51,52]. Although no data exists suggesting that Immunocal® specifically is effective at preventing neuroinflammation, these studies do suggest that increasing GSH levels in glial cells through precursor supplementation may be a viable therapeutic strategy. However, the positive effects of GSH supplementation appear to be at least partially dependent on the ability of GSH to prevent oxidative damage at the level of the mitochondria [49,52]. Thus, mitochondrial GSH transport deficits in ALS, such as those observed in this study, may render supplements, such as Immunocal®, ineffective at attenuating glial inflammation and subsequent neuronal cell death.

Because Immunocal® delayed disease onset, but had no effect on survival, this whey supplement was tested in combination with the anti-glutamatergic compound, riluzole, which displays the opposite effect [30]. As expected, mice treated with riluzole alone displayed a significant extension in survival in comparison to untreated mutant mice, but no effect on disease onset. Mice treated in combination with both agents displayed modest benefits of both Immunocal® and riluzole, developing neuromuscular deficits at a later time point and showing a modest increase in overall survival. Additionally, these results demonstrate that there are no overt adverse effects from the combined administration of these agents, an important consideration when combining therapeutic treatments. These data also show that Immunocal® administered at a known dosage of approximately 660 mg/kg/day recapitulates the modest beneficial effects observed in mutant mice that were given ad libitum access to Immunocal® in their drinking water. For the average adult, this dosage would be equivalent to consuming about four to five packets of Immunocal® each day, or about twice the manufacturer's recommended daily value.

The effect of Immunocal® on delaying disease onset in this ALS mouse model is quite modest. In pre-clinical studies, such as these, it has been recommended that a relatively large number of animals should be tested (~25 per group) to have confidence in the observation of such a small effect [53]. In Table 3, we provide a breakdown of each of the Immunocal® dosing regimens used in this study. In every case, whether Immunocal® was administered ad libitum in drinking water (Group 3) or by oral gavage, either alone (Group 4) or in combination with riluzole (Group 5), we observed a statistically significant delay in disease onset of 7–10 days. Moreover, the mean onset was not significantly different amongst any of the Immunocal® treatment groups, regardless of the method of dosing or whether or not the supplement was given in combination with riluzole (which is known to have no effect on disease onset in the ALS mouse model) [30]. Thus, the data taken as a whole demonstrate a reproducible and statistically significant delay in disease onset with Immunocal® treatment.

Finally, vitamin E displays essentially the same effect in this mouse model of ALS, producing a modest delay in disease onset, but no significant extension of survival [30]. Nonetheless, despite its very modest effects in the ALS mouse model, a pooled analysis of five prospective cohort studies suggests that long-term supplementation with vitamin E is associated with lower ALS rates [54,55]. Thus, even a modest effect in the ALS mouse model may translate into a measurable beneficial effect for some subpopulation of patients, particularly when one considers long-term use with nutritional supplements, such as vitamin E, creatine or Immunocal®.

5. Conclusions

Despite its lack of effect on overall survival, we found that Immunocal® administered orally to $hSOD1^{G93A}$ mice significantly reduced age-associated decline in skeletal muscle function, as measured by the PaGE test. Moreover, Immunocal® significantly delayed the clinical onset of neuromuscular disease in these mutant mice. Finally, Immunocal® prevented depletion of whole blood and spinal cord tissue GSH and maintained the GSH/GSSG ratio at levels indistinguishable from age-matched NonTG mice. Thus, Immunocal® supplementation had a significant, albeit modest, beneficial effect in the $hSOD1^{G93A}$ mutant mouse model of ALS that was positively correlated with the preservation of whole blood and spinal cord tissue GSH levels. Unfortunately, Immunocal® failed to rescue mitochondrial GSH levels in spinal cord of end-stage $hSOD1^{G93A}$ mice. This latter result provides a plausible molecular mechanism for the observed lack of effect of this supplement on overall survival in ALS mice. Moreover, these findings suggest significant limitations to the potential utility of this supplement as a therapeutic agent for ALS. Future studies aimed at elucidating the mechanisms related to dysfunctional GSH transport in spinal cord mitochondria of ALS mice are necessary to further evaluate the pre-clinical effects of Immunocal® in this disease.

Acknowledgments

Supported by a Merit Review grant from the Department of Veterans Affairs to DAL and a grant from the Ludlow-Griffith foundation to DP. We would also like to acknowledge James Fogleman for his guidance regarding statistical analysis. The authors thank Karen Ryan and friends for their generosity and support.

Author Contributions

Substantial contributions to conception and design, acquisition, analysis or interpretation of data: EKR, HMW, ANW, WAS and ND; drafting the article or revising it critically for important intellectual content: EKR, ANW, HMW, DP and DAL; final approval of the version to be published: DAL.

Conflicts of Interest

The authors have received funding from Immunotec Inc. (Quebec, QC, Canada) to support research on the neuroprotective effects of Immunocal®.

References

1. Tandan, R.; Bradley, W.G. Amyotrophic lateral sclerosis: Part 1. Clinical features, pathology, and ethical issues in management. *Ann. Neurol.* **1985**, *18*, 271–280.
2. Barber, S.C.; Shaw, P.J. Oxidative stress in ALS: Key role in motor neuron injury and therapeutic target. *Free Radic. Biol. Med.* **2010**, *48*, 629–641.
3. Kiernan, M.C.; Vucic, S.; Cheah, B.C.; Turner, M.R.; Eisen, A.; Hardiman, O.; Burrell, J.R.; Zoing, M.C. Amyotrophic lateral sclerosis. *Lancet* **2011**, *377*, 942–955.
4. Cozzolino, M.; Carri, M.T. Mitochondrial dysfunction in ALS. *Prog. Neurobiol.* **2012**, *97*, 54–66.

5. Rosen, D.R.; Siddique, T.; Patterson, D.; Figlewicz, D.A.; Sapp, P.; Hentati, A.; Donaldson, D.; Goto, J.; O'Regan, J.P.; Deng, H.X.; *et al.* Mutations in Cu/Zn superoxide dismutase gene are associated with familial amyotrophic lateral sclerosis. *Nature* **1993**, *362*, 59–62.
6. Yim, M.B.; Kang, J.H.; Yim, H.S.; Kwak, H.S.; Chock, P.B.; Stadtman, E.R. A gain-of-function of an amyotrophic lateral sclerosis-associated Cu,Zn-superoxide dismutase mutant: An enhancement of free radical formation due to a decrease in Km for hydrogen peroxide. *Proc. Natl. Acad. Sci. USA* **1996**, *93*, 5709–5714.
7. Ferri, A.; Cozzolino, M.; Crosio, C.; Nencini, M.; Casciati, A.; Gralla, E.B.; Rotilio, G.; Valentine, J.S.; Carri, M.T. Familial ALS-superoxide dismutases associate with mitochondria and shift their redox potentials. *Proc. Natl. Acad. Sci. USA* **2006**, *103*, 13860–13865.
8. Andreassen, O.A.; Ferrante, R.J.; Klivenyi, P.; Klein, A.M.; Shinobu, L.A.; Epstein, C.J.; Beal, M.F. Partial deficiency of manganese superoxide dismutase exacerbates a transgenic mouse model of amyotrophic lateral sclerosis. *Ann. Neurol.* **2000**, *47*, 447–455.
9. Franco, R.; Cidlowski, J.A. Apoptosis and glutathione: Beyond an antioxidant. *Cell Death Differ.* **2009**, *16*, 1303–1314.
10. Griffith, O.W.; Meister, A. Origin and turnover of mitochondrial glutathione. *Proc. Natl. Acad. Sci. USA* **1985**, *82*, 4668–4672.
11. Lash, L.H. Mitochondrial glutathione transport: Physiological, pathological and toxicological implications. *Chem. Biol. Interact.* **2006**, *163*, 54–67.
12. Babu, G.N.; Kumar, A.; Chandra, R.; Puri, S.K.; Singh, R.L.; Kalita, J.; Misra, U.K. Oxidant-antioxidant imbalance in the erythrocytes of sporadic amyotrophic lateral sclerosis patients correlates with the progression of disease. *Neurochem. Int.* **2008**, *52*, 1284–1289.
13. Chi, L.; Ke, Y.; Luo, C.; Gozal, D.; Liu, R. Depletion of reduced glutathione enhances motor neuron degeneration *in vitro* and *in vivo*. *Neuroscience* **2007**, *144*, 991–1003.
14. Pesaresi, M.G.; Amori, I.; Giorgi, C.; Ferri, A.; Fiorenzo, P.; Gabanella, F.; Salvatore, A.M.; Giorgio, M.; Pelicci, P.G.; Pinton, P.; *et al.* Mitochondrial redox signalling by p66Shc mediates ALS-like disease through Rac1 inactivation. *Hum. Mol. Genet.* **2011**, *20*, 4196–4208.
15. Olsson, B.; Johansson, M.; Gabrielsson, J.; Bolme, P. Pharmacokinetics and bioavailability of reduced and oxidized *N*-acetylcysteine. *Eur. J. Clin. Pharmacol.* **1988**, *34*, 77–82.
16. Zeevalk, G.D.; Manzino, L.; Sonsalla, P.K.; Bernard, L.P. Characterization of intracellular elevation of glutathione (GSH) with glutathione monoethyl ester and GSH in brain and neuronal cultures: Relevance to Parkinson's disease. *Exp. Neurol.* **2007**, *203*, 512–520.
17. Bounous, G.; Gold, P. The biological activity of undenatured dietary whey proteins: Role of glutathione. *Clin. Investig. Med.* **1991**, *14*, 296–309.
18. Bounous, G.; Baruchel, S.; Falutz, J.; Gold, P. Whey proteins as a food supplement in HIV-seropositive individuals. *Clin. Investig. Med.* **1993**, *16*, 204–209.
19. De Rosa, S.C.; Zaretsky, M.D.; Dubs, J.G.; Roederer, M.; Anderson, M.; Green, A.; Mitra, D.; Watanabe, N.; Nakamura, H.; Tjioe, I.; *et al.* *N*-acetylcysteine replenishes glutathione in HIV infection. *Eur. J. Clin. Investig.* **2000**, *30*, 915–929.
20. PDR Staff. *Physician's Desk Reference*, 67th ed.; PDR Network: Montvale, NJ, USA, 2013.
21. Baruchel, S.; Bounous, G.; Gold, P. Place for an antioxidant therapy in human immunodeficiency virus (HIV) infection. *J. Nutr.* **1994**, *112*, 1747–1755.

22. Grey, V.; Mohammed, S.R.; Smountas, A.A.; Bahlool, R.; Lands, L.C. Improved glutathione status in young adult patients with cystic fibrosis supplemented with whey protein. *J. Cyst. Fibros.* **2003**, *2*, 195–198.
23. Leitner, M.; Menzies, S.; Lutz, C. *Working with ALS Mice: Guidelines for Preclinical Testing & Colony Management*; Available online: http://jaxmice.jax.org/literature/factsheet/working_with_ALS_mice.pdf (accesssed on 04 June 2014).
24. Weydt, P.; Hong, S.Y.; Kliot, M.; Moller, T. Assessing disease onset and progression in the SOD1 mouse model of ALS. *Neuroreport* **2003**, *14*, 1051–1054.
25. Ludolph, A.C.; Bendotti, C.; Blaugrund, E.; Chio, A.; Greensmith, L.; Loeffler, J.P.; Mead, R.; Niessen, H.G.; Petri, S.; Pradat, P.F.; *et al.* Guidelines for preclinical animal research in ALS/MND: A consensus meeting. *Amyotroph. Lateral Scler.* **2010**, *11*, 38–45.
26. Jarrett, S.G.; Milder, J.B.; Liang, L.P.; Patel, M. The ketogenic diet increases mitochondrial glutathione levels. *J. Neurochem.* **2008**, *106,* 1044–1051.
27. Liang, L.P.; Patel, M. Mitochondrial oxidative stress and increased seizure susceptibility in *Sod2*$^{-/+}$ mice. *Free Radic. Biol. Med.* **2004**, *36*, 542–554.
28. Wilkins, H.M.; Kirchhof, D.; Manning, E.; Joseph, J.W.; Linseman, D.A. Mitochondrial glutathione transport is a key determinant of neuronal susceptibility to oxidative and nitrosative stress. *J. Biol. Chem.* **2013**, *288*, 5091–5101.
29. Miller, R.G.; Mitchell, J.D.; Lyon, M.; Moore, D.H. Riluzole for amyotrophic lateral sclerosis (ALS)/motor neuron disease (MND). *Cochrane Database Syst. Rev.* **2012**, doi:10.1002/14651858.CD001447.pub2.
30. Gurney, M.E.; Cutting, F.B.; Zhai, P.; Doble, A.; Taylor, C.P.; Andrus, P.K.; Hall, E.D. Benefit of Vitamin E, riluzole, and gabapentin in a transgenic model of familial amyotrophic lateral sclerosis. *Ann. Neurol.* **1996**, *39*, 147–157.
31. Pearce, R.K.; Owen, A.; Daniel, S.; Jenner, P.; Marsden, C.D. Alterations in the distribution of glutathione in the substantia nigra in Parkinson's disease. *J. Neural Transm.* **1997**, *104*, 661–677.
32. Calabrese, V.; Sultana, R.; Scapagnini, G.; Guagliano, E.; Sapienza, M.; Bella, R.; Kanski, J.; Pennisi, G.; Mancuso, C.; Stella, A.M.; *et al.* Nitrosative stress, cellular stress response, and thiol homeostasis in patients with Alzheimer's disease. *Antioxid. Redox Signal.* **2006**, *8*, 1975–1986.
33. Iguchi, Y.; Katsuno, M.; Takagi, S.; Ishigaki, S.; Niwa, J.; Hasegawa, M.; Tanaka, F.; Sobue, G. Oxidative stress induced by glutathione depletion reproduces pathological modifications of TDP-43 linked to TDP-43 proteinopathies. *Neurobiol. Dis.* **2012**, *45*, 862–870.
34. Vargas, M.R.; Johnson, D.A.; Johnson, J.A. Decreased glutathione accelerates neurological deficit and mitochondrial pathology in familial ALS-linked hSOD1(G93A) mice model. *Neurobiol. Dis.* **2011**, *43*, 543–551.
35. Lands, L.C.; Grey, V.L.; Smountas, A.A. Effect of supplementation with a cysteine donor on muscular performance. *J. Appl. Physiol.* **1999**, *87*, 1381–1385.
36. Winter, A.W.; Ross, E.K.; Linseman, D.A. University of Denver, Denver, CO, USA. Unpublished work, 2014.
37. Cova, E.; Bongioanni, P.; Cereda, C.; Metelli, M.R.; Salvaneschi, L.; Bernuzzi, S.; Guareschi, S.; Rossi, B.; Ceroni, M. Time course of oxidant markers and antioxidant defenses in subgroups of amyotrophic lateral sclerosis patients. *Neurochem. Int.* **2010**, *56*, 687–693.

38. Muyderman, H.; Hutson, P.G.; Matusica, D.; Rogers, M.L.; Rush, R.A. The human G93A-superoxide dismutase-1 mutation, mitochondrial glutathione and apoptotic cell death. *Neurochem. Res.* **2009**, *34*, 1847–1856.
39. Liu, R.; Li, B.; Flanagan, S.W.; Oberley, L.W.; Gozal, D.; Qiu, M. Increased mitochondrial antioxidative activity or decreased oxygen free radical propagation prevent mutant SOD1-mediated motor neuron cell death and increase amyotrophic lateral sclerosis-like transgenic mouse survival. *J. Neurochem.* **2002**, *80*, 488–500.
40. Ferri, A.; Nencini, M.; Cozzolino, M.; Carrara, P.; Moreno, S.; Carri, M.T. Inflammatory cytokines increase mitochondrial damage in motoneuronal cells expressing mutant SOD1. *Neurobiol. Dis.* **2008**, *32*, 454–460.
41. Wilkins, H.M.; Marquardt, K.; Lash, L.H.; Linseman, D.A. Bcl-2 is a novel interacting partner for the 2-oxoglutarate carrier and a key regulator of mitochondrial glutathione. *Free Radic. Biol. Med.* **2012**, *52*, 410–419.
42. Mu, X.; He, J.; Anderson, D.W.; Trojanowski, J.Q.; Springer, J.E. Altered expression of Bcl-2 and bax mRNA in amyotrophic lateral sclerosis spinal cord motor neurons. *Ann. Neurol.* **1996**, *40*, 379–386.
43. Pasinelli, P.; Belford, M.E.; Lennon, N.; Bacskai, B.J.; Hyman, B.T.; Trotti, D.; Brown, R.H., Jr. Amyotrophic lateral sclerosis-associated SOD1 mutant proteins bind and aggregate with Bcl-2 in spinal cord mitochondria. *Neuron* **2004**, *43*, 19–30.
44. Xu, F.; Putt, D.A.; Matherly, L.H.; Lash, L.H. Modulation of expression of rat mitochondrial 2-oxoglutarate carrier in NRK-52E cells alters mitochondrial transport and accumulation of glutathione and susceptibility to chemically induced apoptosis. *J. Pharmacol. Exp. Ther.* **2006**, *316*, 1175–1186.
45. Papadimitriou, D.; Le Verche, V.; Jacquier, A.; Ikiz, B.; Przeborski, S.; Re, D.B. Inflammation in ALS and SMA: Sorting out the good from the evil. *Neurobiol. Dis.* **2010**, *37*, 493–502.
46. Philips, T.; Robberecht, W. Neuroinflammation in amyotrophic lateral scelerosis: Role of glial activation in motor neuron disease. *Lancet Neurol.* **2011**, *10*, 253–263.
47. Lee, M.; Cho, T.; Jantaratnotai, N.; Wang, Y.T.; McGeer, E.; McGeer, P.L. Depletion of GSH in glial cells incudces neurotoxicity: Relevance to aging and degenerative neurological diseases. *FASEB J.* **2010**, *24*, 2533–2545.
48. Lee, M.; Kwon, B.M.; Suk, K.; McGeer, E.; McGeer, P.L. Effects of obovatol on GSH depleted glia-mediated neurotoxicity and oxidative damage. *J. Neuroimmune Pharmacol.* **2012**, *7*, 173–186.
49. Moss, D.W.; Bates, T.E. Activation of murine microglial cells lines by lipopolysaccharide and interferon-γ causes NO-mediated decreases in mitochondrial and cellular function. *Eur. J. Neurosci.* **2001**, *13*, 529–538.
50. Barger, S.W.; Goodwin, M.E.; Porter, M.M.; Beggs, M.L. Glutamate release from activated microglia requires the oxidative burst and lipid peroxidation. *J. Neurochem.* **2007**, *101*, 1205–1213.
51. Seib, T.M.; Patel, S.A.; Bridges, R.J. Regulation of the system xc^- cystine/glutamate exchanger by intracellular glutathione levels in rat astrocytes primary cultures. *Glia* **2011**, *59*, 1387–1401.

52. Gabryel, B.; Malecki, A. Ebselen attenuates oxidative stress in ischemic astrocytes depleted of glutathione. Comarpison with glutathione precursors. *Pharmacol. Rep.* **2006**, *58*, 381–392.
53. Scott, S.; Kranz, J.E.; Cole, J.; Lincecum, J.M.; Thompson, K.; Kelly, N.; Bostrom, A.; Theodoss, J.; Al-Nakhala, B.M.; Vieira, F.G.; *et al.* Design, power, and interpretation of studies in the standard murine model of ALS. *Amyotroph. Lateral Scler.* **2008**, *9*, 4–15.
54. Wang, H.; O'Reilly, E.J.; Weisskopf, M.G.; Logroscino, G.; McCullough, M.L.; Schatzkin, A.; Kolonel, L.N.; Ascherio, A. Vitamin E intake and risk of amyotrophic lateral sclerosis: A pooled analysis of data from 5 prospective cohort studies. *Am. J. Epidemiol.* **2011**, *173*, 595–602.
55. Michal Freedman, D.; Kuncl, R.W.; Weinstein, S.J.; Malila, N.; Virtamo, J.; Albanes, D. Vitamin E serum levels and controlled supplementation and risk of amyotrophic lateral sclerosis. *Amyotroph. Lateral Scler. Front. Degener.* **2013**, *14*, 246–251.

12

Phenolic Content of *Hypodaphnis Zenkeri* and Its Antioxidant Effects against Fenton Reactions' Mediated Oxidative Injuries on Liver Homogenate

Bruno Moukette Moukette [1], Constant Anatole Pieme [1,*], Prosper Cabral Nya Biapa [2], Jacques Romain Njimou [3], Vicky Jocelyne Ama Moor [1], Marco Stoller [3], Marco Bravi [3] and Jeanne Yonkeu Ngogang [1]

[1] Laboratory of Biochemistry, Department of Biochemistry and Physiological Sciences; Faculty of Medicine and Biomedical Sciences, University of Yaoundé I, P.O. Box 1364 Yaounde, Cameroon; E-Mails: mouket2006@yahoo.fr (B.M.M.); movicky@yahoo.fr (V.J.A.M.); jngogang@yahoo.fr (J.Y.N.)

[2] Laboratory of Medecinal plant Biochemistry, Food Science and Nutrition, Department of Biochemistry, Faculty of Science, University of Dschang, P.O. Box 67 Dschang, Cameroon; E-Mail: brbiapa@yahoo.fr

[3] Department of Chemical Materials Environmental Engineering, Via Eudossiana 18, University of Rome "La Sapienza", 00185 Rome, Italy; E-Mails: jnjmou@yahoo.fr (J.R.N.); marco.stoller@uniroma1.it (M.S.); marco.bravi@uniroma1.it (M.B.)

* Author to whom correspondence should be addressed; E-Mail: apieme@yahoo.fr

External Editors: Antonio Segura-Carretero and David Arráez-Román

---

Abstract: Under oxidative stress conditions, endogenous antioxidant defenses are unable to completely inactivate the free radicals generated by an excessive production of reactive oxygen species (ROS). This state causes serious cell damage leading to a variety of human diseases. Natural antioxidants can protect cells against oxidative stress. *Hypaodaphnis zenkeri* (*H. zenkiri*) is a plant consumed as a spice in the Cameroonian diet, and its bark has been used in traditional medicine for the treatment of several diseases. The present study aims at investigating the antioxidant activity, which includes free radical scavenging and protective properties of an extract from *H. Zenkiri* against oxidative damage on a liver homogenate. The free radical assays determined the scavenging activities of

2,2-diphenyl-1-picrylhydrazyl (DPPH), hydroxyl (OH), nitrite oxide (NO) and 2,2-azinobis(3-ethylbenzthiazoline)-6-sulfonic acid (ABTS) radicals and the enzymes, whose protection was to be considered in the liver homogenate, including superoxide dismutase, catalase, and peroxidase. The antioxidative activities were studied using the ferric reducing antioxidant power (FRAP), reductive activity, and phosphomolybdenum antioxidant power (PAP) methods. In addition, the phenolic contents of the extracts were examined. The results showed that these extracts demonstrated significant scavenging properties and antioxidant activities, with the hydro-ethanolic extract of the bark of *H. zenkeri* (EEH) being the most potent. This extract had the highest total polyphenol (21.77 ± 0.05 mg caffeic acid (CAE)/g dried extract (DE)) and flavonoids (3.34 ± 0.13 mg quercetin (QE)/g dried extract) content. The same extract had significantly greater protective effects on enzyme activities compared to other extracts. The high performance liquied chromatography (HPLC) profile showed higher levels of caffeic acid, OH-tyrosol acid, and rutin in the leaves compared to the bark of *H. zenkeri*. In conclusion, the ethanolic and hydro-ethanolic extracts of the bark and leaves from *H. zenkeri* showed an antioxidant and protective potential against oxidative damage.

Keywords: *Hypodaphnis zenkeri*; polyphenols profile; antioxidant; liver homogenate

---

Abbreviations

MDA: malonaldialdehyde, DPPH: 2,2-diphenyl-1-picrylhydrazyl, FRAP: ferric reducing ability of plasma, Vit C: Vitamine C, ABTS: 2,2-azinobis(3-ethylbenzthiazoline)-6-sulfonic acid, BHT: butylated hydroxyl toluene, ROS: reactive oxygen species, FRAP: Ferric reducing antioxidant power, MDA: malon-dialdehyde, H_2O_2: hydrogen peroxide.

1. Introduction

Reactive oxygen species (ROS) are by-products of normal metabolism. They are produced in cells as a response to several factors, including oxidative and thermal stresses, ultraviolet light, chemical agents, and ionizing radiation. These species are known to play a dual role in biological systems, since they can be either harmful or beneficial to living systems [1]. Positive effects of ROS involve physiological roles in cellular responses, such as in defense against infectious agents and in the function of a number of cellular signaling systems. One further beneficial example of ROS at low concentrations is the induction of a mitogenic response [1].

A negative effect is that, in high concentrations, they lead to oxidative stress. This is described as a condition in which cellular antioxidant defenses are inadequate to completely inactivate the free radicals generated by an excessive production of ROS, loss of antioxidant defenses, or both [2]. Oxidative stress can cause DNA damage, cell functions inhibition, lipid and protein peroxidation, and disturbance of glutathione levels. In addition, ROS contribute to the development of cancer, diabetes, atherosclerosis, inflammatory diseases, and ageing [3].

It has been estimated that one human cell is exposed to approximately 1.5×10^5 oxidative hits a day from hydroxyl radicals and other such reactive species [3]. The generation of various free radicals is closely linked with the participation of redox-active metals [4]. The release of iron in the oxidative process is facilitated by $^{\bullet}O_2$, and the free ion participates in the Fenton reaction, generating the highly reactive hydroxyl radical [1,5]. Iron-mediated formation of ROS leads to DNA damage and, therefore, appears to be important for the development of cancer, since cancer cells are known to grow rapidly in response to iron [6]. Metal-induced generation of oxygen radicals results in the attack of not only DNA in the cell nucleus but also other cellular components involving polyunsaturated fatty acid residues of phospholipids, which are extremely sensitive to oxidation [7]. Lipid peroxidation is an oxidative deterioration of polyunsaturated lipids, and it involves ROS and transition metal ions, leading to the yielding of a wide range of cytotoxic products, most of which are aldehydes, like malon-dialdehyde (MDA) and 4-hydroxynonrnal (HNE) [8]. The oxidative state created by free radicals also deteriorates proteins with the introduction of carbonyl groups and the formation of protein-centered alkyl groups.

In order to contain the harmful effects of ROS, the body has natural antioxidants that are the cell's defense mechanisms such as glutathione, alpha-lipoic acid, coenzyme Q, ferritin, uric acid, bilirubin, metallothionein, L-carnitine, melatonin, enzymatic superoxide dismutase (SOD), catalase (CAT), glutathione peroxidases (GPXs), thioredoxins (TRX) and peroxiredoxins (PRXs) which scavenge reactive species [9–13]. Despite the presence of the cell's antioxidant defense system to counteract oxidative damage from ROS, oxidative damage accumulates during the life cycle and the natural defense could be overcome by the ROS [9]. There is currently immense interest in natural antioxidants and their role in human health and nutrition [14–16]. Considerable amount of data has been generated on antioxidant properties of food plants around the globe [12,17,18]. Fruits, vegetables, and herbs attract great attention due to their high content of bioactive compounds with antioxidant characteristics such as phenolic compounds [19,20]. Phenolic compounds are large and heterogeneous groups of secondary plant metabolites that are distributed throughout the plant kingdom. Phenolic compounds include flavonoids, tannins, and phenolic acids [21]. They have been implicated in a number of varied roles including ultra-violet (UV) protection, pigmentation, disease resistance, and nodule production.

Hypodaphnis zenkeri is a medium-sized tree of the Lauraceae family found mainly in tropical rain forests in Central and West Africa. *H. zenkiri* is a tree reaching a height of 20 to 25 m [22,23]. Its bark is consumed as a spice in Cameroon and is also used in traditional medicine [23,24]. The aqueous/ethanol extract of the bark of *H. zenkiri* have been postuled to possess quinones, tannins, terpenoids and reducing sugars with a great polyphenolic content and an antioxidant power in the 2,2-azinobis(3-ethylbenzthiazoline)-6-sulfonic acid (ABTS) assay [22–24]. A previous study demonstrated that the bark of *H. zenkiri* lowered blood glucose and ameliorated the lipid profile in triton W-1339 induced acute hyperlipidemic rats and rats fed with a high fat and high glucose diet [23]. However the different phenolic compounds are still unknown and the mechanism that is responsible for the antioxidant and the protective effect on hepatic enzymes is not yet elucidated.

The present study aims at determining the phenolic profile of *H. zenkiri* by high performance liquid chromatography (HPLC), investigating the free radical scavenging potential on various free radicals, providing further information on its antioxidant potential and studying its protective effect against oxidative mediated free radical damage on a liver homogenate.

2. Material and Methods

2.1. Plant Material

The leaves and barks of *H. zenkiri* were collected at the Kala Mountain in the central region of Cameroon. They were authenticated by Nana Pierre, a botanist at the National Herbarium of Cameroon, who compared them to the voucher specimens (16419/SFR/CAM).

2.2. Preparation of Plant Extracts

The collected leaves and barks were dried at ambient temperature, crushed, and sifted. The powders were then macerated at the ratio of 1:10 (w/v) for 48 h in ethanol for the ethanolic extract and in a mixture of water/ethanol (30/70; pH = 3) for the hydro-ethanolic extract. The mixtures were then filtered using a Buchner funnel (Thermo Fisher Scientific Inc., Waltham, MA, USA) and Whatman No. 1 filter paper (Whatman International, Maidstone, UK). This process was repeated once on the residue after 48 h. The supernatant was concentrated using a rotavaporator (Janke & Kunkel, Freiburg, Germany), and the extract was dried in an oven at 55 °C for two days. Each crude extract obtained was labeled using the following codes: EEE: *H. zenkeri* (bark) ethanolic extract; EFE: *H. zenkeri* (leaves) ethanolic extract; EEH: *H. zenkeri* (bark) hydro-ethanolic extract; EFH: *H. zenkeri* (leaves) hydro-ethanolic extract. The different samples were then kept at 4 °C. Prior to the experimentation, the samples of the four plant extracts were reconstituted using the appropriate solvent and different dilutions (25, 50, 75, 150, 300 μg/mL, respectively).

2.3. Determination of the Free Radical Scavenging and Antioxidant Properties

2.3.1. Determination of the Free Radical Scavenging Potential of the Samples

2.3.1.1. Scavenging Activity of the 2,2-Diphenyl-1-Picrylhydrazyl (DPPH) Radical

This assay measures the free radical scavenging capacity of the investigated extracts [25]. Briefly, in 3 mL of each diluted extract or vitamin C used as standard, 1 mL of methanol solution of DPPH 0.1 mM was added. The mixture was kept in the dark at room temperature for 30 min and the absorbance was measured at 517 nm against a blank. The following equation was used to determine the percentage of the radical scavenging activity of each extract.

$$Scavenging\ effect\ (\%) = 100 \times (A_o - A_s)/A_o \quad (1)$$

where A_o is the absorbance of the blank and A_s the absorbance of the sample.

2.3.1.2. Scavenging Effect of the $ABTS^+$ Radical

The ABTS assay was based on a previously described method [26] with slight modifications. The ABTS radical cation ($ABTS^+$) was produced by the reaction of a 7 mM ABTS solution with 2.45 mM potassium persulfate. The mixture was stored in the dark at room temperature for 12 h before use. The $ABTS^+$ solution was diluted with ethanol to obtain an absorbance of 0.70 ± 0.05 at 734 nm. After addition of 25 μL of extract samples or vitamin C used as standard to 2 mL of diluted $ABTS^+$

solution, absorbance was measured at 734 nm after exactly 6 min. The decrease in absorption was used for calculating scavenging effect values. The following equation was used to determine the percentage of the radical scavenging activity of each extract.

$$Scavenging\ effect\ (\%) = 100 \times (A_o - A_s)/A_o \quad (2)$$

where A_o is the absorbance of the blank; A_s is the absorbance of the sample.

2.3.1.3. Nitric Oxide Scavenging Activity

Nitric oxide scavenging activity was determined according to the Griess Illosvoy reaction [27]. The reaction mixture contained 2 mL of 10 mM SNP (sodium nitro-prusside) in 0.5 mL of phosphate buffer (0.5 M; pH 7.4). Various concentrations (25, 50, 75, 150, 300 µg/mL) of the extracts (0.5 mL) were added in a final volume of 3 mL. After incubation for 60 min at 37 °C, Griess reagent (0.1% α-napthyl-ethylenediamine in water and 1% sulfanilic acid in 5% H_3PO_4) was added. The pink chromophore generated during diazotization of nitrite ions with sulfanilamide and subsequent coupling with α-napthyl-ethylenediamine was measured spectrophotometrically at 540 nm. Ascorbic acid was used as a positive control. Nitric oxide scavenging ability (%) was calculated using the formula:

$$\text{Percentage of NO radical scavenging activity (\%)} = 100 \times (A_o - A_s)/A_o \quad (3)$$

where A_o is the absorbance of the blank and A_s the absorbance of the sample.

2.3.1.4. Hydroxyl Radical Scavenging Activity

The scavenging activity of the extracts on the hydroxyl radical was measured according to a previously described method [28]. In 1.5 mL of each diluted extract, 60 µL of $FeCl_3$ (1 mM), 90 µL of 1,10-Phenanthroline (1 mM), 2.4 mL of 0.2 M phosphate buffer, (pH 7.8) and 150 µL of H_2O_2 (0.17 M) were added, respectively. The mixture was then homogenized and incubated at room temperature for 5 min. The absorbance was read at 560 nm against the blank. The percentage of the radical scavenging activity of each extract was calculated from the equation below:

$$\text{Percentage of OH radical scavenging activity (\%)} = 100 \times (A_o - A_s)/A_o \quad (4)$$

where A_o is the absorbance of the blank and A_s the absorbance of the sample.

2.3.2. Determination of the Total Antioxidant Potential of the Different Samples

2.3.2.1. Total Antioxidant Activity by Ferric Reducing Antioxidant Power Assay (FRAP)

The FRAP was determined using a previously described method [29] with slight modifications. The fresh FRAP reagent consisted of 500 mL of acetate buffer (300 mM pH 3, 6), 50 mL of 2,4,6-Tri (2-pyridyl)-*s*-triazin (TPTZ) (10 mM), and 50 mL of $FeCl_3 \cdot 6H_2O$ (50 mM). The colorimetric measurement was performed at 593 nm, and the reaction was monitored up to 12 min using the mixture of 75 µL of each extract and 2 mL of FRAP reagent. The ascorbic acid was used to draw a standard curve and the butylated hydroxyl toluene (BHT) was used for the comparison. The absorbance was read at 593 nm. The result where expressed as mg equivalent vitamin C/g of dried extract (mg eq Vit C/g DE).

2.3.2.2. Phosphomolybdenum Antioxidant Power (PAP)

The total antioxidant activity of extracts was evaluated by green phosphomolybdenum complex according to a described method [30]. An aliquot of 10 μL of extract samples solution was mixed with 900 μL of reagent solution (0.6 M sulphuric acid, 28 mM sodium phosphate and 4 mM ammonium molybdate) in a micro centrifuge tube for a final volume of 1 mL. Tubes were incubated in a dry thermal bath at 95 °C for 90 min. After cooling, the absorbance of the mixture was measured at 695 nm against a blank. Ascorbic acid was used as reference to draw the standard curve and BHT was used as comparison. The reducing capacities of the analyzed extracts were expressed as mg of ascorbic acid (AS) equivalents/g of dried extract (mg eq AS/g DE).

2.3.2.3. Reducing Power Assay

The reducing power of the extracts was determined by a method described by Oyaizu (1996) [31]. Different concentrations (25, 50, 75, 150, 300 μg/mL) of extracts in 1 mL of distilled water were mixed with 2.5 mL of phosphate buffer (0.2 M, pH 6.6) and 2.5 mL of potassium ferrocyanide (1%). The mixture was incubated at 50 °C for 20 min. Aliquots (2.5 mL) of trichloroacetic acid (10%) were added to the mixture and centrifuged at 3000 rpm for 10 min. The upper layer of the solution (2.5 mL) was mixed with 2.5 mL of distilled water and 0.5 mL of $FeCl_3$ (0.1%). Increasing absorbance was measured at 700 nm against the blank indicates increased reducing power.

2.3.3. Determination of the Phenolic Content of Extracts

2.3.3.1. Total Phenol Determination

The total phenol was determined by the Folin–Ciocalteu method [32], the reaction mixture contained 200 μL of diluted extracts, 800 μL of freshly prepared diluted Folin Ciocalteu reagent and 2 mL of 7.5% sodium carbonate. The final mixture was diluted to 7 mL with deionized water and kept in the dark at ambient conditions for 2 h to complete the reaction. The absorbance at 765 nm was measured. Caffeic acid was used as standard, and the results were expressed as mg caffeic acid/g dried extract (mg CAE/g DE).

2.3.3.2. Determination of Total Flavonoid Content

Total flavonoid content was determined using aluminum chloride ($AlCl_3$) according to a known method [33] using quercetin as a standard. Extract (0.1 mL) was added to 0.3 mL distilled water followed by 0.03 mL of $NaNO_2$ (5%). After incubation of 5 min at 25 °C, 0.03 mL of $AlCl_3$ (10%) was added. After a further 5 min, the reaction mixture was treated with 0.2 mL of 1 mM NaOH. Finally, the reaction mixture was diluted to 1 mL with water and the absorbance was measured at 510 nm. The results were expressed as mg quercetin (QE) of dried extract (mg QE/g DE).

2.3.3.3. Determination of Total Flavonols

Total flavonols in the plant extracts were estimated using a known method [34] with modifications. To 2.0 mL of sample or standard, 2.0 mL of $AlCl_3$ (2%) and 3.0 mL of sodium acetate solution

(50 g/L) were added. The mixture was incubated for 2.5 h at 20 °C and the absorption was read at 440 nm. Extract samples were evaluated at a final concentration of 0.1 mg/mL. Total flavonols content was calculated as quercetin (mg/g) using the equation $y = 5.3911\,x + 0.0313$; $R^2 = 0.9967$, where x is the absorbance and y, the concentration of quercetin equivalent of dried extract (mg QE/g DE).

2.3.4. Quantification of Phenolics by HPLC

High Performance Liquid Chromatography (HPLC) with ultra violet (UV) detection is frequently used for the separation and detection of phenolic compounds present in extracts. Samples were dissolved in pure water according to the ratio (0.3 g/10mL) and centrifuged at 4706 rpm for 10 min. The supernatant was filtered through a cellulose acetate membrane filter (0.20 μm or 0.45 μm, Schleicher & Schuell, Roma, Italy) and used for analysis. A portion of 25 μL of the filtrate was injected into the HPLC system and eluted as described below. The analysis was performed on an Agilent Technologies 1200 HPLC system fitted with a SUPELCOSIL LC-18 column (length 250 mm, diameter 4.6 mm, packaging size 5 mm, (TK mediterranea™ Sea 18, Roma, Italy). The column temperature was set at 20 °C. The mobile phase consisted of a mixture of an aqueous solution of acetic acid at 0.5% by volume (A) and acetic nitrile (B). Elution was performed by according to the following protocol:

- At start and for the first 2 min of the run, 100% of A.
- From 2 min to 60 min after the run start, a linear composition ramp was used, targeting 40% of A and 60% of B.

The flow rate was set equal to 1 mL/min. Polyphenols were detected by a UV detector (280 nm, TK mediterranea™ Sea 18, Roma, Italy). Beforehand, the retention times of the identified polyphenolic compounds of interest available were measured by using of single standard solution at a concentration of 100 mg/L.

2.3.5. Protective Properties of the Plant against Oxidative Damage

2.3.5.1. Preparation of Liver Homogenate

The liver was isolated from three normal albino *Wistar* rats. The organs were weighed and 10% (w/v), the homogenate was prepared in phosphate buffer (0.1 M, pH 7.4 having 0.15 M KCl) using the homogenizer at 4 °C [35]. The homogenate was centrifuged at 3000 rpm for 15 min and the clear cell-free supernatant obtained was used for the study.

2.3.5.2. Preparation of the Pro-Oxidative Solution

The oxidant solution was prepared immediately before its utilization by adding a solution of ferric chloride 100 mM to H_2O_2 0.50% prepared in phosphate buffer (0.1 M, pH 7.4). This solution was used for the investigation of the protective assays on liver enzymes.

2.3.5.3. Total Protein Content

The total protein content of the mixture of liver was measured according to the protein kit supplier method (Human Kit-Hu102536, Humann, Wiesbaden, Germany). This result was used to express the activities of the different enzymes per gram of organs.

2.3.5.4. *In Vitro* Lipid Peroxidation Assay

Lipid peroxidation assay was performed by a formerly described protocol [10]. Phosphate buffer 0.58 mL (0.1 M; pH 7.4), 200 µL sample, 200 µL liver homogenate, and 20 µL ferric chloride (100 mM) were combined to form a mixture, which was placed in a shaking water bath for 1 h at 37 °C. The reaction was terminated by adding 1 mL trichloroacetic acid (10%), 2-thiobarbituric acid 1 mL (0.67%) to all the tubes, which were placed in a boiling water bath for 20 min. Then the test tubes were shifted to a crushed ice bath and were centrifuged at 3000 rpm for 10 min. Absorbance of the supernatant was checked at 535 nm and was calculated as nM of MDA tissue using a molar extinction coefficient of 1.56×10^5/M.cm.

2.3.5.5. Determination of Peroxidase Activity

Peroxidase activity was determined by the peroxidase kit (CAS Number 7722-84-1, Munich, Germany) supplier with modifications. A solution containing the mixture of 1 mL of the oxidant solution ($FeCl_3$, 100 mM) and extract or vitamin C (standard) for a final concentration of 100 µg/mL was incubated for 1 h in a water bath at 37 °C. An aliquot of phosphase buffered saline (PBS) (0.1 mL), hydrogen peroxide (50 µL), and pyrogallol solution (110 µL) were added to distilled water (625 µL) that had been dispensed into an Eppendorf tube (Fisher Scientific, Wohlen, Switzerland). The plant extract (75 µL) from the mixture was thereafter added. For the blank, the control oxidant solution and the vitamin C as standard, the same reagents were used, except the extract, which was replaced by distilled water (75 µL). The reaction was mixed and incubated for at least 10 min. The solution containing 100 mM, pH 6.0 PBS (40 µL) and 0.002% (v/v) diluted liver homogenate (40 µL) was added to the blank and test mixtures, respectively. These were mixed, and the increase in absorbance at 420 nm was measured every 10 s for 3 min using a spectrophotometer (BioMate 3S UV-Visible, Thermo Scientific™, Wohlen, Switzerland). One unit of peroxidase was defined as the change in absorbance/seconds/mg of protein at 420 nm using molar extinction coefficient of 12/M.cm.

2.3.5.6. Determination of Catalase Activity

Prior to the test, a solution containing a mixture of 1 mL of total volume of the oxidant solution and extract or vitamin C (standard) for a final concentration of 100 µg/mL was incubated for 1 h in a water bath at 37 °C. The catalase activity of liver homogenate was assayed as previously described with modifications [10]. An aliquot of hydrogen peroxide (0.8 mL) was dispensed into an Eppendorf tube. Phosphate buffer (1.0 mL), extracted sample/vitamin C/oxidant solution (75 µL) and (0.002% v/v) diluted homogenate (125 µL) were added. The reaction mixture (0.5 mL) was dispensed into 5% dichromate reagent (1.0 mL) and vigorously shaken. The mixture was heated in a Clifton water bath for 10 min, and allowed to cool. The absorbance at 570 nm was taken using spectrophotometer

(BioMate 3S UV-Visible, Thermo Scientific™, Wohlen, Switzerland). The absorbance obtained was extrapolated from the following standard curve: $y = 0.0028\ x + 0.0132$. The catalase activity was thereafter expressed as Unit/min/mg of protein (UI/mg Prot.).

$$CAT(unit/mg\ protein) = (Abs/min \times 30000\ units)/(40cm/M \times mg\ protein) \times df \quad (5)$$

where df = dilution factor, Abs = absorbance.

2.3.5.7. Superoxide Dismutase (SOD) Activity

The measurement of total SOD activity was performed according to the Misra and Fridovich method [36] with some slight modifications. The principle of this method is based on the inhibition of epinephrine autoxidation. Distilled water (0.2 mL) and 2.5 mL sodium carbonate buffer 0.05 M, pH 10.2 were added to the 0.3 mL buffered epinephrine to initiate the reaction. The absorbance at 480 nm was read for 150 s at 30 s intervals against a blank made up of 2.5 mL buffer, 0.3mL epinephrine and 0.2 mL distilled water. The following equation allowed the calculation of the SOD activity:

$$SOD(unit/mg\ protein) = SOD(units/mL/min)/protein(mg/mL) \times df \quad (6)$$

where df = dilution factor. The SOD activity was there after expressed as Unit/min/mg of protein (UI/mg Prot.).

2.3.6. Statistical Analysis

The results were presented as mean ± SEM of triplicate assays. Analyses of data were conducted using one-way ANOVA (Analysis of variance) followed by the Kruskal Wallis test and Dunnett's multiple test (SPSS program version 18.0 for Windows, IBM Corporation, New York, NY, USA). The Log probit was used to determinate the IC_{50} using the software XLstat version 7 (Addinsoft, New York, NY, USA) were used to achieve the Pearson Correlation Analysis (PCA). The differences were considered as significant at $p < 0.05$.

3. Results and Discussion

In order to reduce the oxidative damage induced by free radicals in biological systems, several dietary sources of antioxidants have been investigated. Phytochemicals such as phenolic compounds and some amino acids, have been found to have outstanding antioxidant properties against some free radical species [37]. Regarding the increase of interest in natural antioxidant supplements from foods, medicinal plants, and spices, this study was designed to investigate the antioxidant properties of *H. zenkiri* used in Cameroon as a spice in several dishes. Antioxidant activity cannot be measured directly but rather by the effects of the antioxidant in controlling the extent of oxidation [38]. A rapid, simple, and inexpensive method to measure antioxidant capacity of food involves the use of the free radical 2,2-diphenyl-1-picrylhydrazyl (DPPH). The results of the scavenging activity using DPPH has shown that EEH extract has the highest and most significant ($p < 0.05$) scavenging potential among the extracts with a percentage of inhibition of 27.27% ± 0.45% at the concentration of 25 µg/mL to 81.61% ± 0.66% at 300 µg/mL followed by EEE (Figure 1). However, this result is lower than the activity vitamin C, which was used as control. EFE and EFH showed the lowest scavenging powers at all the concentrations. Our results corroborate previous findings that stated that phenolic compounds generally exhibited significant scavenging effects against the DPPH free radical [9,38]. DPPH is widely used to test the ability of compounds to act as free radical scavengers or hydrogen donors. It has been used to quantify the antioxidants in complex biological systems. The DPPH method can be used for solid or liquid samples, and it is not specific to any particular antioxidant component, but applies to the overall antioxidant capacity of the sample. A measure of total antioxidant capacity helps in the understanding of functional properties of foods [13]. The hydroxyl radical scavenging potential of the different extracts displayed in Figure 2 demonstrated that all the tested extracts scavenged the OH radical with variable scavenging powers depending on the type of extract and the concentration. The inhibitory properties of EEE and EEH extracts increased from 23.86% ± 0.28% to 86.61% ± 1.25% and from 17.37% ± 5.42% to 82.61% ± 0.28%, respectively, demonstrating that they have almost similar and the highest scavenging power of the substances tested. Vitamin C showed the significant < highest ($p < 0.05$) overall potential. Our results show that these plant extracts have the ability to inhibit the non-specific hydroxyl radical, preventing it from reacting with polyunsaturated fatty acid moieties of cell membrane phospholipids and thereby causing damage to cells [39].

Figure 1. 2,2-diphenyl-1-picrylhydrazyl (DPPH) scavenging potential of the different plant extracts. Values are expressed as mean ± standard deviation (SD) of three replicates. In the same concentration the values affected with different letter are significantly different at $p < 0.05$. EEE: *H. zenkeri (*bark) ethanolic extract; EFE: *H. zenkeri* (leaves) ethanolic extract; EEH: *H. zenkeri* (bark) hydro-ethanolic extract; EFH: *H. zenkeri* (leaves) hydro-ethanolic extract; Vit C: Vitamin C.

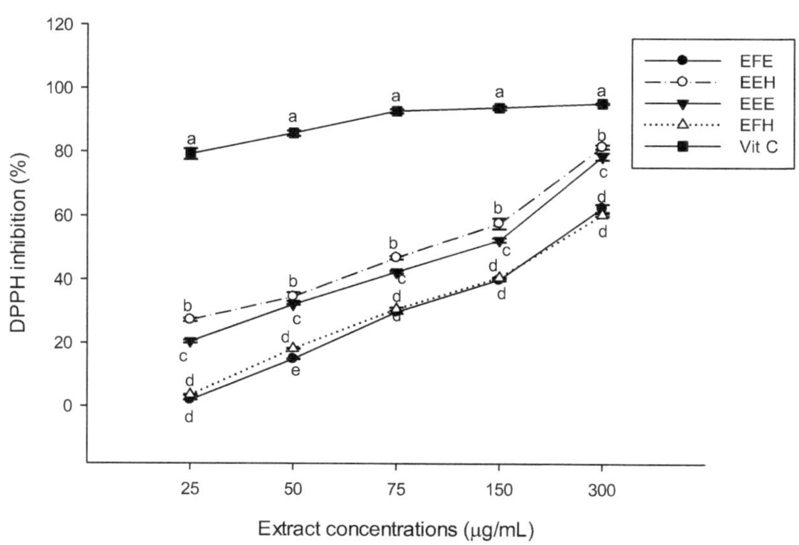

Figure 2. Hydroxyl radical (OH) scavenging potential of the different plant extracts. Values are expressed as mean ± SD of three replicates. In the same concentration the values affected with different letter are significantly different at $p < 0.05$. EEE: *H. zenkeri (*bark) ethanolic extract; EFE: *H. zenkeri* (leaves) ethanolic extract; EEH: *H. zenkeri* (bark) hydro-ethanolic extract; EFH: *H. zenkeri* (leaves) hydro-ethanolic extract; Vit C: Vitamin C.

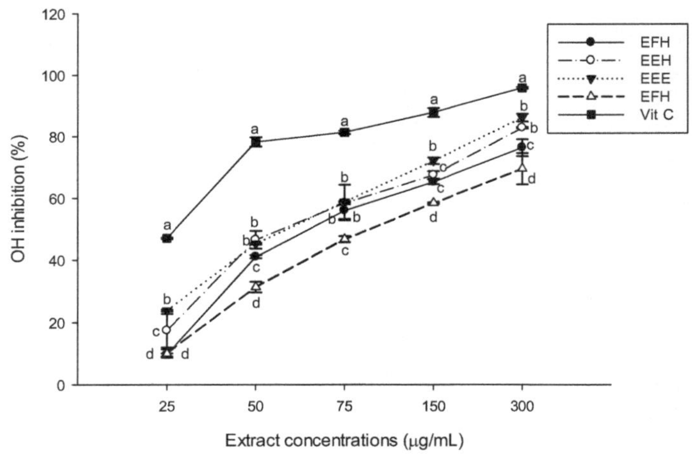

The nitric oxide (NO) scavenging assay measures the ability of the extract to chelate NO using the Griess reaction. The nitrite ions were generated from sodium nitroprusside in aqueous solution at a physiological pH, which reacted with oxygen [39]. The different extracts scavenged the NO radical in a concentration-dependent manner (Figure 3). Among the tested extracts, EEE and EEH were the significantly ($p < 0.05$) most potent at all the concentrations but their NO scavenging capacities were lower than that of vitamin C. The lowest scavenging activity was shown by EFE. EFE therefore demonstrates the ability of *H zenkiri* to be a potential free radical quencher.

Figure 3. Nitric oxide radical (NO) scavenging potential of the different plant extracts. Values are expressed as mean ± SD of three replicates. In the same concentration the values labeled with different letters differ significantly at $p < 0.05$. EEE: *H. zenkeri* (bark) ethanolic extract; EFE: *H. zenkeri* (leaves) ethanolic extract; EEH: *H. zenkeri* (bark) hydro-ethanolic extract; EFH: *H. zenkeri* (leaves) hydro-ethanolic extract; Vit C: Vitamin C.

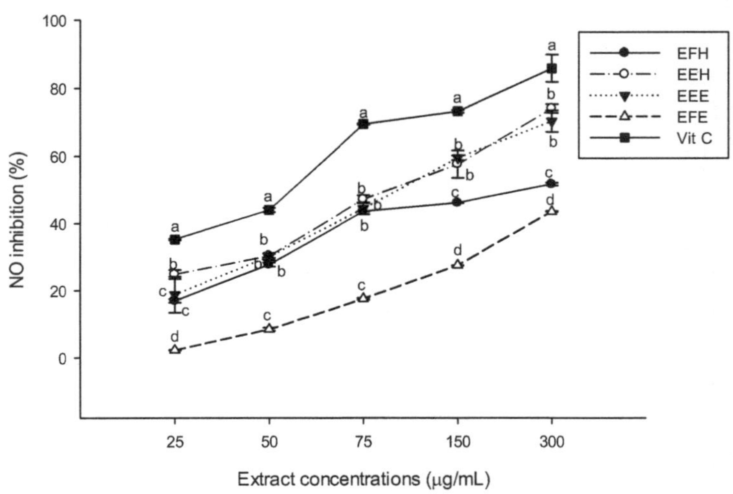

The ABTS method has the extra flexibility in that it can be used at different pH levels and is thus useful when studying the effect of pH on antioxidant activity of various compounds. It is also useful for measuring antioxidant activity of samples extracted in acidic solvents [13]. The inhibitory potential on the ABTS radical of the extracts showed that all the tested samples inhibited the ABTS radical, and the inhibition percentage increased with concentration (Figure 4). The extract EEH had a significantly ($p < 0.05$) more powerful inhibitory potential while the EFH and EFE extracts had the lowest scavenging potentials at all the concentrations. This result suggests that our extracted phytochemicals could act as radical scavengers owing to their hydrogen and electron donating capacity and their ability to delocalize/stabilize the resulting phenoxyl radical within the structure [40].

Figure 4. The 2,2-azinobis(3-ethylbenzthiazoline)-6-sulfonic acid (ABTS) scavenging potential of the different plant extracts. Values are expressed as mean ± SD of three replicates. In the same concentration the values labeled with different letters differ significantly at $p < 0.05$. EEE: *H. zenkeri (*bark) ethanolic extract; EFE: *H. zenkeri* (leaves) ethanolic extract; EEH: *H. zenkeri* (bark) hydro-ethanolic extract; EFH: *H. zenkeri* (leaves) hydro-ethanolic extract; Vit C: Vitamin C.

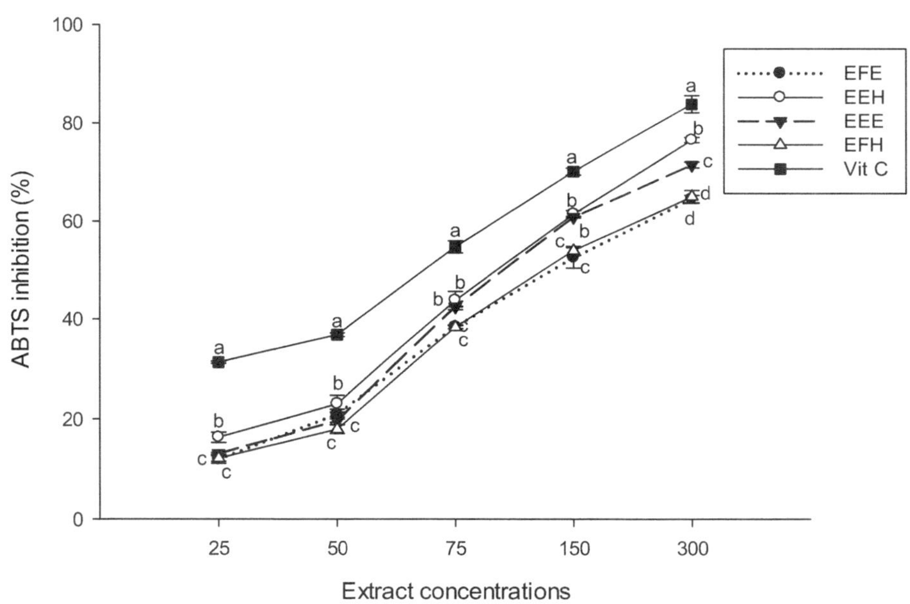

The reducing capacity of extracts may serve as an indicator of their potential antioxidant activity. Higher absorbance indicates a higher reducing power and higher antioxidant activity [37]. The results of the reductive power of the different extracts revealed that the extract EEE had the highest activity of all extracts (Figure 5). The other extracts exhibited poor activity and were not significantly ($p < 0.05$) different at the concentrations that were used in this study. Vitamin C that was used as standard showed the highest activity at all the concentrations. This activity could be attributed to phenolic compounds that have been identified in these extracts.

The ferric reducing antioxidant power (FRAP) method is based on the reduction of a ferroin analog, the Fe^{3+} complex of tripyridyltriazine $Fe(TPTZ)^{3+}$, to the intensely blue colored Fe^{2+} complex $Fe(TPTZ)^{2+}$ by antioxidants in acidic medium. The resulting FRAP activity is shown by the increase of the absorbance at 593 nm [38]. The FRAP anti-oxidative power of the different tested extracts is represented in Figure 6. These results show that EEH has the significantly ($p < 0.05$) highest antioxidant power among the tested extracts (32.79 ± 1.46 mg eq Vit C/g DE) followed by EEE (28.05 ± 0.24 mg eq Vit C/g DE). The amount of Fe^{3+} ions reduced to Fe^{2+} ions varied with the concentration of phenols. The BHT used as standard had the highest and most significant ($p < 0.05$) FRAP antioxidant power.

Figure 5. Reductive activity of the different plant extracts. Values are expressed as mean ± SD of three replicates. In the same concentration the values labeled with different letters differ significantly at $p < 0.05$. EEE: *H. zenkeri (*bark) ethanolic extract; EFE: *H. zenkeri* (leaves) ethanolic extract; EEH: *H. zenkeri* (bark) hydro-ethanolic extract; EFH: *H. zenkeri* (leaves) hydro-ethanolic extract; Vit C: Vitamin C.

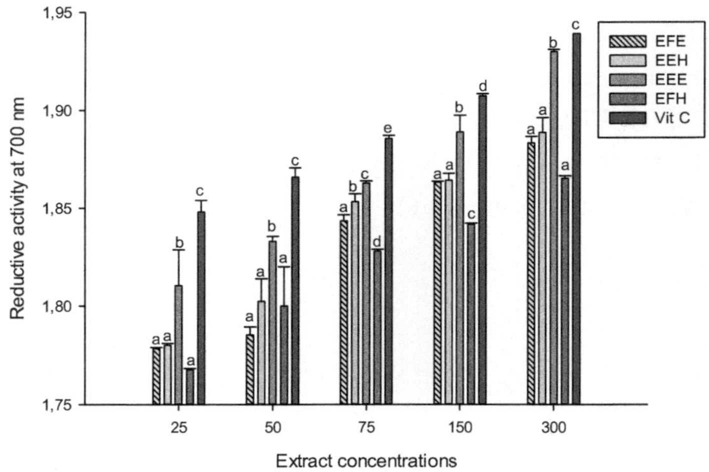

Figure 6. Ferric reducing antioxidant power (FRAP) antioxidant activities of the different plant extracts. Values are expressed as mean ± SD of three replicates. The values labeled with different letters differ significantly different at $p < 0.05$. EEE: *H. zenkeri (*bark) ethanolic extract; EFE: *H. zenkeri* (leaves) ethanolic extract; EEH: *H. zenkeri* (bark) hydro-ethanolic extract; EFH: *H. zenkeri* (leaves) hydro-ethanolic extract; BHT: butylated hydroxyl toluene.

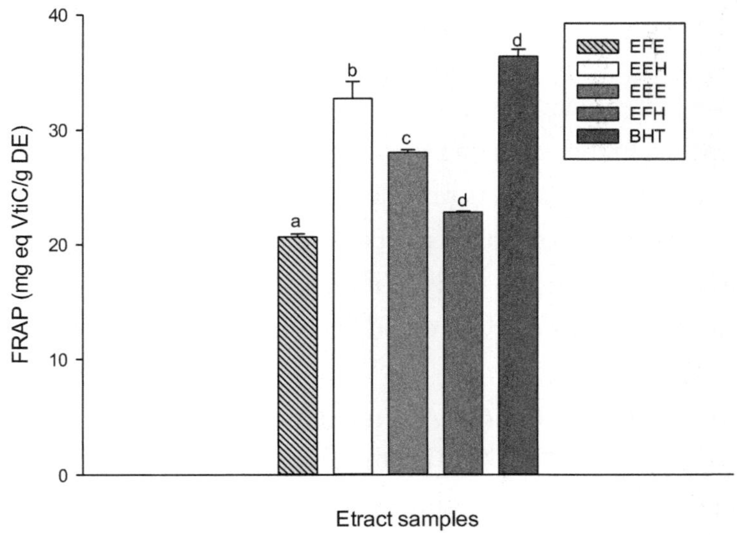

The results of the phosphomolybdenum antioxidative power (PAP) of the different samples presented in Figure 7 showed that all the tested extracts had a PAP and that this property varied with the type of extract. The EEH extract showed the higher PAP among the extracts (173.58 ± 9.37 mg eq Vit C/g DE). The above results are similar to that of the BHT (178.26 ± 2.42 mg eq Vit C/g DE). These results support the hypothesis that our extract could act also as ion chelator.

Phenolic compounds are involved in repair and adaptive systems and can act preventively or therapeutically in various diseases [40,41]. Table 1 presents the phenolic composition of the different extracts. These results show that the extract EEH (21.77 ± 0.05 caffeic acid (CAE)/g DE) has the highest total phenol concentration followed by EEE (18.38 ± 0.09 CAE/g DE). Similar results were noted for flavonoids and flavonols. These results underline the high antioxidant activities observed in EEH and EEE extracts. There is a strong relationship between total phenolic and flavonoid contents and antioxidant, free radical scavenging activities in many plants although this depends on their proportions in the plants [40].

Figure 7. Phosphomolybdenum antioxidative power (PAP) of the different plant extracts. Values are expressed as mean ± SD of three replicates. The values labeled with different letters differ significantly at $p < 0.05$. EEE: *H. zenkeri (*bark) ethanolic extract; EFE: *H. zenkeri* (leaves) ethanolic extract; EEH: *H. zenkeri* (bark) hydro-ethanolic extract; EFH: *H. zenkeri* (leaves) hydro-ethanolic extract; BHT: butylated hydroxyl toluene.

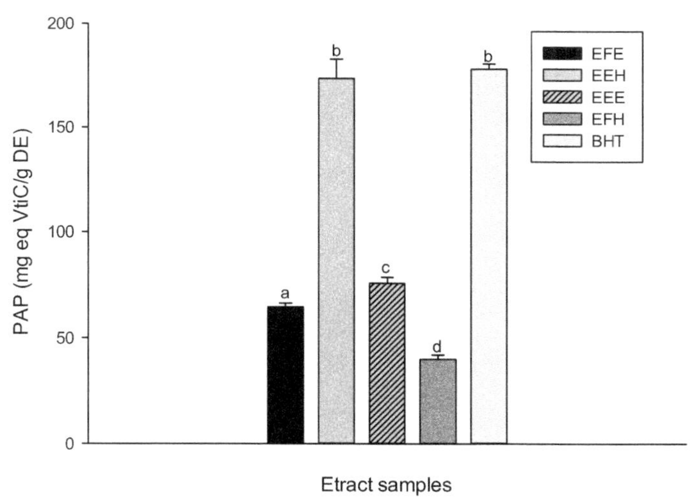

Table 1. Total phenol, flavonoid, and flavonol contents of the different plant extracts.

Samples	Phytochemicals		
	Total Phenols (mg CAE/g DE)	Flavonoids (mg QE/g DE)	Flavonols (mg CAE/g DE)
EEE	18.38 ± 0.09 [a]	2.58 ± 0.57 [a]	1.10 ± 0.41 [a]
EEH	21.77 ± 0.05 [b]	3.34 ± 0.13 [a]	1.47 ± 0.03 [a]
EFH	10.70 ± 0.01 [c]	1.40 ± 0.35 [b]	0.71 ± 0.06 [b]
EFE	7.21 ± 0.05 [d]	0.50 ± 0.18 [c]	0.27 ± 0.01 [c]

Values are expressed as mean ± SD of three replicates. The values labeled with different letters differ significantly at $p < 0.05$. EEE: *H. zenkeri (*bark) ethanolic extract; EFE: *H. zenkeri* (leaves) ethanolic extract; EEH: *H. zenkeri* (bark) hydro-ethanolic extract; EFH: *H. zenkeri* (leaves) hydro-ethanolic extract. DE: dried extract; QE: quercetin; CAE; caffeic acid.

Lipid peroxidation is one of the major ways by which ROS cause cell damage since peroxidation results in changes in fluidity, membrane permeability, and alteration of functions of proteins that are embedded in the membrane [42]. Natural products from medicinal plants can reduce this deleterious process [10]. The protective effects of the extracts tested against lipid peroxidation are presented in Figure 8. This result shows a significant ($p < 0.05$) increase of the oxidant level (positive) (122.95 ± 2.42 nM) compared to the normal (negative) (65.13 ± 0.72 nM). The different tested extracts have shown the reduction in MDA level. The extract EEH has the most significant and highest inhibition (73.21 ± 3.02 nM) as demonstrated by its lowest MDA level. This result suggests that the polyphenol compounds present in the extract may either delay or inhibit the initiation step of lipid peroxidation by reacting with a lipid radical or by inhibiting their propagation step or by reacting with peroxyl or alkoxyl radicals [38,43]. Also, the antioxidants from the extracts may further interfere with chain propagation reactions by forming peroxy-antioxidant stable compounds [38]. ROS damage macromolecules in cells and have been involved in the etiologies or manifestations of several pathological processes [2,44]. Antioxidant enzymes are capable of eliminating ROS and lipid peroxidation products, therefore, they can protect cells and tissues from oxidative damage. Antioxidant enzymes include SOD, catalase and peroxidases. SOD is a key enzyme in the natural defense against free radicals, and its determinant role has been described [45]. It is well known that the superoxide ion (O_2^-) is the starting point in the chain production of free radicals. At this early stage, superoxide dismutase inactivates the superoxide ion by transforming it into hydrogen peroxide (H_2O_2) [45]. The SOD activity of the different tested samples showed an increase of the SOD activity of the different extracts compared to the oxidant 2.22 ± 0.16 UI/mg Prot. (Figure 9). The extracts EEE and EEH showed the highest activities with values of 5.79 ± 0.02 UI/mg Prot and 6.13 ± 0.03 UI/mg Prot., respectively). This result suggests that our extracts contain molecules that enable them to act as secondary or preventative antioxidants that retard the rate of oxidation. These extracts may achieve this activity through several ways including the removal of substrate or singlet oxygen quenching therefore protecting the enzymes [38]. Hydrogen peroxide (H_2O_2), a highly ROS, is produced as the result of SOD reactions [46]. The catalase activity recorded in the different groups is displayed in Figure 10. This result shows a significant ($p < 0.05$) decrease of the catalase activity in the oxidant (positive) (5.22 ± 0.92 UI/mg Prot.) compared to the negative (40.88 ± 2.66 UI/mg Prot.). This activity increases in the different extracts tested with the EEH extract showing the significant and higher activity (101.67 ± 0.92 UI/mg Prot.). The catalases provide protection against the toxic effects of H_2O_2 that is generated in respiring cells due to its catalytic function [44,47].
This protective potential of plant extracts against enzyme depletion has been attributed to phenolic compounds [41]. Functionally, catalases are related to peroxidases which both degrade H_2O_2 to O_2 and H_2O [44]. The protective effect of the different plant extracts on peroxidase activity is presented in Figure 11. This result shows the increase of the peroxidase activity of different extracts compared to the oxidant (positive) control. Among the tested samples, the extracts EEH (9.25 ± 0.40 UI/mg Prot.) and EEE (8.97 ± 0.19 UI/mg Prot.) show similar results to vitamin C (9.38 ± 0.14 UI/mg Prot.). This result confirms that phenolic compounds can act as ion chelators and can, therefore, prevent the involvement of hydroxyl radical in Fenton reactions, which can generate higher concentrations of hydroxyl radicals that could in turn injure macromolecules such as enzymes [10,40].

Figure 8. Protective properties of plant extracts against lipid peroxidation. Values are expressed as mean ± SD of three replicates. In the same column the values labeled with different letters differ significantly at $p < 0.05$. EEE: *H. zenkeri (*bark) ethanolic extract; EFE: *H. zenkeri* (leaves) ethanolic extract; EEH: *H. zenkeri* (bark) hydro-ethanolic extract; EFH: *H. zenkeri* (leaves) hydro-ethanolic extract; Vit C: Vitamin C. Pos Control: oxidant (positive) control. Neg Control: Normal (negative) control.

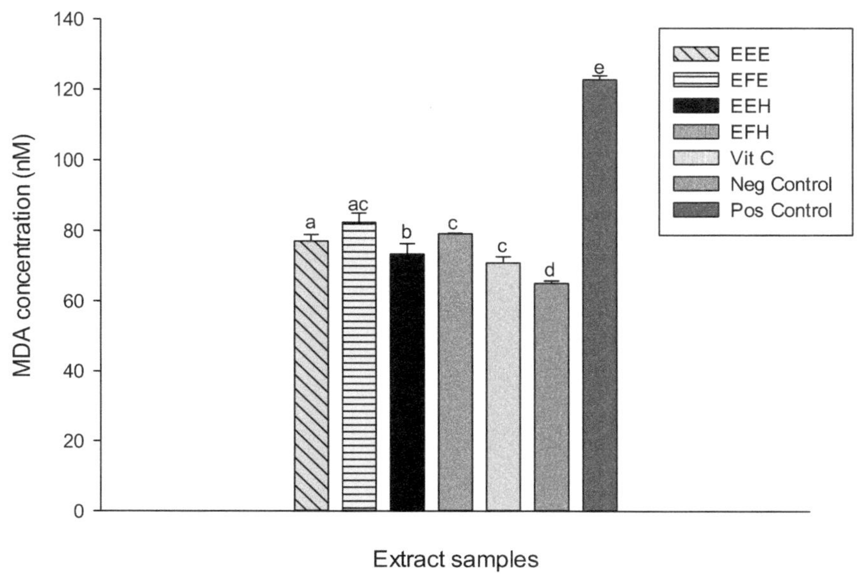

Figure 9. Protective properties of plant extracts: SOD activity. Values are expressed as mean ± SD of three replicates. In the same column the values labeled with different letters differ significantly at $p < 0.05$. EEE: *H. zenkeri (*bark) ethanolic extract; EFE: *H. zenkeri* (leaves) ethanolic extract; EEH: *H. zenkeri* (bark) hydro-ethanolic extract; EFH: *H. zenkeri* (leaves) hydro-ethanolic extract; Vit C: Vitamin C. Pos Control: oxidant (positive) control. Neg Control: Normal (negative) control.

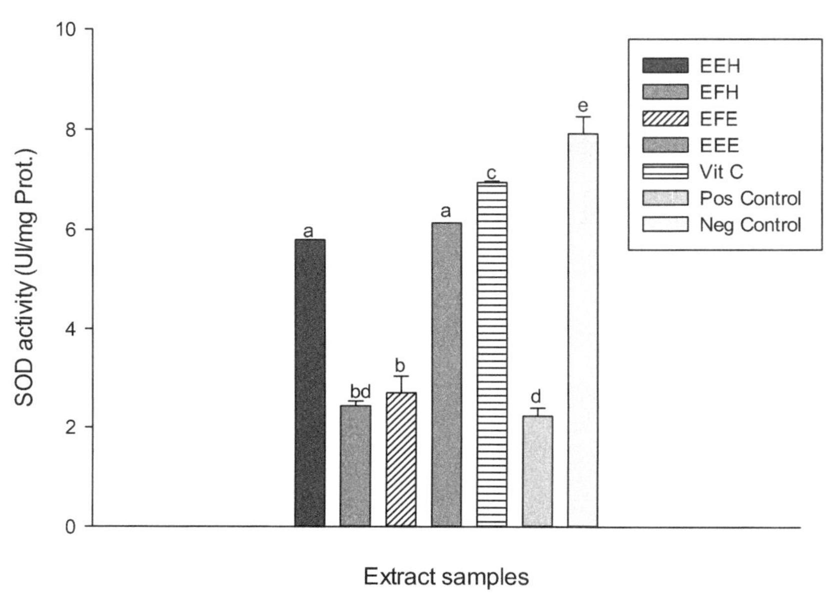

Figure 10. Protective properties of plant extracts: catalase activity. Values are expressed as mean ± SD of three replicates. In the same column the values labeled with different letters differ significantly at $p < 0.05$. EEE: *H. zenkeri (*bark) ethanolic extract; EFE: *H. zenkeri* (leaves) ethanolic extract; EEH: *H. zenkeri* (bark) hydro-ethanolic extract; EFH: *H. zenkeri* (leaves) hydro-ethanolic extract; Vit C: Vitamin C. Pos Control: oxidant (positive) control. Neg Control: Normal (negative) control.

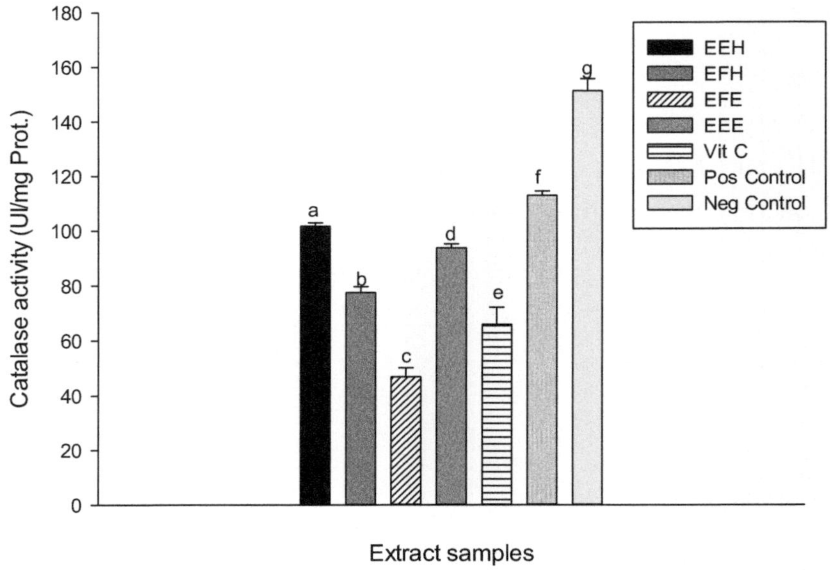

Figure 11. Protective properties of plant extracts: peroxidase activity. Values are expressed as mean ± SD of three replicates. In the same column the values labeled with different letters differ significantly at $p < 0.05$. EEE: *H. zenkeri (*bark) ethanolic extract; EFE: *H. zenkeri* (leaves) ethanolic extract; EEH: *H. zenkeri* (bark) hydro-ethanolic extract; EFH: *H. zenkeri* (leaves) hydro-ethanolic extract; Vit C: Vitamin C. Pos Control: oxidant (positive) control. Neg Control: Normal (negative) control.

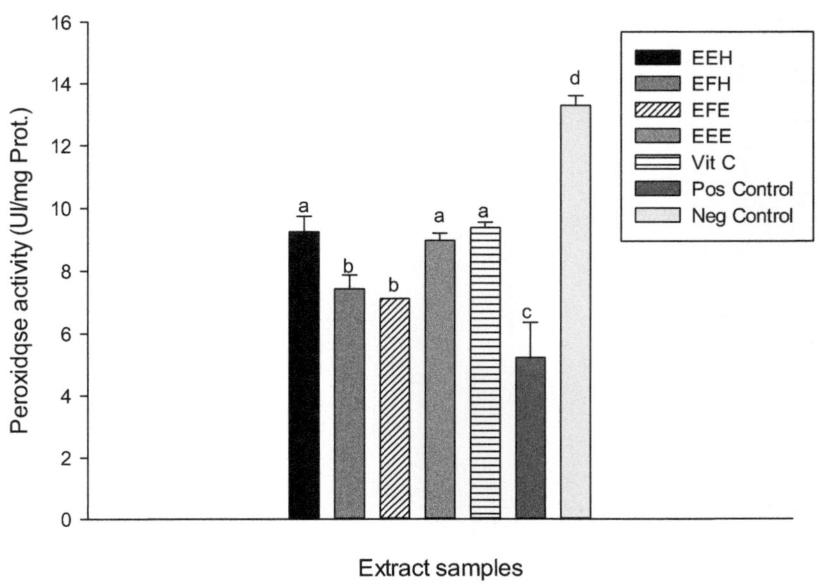

Various plants have been investigated to identify the presence of phenolic compounds using HPLC methods. The determination of phenolic compounds in the plant extracts helps to characterize them and to recognize their efficient uses as important plant resources [48]. The identification of phenolic compounds in extracts of *H. zenkeri* was carried out in this study and the phenolic compounds profile of the leaves and bark extracts are presented in Figures 12 and 13 while the level of each identified phenol is shown in Table 2. The results demonstrated that the levels of phenolic molecules were higher in the bark than the leaves (Table 2). Three groups of polyphenols have been identified in the two samples. These include caffeic acid, OH-tyrosol acid, and Rutin, which were higher in the bark than in the leaves. The bark also possesses Quercetin, 3,4-OH benzoic acid, Eugenol, and Apigenin in higher concentrations than are found in the leaves. This result may explain the higher antioxidants potential observed in the bark samples of EEH and EEE compared to those of the leaves samples of EFH and EFE. However numerous pics that characterized other compounds have not been identified this could explain the activities observed in the leaves.

Table 2. Level of phenolic compounds in the different plant parts.

Standards Polyphenols	***H. zenkeri* (Barks)**		***H. zenkeri* (Leaves)**	
Characteristics	A (mUA)	Conc (mg/g DW)	A (mUA)	Conc (mg/g DW)
3,4-OH Benzoic Acid	46.54 ± 0.00	184 ± 0.00	0.00 ± 0.00	0.00 ± 0.00
Apigenin	96.31 ± 0.00	0.02 ± 0.00	0.00 ± 0.00	0.00 ± 0.00
Caffeic Acid	323.24 ± 0.00	6.06 ± 0.00	29.84 ± 0.00	0.56 ± 0.00
Catechine	132.8 ± 0.00	9.65 ± 0.00	0.00 ± 0.00	0.00 ± 0.00
Eugenol	52.9 ± 0.00	15.29 ± 0.00	0.00 ± 0.00	0.00 ± 0.00
Gallic Acid	25.15 ± 0.00	0.64 ± 0.00	0.00 ± 0.00	0.00 ± 0.00
O-Coumaric Acid	97.43 ± 0.00	3.01 ± 0.00	0.00 ± 0.00	0.00 ± 0.00
OH-Tyrosol	71.4 ± 0.00	6.60 ± 0.00	16.87 ± 0.00	1.56 ± 0.00
P-Coumaric acid	122.74 ± 0.00	2.40 ± 0.00	0.00 ± 0.00	0.00 ± 0.00
Quercetin	233.88 ± 0.00	21.97 ± 0.00	0.00 ± 0.00	0.00 ± 0.00
Rutin	131.5 ± 0.00	11.07 ± 0.00	22.9 ± 0.00	1.93 ± 0.00
Syringic Acid	85.5 ± 0.00	2.12 ± 0.00	0.00 ± 0.00	0.00 ± 0.00
Theobromine	94.73 ± 0.00	3.18 ± 0.00	0.00 ± 0.00	0.00 ± 0.00
Tyrosol	111.02 ± 0.00	6.49 ± 0.00	0.00 ± 0.00	0.00 ± 0.00
Vanillic Acid	148.93 ± 0.00	4.76 ± 0.00	0.00 ± 0.00	0.00 ± 0.00

Conc: concentration; DW: Dried Weight; A: area.

Figure 12. High performance liquid chromatography (HPLC) chromatograms of phenolic extracts from the leaves of *H. zenkeri* recorded at 280 nm (TR: 19.10: 3,4-OH benzoic acid; 33.49: apigenin; 25.67: caffeic acid; 23.48: catechine; 29.43: eugenol; 14.38; gallic acid; 25.11: *O*-coumaric; 21.91:OH-tyrosol; 30.52: *P*-coumaric acid. 42.19: quercetin; 29.45: rutin; 25.55: syringic acid; 17.35: theobromine; 21.77: tyrosol and 25.27: vanillic acid).

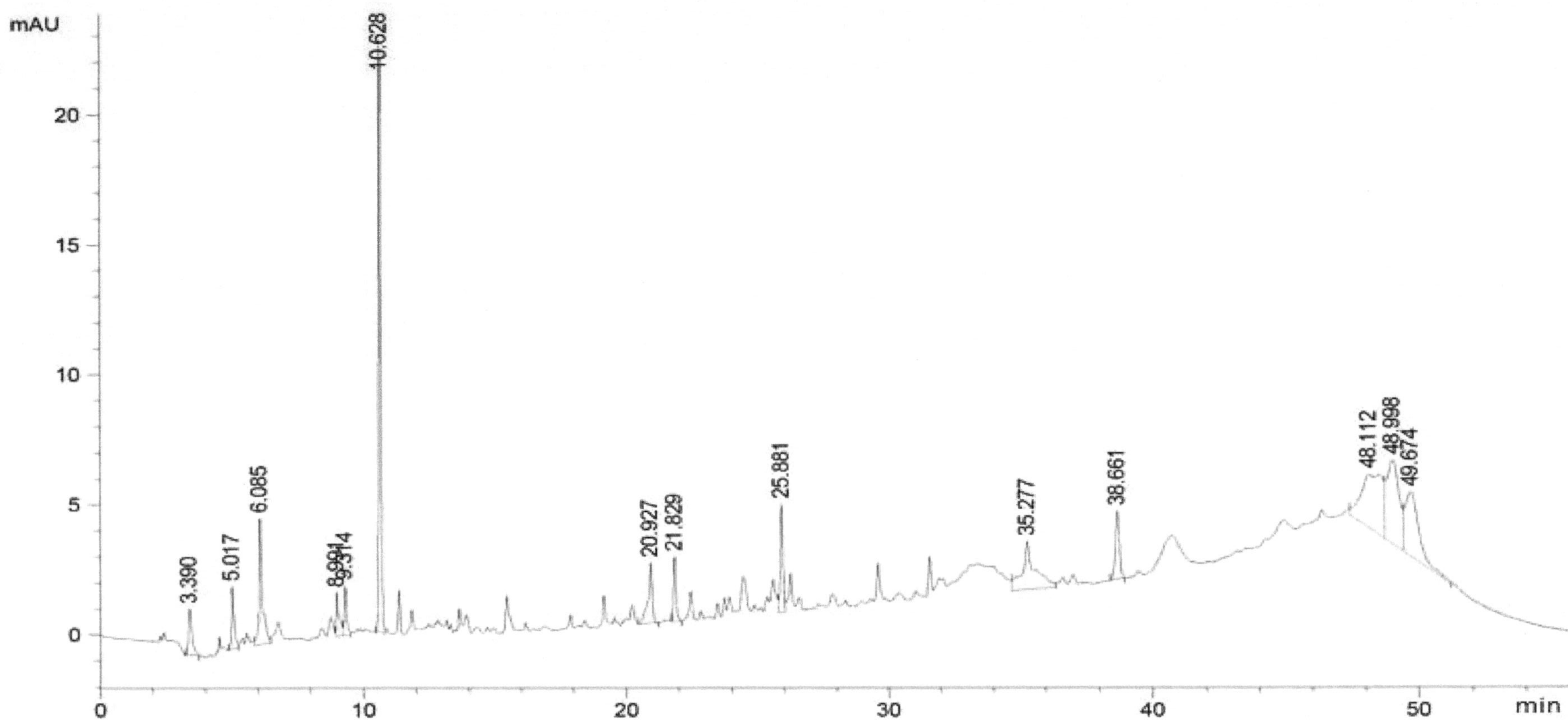

Figure 13. HPLC chromatograms of phenolic extracts from the barks of *H. zenkeri* recorded at 280 nm (TR: 19.10: 3,4-OH benzoic acid; 33.49:apigenin; 25.67: caffeic acid; 23.48: catechine; 29.43: eugenol; 14.38; gallic acid; 25.11: *O*-coumaric; 21.91:OH-tyrosol; 30.52: *P*-coumaric acid. 42.19: quercetin; 29.45: rutin; 25.55: syringic acid; 17.35: theobromine; 21.77: tyrosol and 25.27: vanillic acid.).

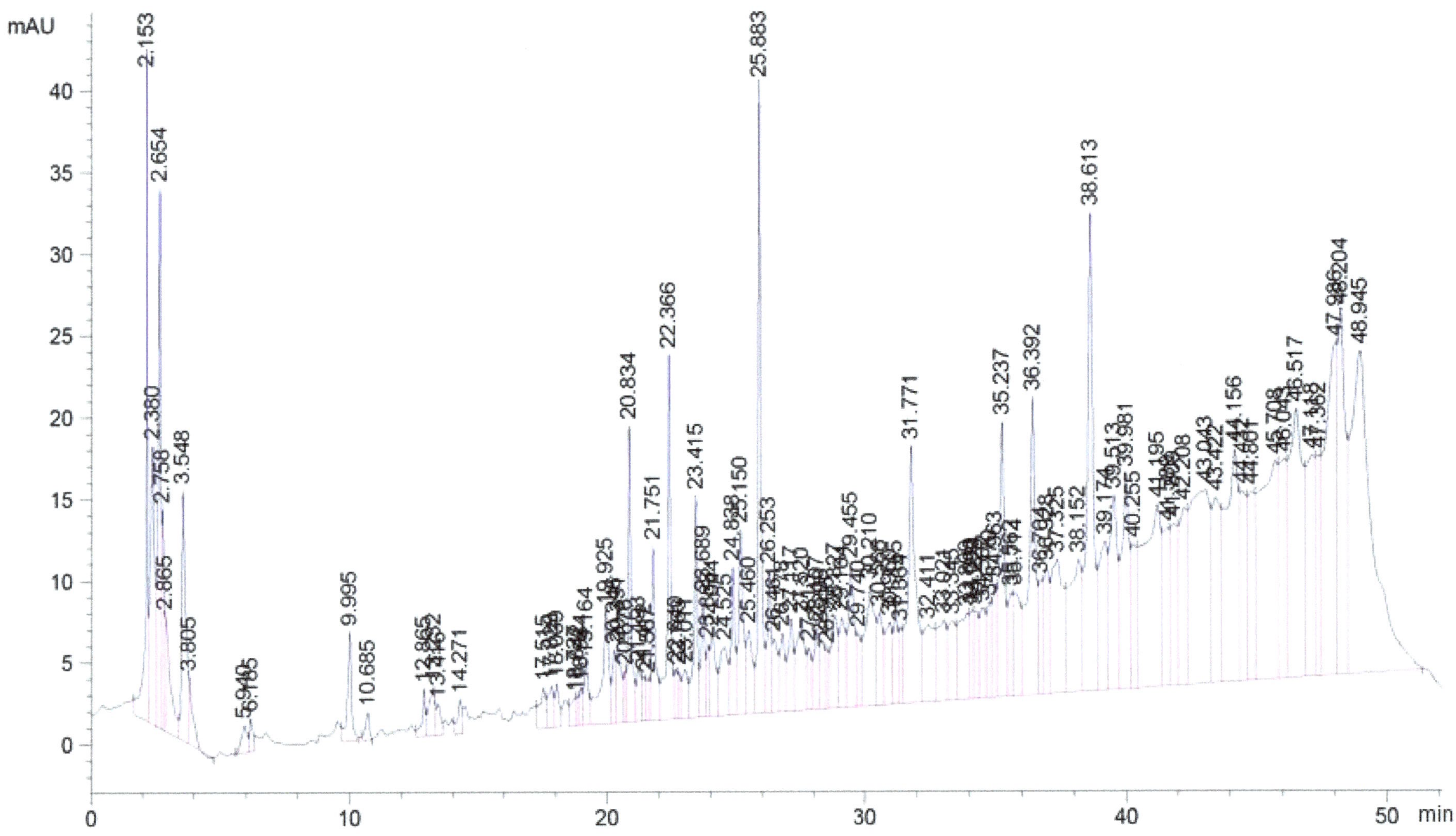

4. Conclusions

In conclusion, the ethanolic and hydro-ethanolic extract of the bark and leaves of *H. zenkeri* showed an antioxidant and protective potential against oxidative damage. The hydro-ethanolic extract of the bark EEH exhibited the most significantly elevated activities among the tested extracts. The HPLC based phenolic profile of the samples showed a higher amount of phenolic compounds in the bark than in the leaves. Nevertheless, additional experiments need to be conducted to purify and identify the active compounds as well as to elucidate the other biological effects on *in vivo* experimental models.

Acknowledgments

We are grateful to Nana Pierre from the National Herbarium for helping with the collection and identification of the plant material. We acknowledge the Department Chemical Engineering Materials Environment of Sapienza University of Rome for their hospitality and access to scientific instrumentation.

Author Contributions

Bruno Moukette Moukette conducted the study; Prosper Cabral Nya Biapa conducted the statistical analysis and assisted with the HPLC study; Jacques Romain Njimou conducted the HPLC assay; Vicky Jocelyne Ama Moor, Marco Stoller and Marco Bravi supervised the HPLC assay, helped with building and correction of the manuscript; Constant Anatole Pieme designed the research and co-directed the research work with Jeanne Yonkeu Ngogang and provided reagents. All the authors read and approved the final manuscript.

Conflicts of Interest

The authors declare that there are no a conflict of interests

References

1. Valko, M.; Rhodes, J.; Moncol, J.; Izakovic, M.; Mazur, M. Free radicals, metals and antioxidants in oxidative stress-induced cancer. *Chem. Biol. Interact.* **2006**, *160*, 1–40.
2. Halliwell, B. Antioxidants and human disease: A general introduction. *Nutr. Rev.* **1997**, *55*, 44–49.
3. Beckman, K.; Ames, B. Oxidative decay of DNA. *J. Biol. Chem.* **1997**, *272*, 19633–19636.
4. Valko, M.; Morris, H.; Cronin, M. Metals, toxicity and oxidative stress. *Curr. Med. Chem.* **2005**, *12*, 1161–1208.
5. Halliwell, B.; Gutteridge, J. The importance of free radicals and catalytic metal ions in human diseases. *Mol. Asp. Med.* **1985**, *8*, 89–193.
6. Ullen, H.; Augustsson, K.; Gustavsson, C.; Steineck, G. Supplementary iron intake and risk of cancer: Reversed causality? *Cancer Lett.* **1997**, *114*, 215–216.
7. Esterbauer, H.; Schaur, R.; Zollner, H. Chemistry and biochemistry of 4-hydroxynonenal, malonaldehyde and related aldehydes. *Free Radic. Biol. Med.* **1991**, *11*, 81–128.
8. Harman, D. Aging: Overview. *Ann. N. Y. Acad. Sci.* **2000**, *928*, 1–21.

9. Biapa, N.; Oben, J.; Ngogang, J. Scavenging radical kinetic and antianaemic screening properties of some medicinal plants used in Cameroon. *Int. J. Appl. Res. Nat. Prod.* **2011**, *4*, 29–35.
10. Biapa, P.; Matei, H.; Bâlici, S.; Oben, J.; Ngogang, J. Protective effects of stem bark of *Harungana madgascariensis* on the red blood cell membrane. *BMC Complement. Altern. Med.* **2013**, *13*, 1–9.
11. Djacbou, D.; Pieme, C.; Biapa, P.; Beng, B.P. Comparison of *in vitro* antioxidant properties of extracts from three plants used for medical purpose in Cameroon: *Acalypha racemosa, Garcinia lucida* and *Hymenocardia lyrata*. *Asian Pac. J. Trop. Biomed.* **2014**, *4*, 745–752.
12. Nanfack, P.; Biapa, N.; Pieme, C.; Moor, V.A.; Moukette, B.; Ngogang, Y. The *in vitro* antisickling and antioxidant effects of aqueous extracts *Zanthoxyllum heitzii* on sickle cell disorder. *BMC Complement. Altern. Med.* **2013**, *13*, 162.
13. Shalaby, E.; Shanab, S. Antioxidant compounds, assays of determination and mode of action. *Afr. J. Pharm. Pharmacol.* **2013**, *7*, 528–539.
14. Assam, J.; Dzoyem, J.; Pieme, C.; Penlap, V. *In vitro* antibacterial activity and acute toxicity studies of aqueous-methanol extract of *Sida rhombifolia* Linn. (Malvaceae). *BMC Complement. Altern. Med.* **2010**, *10*, 1–7.
15. Choumessi, A.; Danel, M.; Chassaing, S.; Truchet, I.; Penlap, V.; Pieme, A.; Asonganyi, T.; Ducommun, B.; Valette, A. Characterization of the antiproliferative activity of *Xylopia aethiopica*. *Cell Div.* **2012**, *7*, 8.
16. Dongmo, F.; Oben, E.; Momo, N.; Mandob, E. Phytochemical contituents and antioxydant potential of some Cameroonian medicinal plants. *Pharmacologyonline* **2007**, *2*, 436–452.
17. Nguefack, J.; Leth, V.; Zollo, P.A.; Mathur, S. Evaluation of live essential oils from aromatic plants of Cameroon for controlling food spoilage and mycotoxin producing fungi. *Int. J. Food Microbiol.* **2004**, *94*, 329–334.
18. Noumi, E. Les Plantes à Epices, à Condiments et à Aromates du Cameroun. Ph.D Thesis, Université de Yaoundé, Yaoundé, Cameroon, September 1984.
19. Tchamadeu, M.; Dzeufiet, P.; Nougaa, C.K.; Azebazeb, A.G.; Allard, J.; Girolami, J.; Tackc, I.; Kamtchouinga, P.; Dimo, T. Hypoglycaemic effects of *Mammea africana* (Guttiferae) in diabetic rats. *J. Ethnopharmacol.* **2010**, *127*, 368–372.
20. Titanji, P.V.; Zofou, D.; Ngemenya, M. The antimalarial potential of medicinal plants used for the treatment of malaria in Cameroonian folk medicine. *Afr. J. Tradit. Complement. Altern. Med.* **2008**, *5*, 302–321.
21. Maestri, D.; Nepote, V.; Lamarque, A.; Zygadlo, J. Natural products as antioxidants. *Phytochem. Adv. Res.* **2006**, *2*, 105–135.
22. Momo, I.; Dufat, T.; Wandji, J.; Michel, S.; Chiozem, D. New triterpenoids from the stem bark of *Hypodaphnis zenkeri*. *Nat. Prod. Res.* **2013**, *27*, 137–145.
23. Etoundi, O.; Kuate, D.; Ngondi, J.; Oben, E. Effects of extracts of *Hypodaphnis Zenkiri* and *Xylopia Aethiopica* on blood lipids, glycemia and body weight of roton W-1339 and insulino resistant rats. *Int. J. Res. Ayurveda Pharm.* **2013**, *4*, 736–741.
24. Etoundi, C.; Kuaté, D.; Ngondi, J.; Oben, J. Anti-amylase, anti-lipase and antioxidant effects of aqueous extracts of some Cameroonian spices. *J. Nat. Prod.* **2010**, *3*, 165–171.
25. Molyneux, P. The use of the stable free radical diphenylpicrylhydrazyl (DPPH) for estimating antioxydant activity. *Sonklanokarin J. Sci. Tecnol.* **2004**, *26*, 211–219.

26. Re, R.; Pellegrini, N.; Proteggente, A.; Pannala, A.; Yang, M.; Rice-Evans, C. Antioxidant activity applying an improved ABTS radical cation decolorization assay. *Free Radic. Biol. Med.* **1999**, *26*, 1231–1237.
27. Garratt, D. The quantitative analysis of drugs. *Chapman Hall Ltd. Jpn.* **1964**, *3*, 456–458.
28. Yu, W.; Zhao, Y.; Shu, B. The radical scavenging activities of *radix puerariae* isoflavonoids: A chemiluminescence study. *Food Chem.* **2004**, *86*, 525–529.
29. Benzie, F.; Strain, J. The ferric reducing ability of plasma (FRAP) as a measure of "antioxidant power": The FRAP assay. *Anal. Biochem.* **1996**, *239*, 70–76.
30. Prieto, P.; Pineda, M.; Aguilar, M. Spectophotometric quantitative of antioxidant capacity through the formation of a phosphomolybdenum complex: Specific application to the determination of vitamin E. *Anal. Biochem.* **1999**, *269*, 337–341.
31. Oyaizu, M. Studies on product of browning reaction prepared from glucose amine. *Jpn. J. Nutr.* **1986**, *44*, 307–315.
32. Singleton, V.; Draper, D. The transfer of polyphenolic compuonds from grape seeds into wine. *Am. J. Enol. Vitic.* **1964**, *15*, 34–40.
33. Zhishen, J.; Mengcheng, T.; Jianming, W. The determination of flavonoid contents in mulberry and their scavenging effects on superoxide. *Radic. Food Chem.* **1999**, *64*, 555–559.
34. Kumaran, A.; Karunakaran, R. *In vitro* antioxidant activities of methanol extracts of five *Phyllanthus* species from India. *LWT-Food Sci. Technol.* **2007**, *40*, 344–352.
35. Kumar, S.; Mishra, A.; Pandey, A. Antioxidant mediated protective effect of *Parthenium hysterophorus* against oxidative damage using *in vitro* models. *BMC Complement. Altern. Med.* **2013**, *13*, 120.
36. Misra, H.; Fridovich, I. Estimation of superoxide dismutase. *J. Biochem.* **1972**, *247*, 3170–3178.
37. Cvjetko, M.; Lepojeviæ, Z.; Vidoviæ, S.; Miloševiæ, S. Antioxidant properties of rapeseed. *Zb. Rad. Tehnol. Fak. Leskov.* **2009**, *19*, 27–33.
38. Antolovich, M.; Prenzler, P.; Patsalides, E.; McDonald, S.; Robards, K. Methods for testing antioxidant activity. *Analyst* **2001**, *127*, 183–198.
39. Panda, S.K. Assay guided comparison for enzymatic and non-enzymatic antioxidant activities with special reference to medicinal plants. *Antioxid. Enzym.* **2012**, *14*, 382–400.
40. Biskup, I.; Golonka, I.; Gamian, A.; Sroka, Z. Antioxidant activity of selected phenols estimated by ABTS and FRAP methods. *Postepy Hig. Med. Dosw.* **2013**, *67*, 958–963.
41. Chumark, P.; Khunawat, P.; Sanvarinda, Y.; Phornchirasilp, S.; Morales, N.; Phivthong, P.; Ngam, L.; Ratanachamnong, P.; Srisawat, S.; Pongrapeeporn, U. The *in vitro* and *ex vivo* antioxidant properties, hypolipidaemic and antiatherosclerotic activities of water extract of *Moringa oleifera* Lam. leaves. *J. Ethnopharmacol.* **2008**, *116*, 439–446.
42. Bopanna, K. Antidiabetic and antihyperlipidemic activities in alloxan diabetic rabbits. *Ind. J. Ethnopharmacol.* **1997**, *29*, 162–167.
43. Pieme, C.; Ngoupayo, J.; Nkoulou, C.; Moukette, B.; Nono, B.; Moor, V.; Minkande, J.; Ngogang, J. *Syzyguim guineense* extracts show antioxidant activities and beneficial activities on oxidative stress induced by ferric chloride in the liver homogenate. *Antioxidants* **2014**, *3*, 1–18.

44. Lee, H.; Eum, W.; Kim, D.; Lee, B.; Yoon, C.; Jang, S.; Choi, H.; Choi, S.; Baek, N.; Kang, J.; *et al*. Isolation and identification of an antioxidant enzyme catalase stimulatory compound from *Garnoderma lucidum*. *J. Biochem. Mol. Biol.* **2003**, *36*, 450–455.
45. Menvielle-Bourg, F. Superoxide Dismutase (SOD), a powerful antioxidant, is now available orally. *Phytothérapie* **2005**, *3*, 118–121.
46. Halliwell, B. Free radicals, antioxidants and human disease: Curiosity, cause or consequences. *Lancet* **1994**, *344*, 721–724.
47. Israhad, M.; Chaudhuri, P. Oxidant—Antioxydant system: Role and significance in human body. *Indian J. Exp. Biol.* **2002**, *40*, 1233–1239.
48. Alam, N.; Hossain, M.; Khali, M.; Moniruzzaman, M.; Sulaiman, S.; Gan, S. High catechin concentrations detected in *Withania somnifera* (ashwagandha) by high performance liquid chromatography analysis. *BMC Complement. Altern. Med.* **2011**, *11*, 65.

13

Curcumin Stimulates the Antioxidant Mechanisms in Mouse Skin Exposed to Fractionated γ-Irradiation

Ganesh Chandra Jagetia [1,*] and Golgod Krishnamurthy Rajanikant [2]

[1] Department of Zoology, Mizoram University, Aizawl-796 004, India

[2] School of Biotechnology, National Institute of Technology, Calicut-673 601, India; E-Mail: rajaniatrb@yahoo.com

* Author to whom correspondence should be addressed; E-Mail: gc.jagetia@gmail.com

Academic Editor: Nikolai Gorbunov

Abstract: Fractionated irradiation is one of the important radiotherapy regimens to treat different types of neoplasia. Despite of the immense therapeutic gains accrued by delivering fractionated irradiation to tumors, the radiation burden on skin increases significantly. Low doses of irradiation to skin adversely affect its molecular and metabolic status. The use of antioxidant/s may help to alleviate the radiation-induced changes in the skin and allow delivering a higher dose of radiation to attain better therapeutic gains. Curcumin is an antioxidant and a free radical scavenging dietary supplement, commonly used as a flavoring agent in curries. Therefore, the effect of 100 mg/kg body weight curcumin was studied on the antioxidant status of mice skin exposed to a total dose of 10, 20 and 40 Gy γ-radiation below the rib cage delivered as a single fraction of 2 Gy per day for 5, 10 or 20 days. Skin biopsies from both the curcumin treated or untreated irradiated groups were collected for the biochemical estimations at various post-irradiation times. The irradiation of animals caused a dose dependent decline in the glutathione concentration, glutathione peroxidase, and superoxide dismutase activities and increased the lipid peroxidation in the irradiated skin. Curcumin treatment before irradiation resulted in a significant rise in the glutathione concentration and activities of both the glutathione peroxidase and superoxide dismutase enzymes in mouse skin, whereas lipid peroxidation declined significantly. The present study indicates that curcumin treatment increased the antioxidant status of mouse exposed to different doses of fractionated γ-radiation.

Keywords: curcumin; mice; skin; irradiation; antioxidant enzymes; lipid peroxidation

1. Introduction

Skin is the outer most covering of the body, which protects the body against the invading pathogens, evaporation, and degradation of folate. It also insulates the body against the external environment, regulates body temperature, synthesizes Vitamin D, and provides a waterproof covering to the body [1]. Ionizing radiation is an important treatment modality in the management of various neoplastic disorders, where cancer patients are usually exposed to 20–30 fractions of 1.5–2 Gy each spread over a period of 5–6 weeks so as to spare the normal tissues and at the same time increase the radiotoxicity of tumors. Despite immense therapeutic benefit, the normal skin invariably suffers from the cytotoxic effect of radiation. According to the classification of the detrimental somatic effects of ionizing radiation, the radiation-induced damage to the skin can be both stochastic and non-stochastic [2].

Consistent with this view, ionizing radiation interacts with skin and undoubtedly damages it by direct or indirect processes by generating numerous radiolytic reactive oxygen products including $^{\bullet}OH$, $H^{\bullet}$, $O_2^{\bullet-}$, $HOO^{\bullet}$ free radicals and H_2O_2 in aqueous milieu of the skin cells [3]. A plethora of defense mechanisms exists in skin [4–7] that can deal with the onslaught of reactive oxygen species (ROS) under normal conditions; however, an additional oxidative stress generated after exposure to ionizing radiation may not be efficiently handled by it [8]. The management of skin reactions after radiotherapy is a challenging task after radiotherapy as –the low level of fractionated irradiation has been linked to the induction of basal and squamous cell skin carcinomas [9]. It is also associated with radiation-induced oedema, erythema, pigmentation, fibrosis, ulceration, pain, warmth, burning, itching of the skin, dermatitis and dry and moist desquamation [10,11]. Skin irradiation to low doses of radiation has been found to alter its metabolic profile [12]. Some of the general events associated with early phase of oxidative stress response in the skin are depletion of endogenous intra- and inter-cellular antioxidants, enhancement of intracellular lipid peroxidation levels and the induction of specific signal transduction pathways that can modulate inflammatory, immune suppressive or apoptotic processes in the skin [13–15]. It is necessary to counter the additional oxidative stress induced by ionizing radiation by exogenous supply of antioxidants, which could act as safe and effective skin protectants in the irradiated skin. The introduction of exogenous antioxidants that scavenge ROS and restore normal redox state may be beneficial in such a situation [16–19]. Application of such antioxidants to protect normal tissues like skin from radiation injury might allow one to increase the radiation dose to the tumor thus increasing the probability of better tumor control in clinics.

The polyphenol curcumin or diferuloylmethane (1,7-bis (4-hydroxy-3-methoxy-phenyl) hepta-1, 6-diene-3, 5-dione) is one of the most active molecules present in the turmeric rhizome (family: Zingiberaceae) that imparts the characteristic yellow color to curry powder, the turmeric [20]. Curcumin is widely used as a spice, dietary pigment, and as an Indian folk medicine for the treatment of various illnesses including cough, common cold, sore throat and healing of wounds. Traditional medicinal practitioners prescribe turmeric to treat rheumatism, body pain, skin diseases, intestinal worms, diarrhea, intermittent, fevers, hepatic disorders, biliousness, urinary discharges, dyspepsia, inflammations, constipation, leucoderma, amenorrhea, and colic. Turmeric is an emmenagogue, diuretic, carminative, and it is applied externally against bruises, pains, sprains, boils, swellings, and skin diseases [21]. In China, turmeric is used to treat angina pectoris, stomachache, postpartum abdominal pain, and gallstones [22]. Current traditional Indian medicine uses turmeric to treat biliary disorders, anorexia, cough, diabetic wounds, hepatic disorders, rheumatism, and sinusitis. This nonnutritive curry flavoring phytochemical is pharmacologically safe, since it has been used as a dietary spice up to a dose of 100 mg/day, for centuries [23,24]. Humans can tolerate a dose as high as 12 g/day of curcumin without any untoward toxic side effects [25], which reaffirms its nontoxic nature.

Curcumin and related compounds have the ability to induce glutathione-*S*-transferase, inhibit free radical generation and act as a free radical scavengers and antioxidants, inhibiting lipid peroxidation [26–30]. Because ROS have been known to play an important role in radiation-induced skin injury, one might expect that curcumin, as an antioxidant, radioprotector and free radical scavenger, would protect skin from radiation damage by increasing the antioxidant status of the skin. Earlier studies have revealed that curcumin pretreatment protected mouse against the deep dermal irradiated wound after whole body, hemi-body and fractionated irradiation [19,31–33]. Recently, curcumin has been reported to enhance re-epithelialization in CO_2 laser-induced incision wounds in mice [34]. Curcumin is a dietary supplement and is not synthesized in the body. Therefore, the present study was carried out to obtain an insight into the effect of curcumin on antioxidant status and lipid peroxidation in the mouse skin exposed to 10, 20 and 40 Gy of fractionated γ- radiation.

2. Materials and Methods

The animal care and handling were carried out according to the guidelines issued by the World Health Organization, Geneva, Switzerland and the INSA (Indian National Science Academy, New Delhi). Usually, eight to 10-week old male and female (1:1 ratio) Swiss albino mice weighing 30–36 g were selected from an inbred colony maintained under the controlled conditions of temperature (23 ± 2 °C), humidity (50% ± 5%) and light (12 h of light and dark cycle, respectively). The animals were given sterile food and water throughout the experiment. The food consisted of 50% cracked wheat, 40% Bengal gram, 4% milk powder, 4% yeast powder, 0.75% sesame oil, 0.25% cod liver oil, and 1% salt. Four animals were housed in a sterile polypropylene cage containing sterile paddy husk (procured locally) as bedding during the experimentation. The study had been approved by the institutional animal ethical committee of Kasturba Medical College, Manipal, India, where the whole study was carried out.

2.1. Preparation of Drug and Mode of Administration

Curcumin (Catalog No: C1386) was procured from Sigma Chemical Co. (St. Louis, MO, USA). The required amount of curcumin was suspended in 0.5% carboxymethylcellulose (CMC) and the animals were administered with 0.01 mL/g body weight of CMC or curcumin (CUM) orally.

2.2. Experimental Protocol

The animals were divided into the following groups:

CMC + Sham-Irradiation (SIR): The animals of this group received 0.01 mL/g body weight of 0.5% CMC daily, consecutively for 5, 10 and 20 days, respectively, before sham-irradiation.

CUM + SIR: The animals of this group received 100 mg/kg body weight of curcumin daily, consecutively for 5, 10 and 20 days, respectively, before sham-irradiation.

CMC + irradiation (IR): The animals of this group received 0.01 mL/g body weight of 0.5% CMC once daily before exposure to 2 Gy/day consecutively for 5, 10 or 20 days, respectively.

CUM + IR: The animals of this group received 100 mg/kg body weight of curcumin once daily before exposure to 2 Gy/day consecutively for 5, 10 or 20 days, respectively [19].

2.3. Irradiation

One hour after each administration of CMC or curcumin, each animal was placed into a specially designed well-ventilated acrylic restrainer and the lower half of the animal body (below the rib cage) was exposed to 0 or 2 Gy once daily, delivered at a dose rate of 1.35 Gy/min from a ^{60}Co Teletherapy source (Theratron, Atomic Energy Agency, Ontario, Canada). Treatments were given once daily for 5, 10 or 20 days resulting in a cumulative dose of 10 Gy (a total of 5 fractions of 2 Gy each), 20 Gy (a total of 10 fractions of 2 Gy each) or 40 Gy (a total of 20 fractions of 2 Gy each), respectively. A two-day gap was allowed after the delivery of fifth, 10th and 15th fractions of radiation for mice receiving total doses of 20 or 40 Gy.

2.4. Preparation of Animals

The hairs were depilated from the lower half of the dorsum of the animals before the last exposure. Skin biopsies from each dose of all groups were collected at 0, 1.5, 3, 6, 12, 24, 48, 72 and 144 h after the last exposure. The skin was freed from *panniculus carnosus* and flash frozen in the liquid nitrogen. The skin was weighed and homogenized in the phosphate buffered saline. Four animals were used for each irradiation dose at each time point in all concurrent groups.

2.5. Biochemical Parameters

2.5.1. Glutathione (GSH)

GSH content was measured by the method of Moron *et al.*, [35]. Briefly, proteins were precipitated by 25% TCA, centrifuged and the supernatant was collected. The supernatant was mixed with 0.2 mol sodium phosphate buffer pH 8.0 and 0.06 mmol DTNB and incubated for 10 min at room temperature. The absorbance of the sample/s was read against the blank at 412 nm in a UV-Visible Spectrophotometer (Shimadzu UV-260, Shimadzu Corp., Tokyo, Japan) and the GSH concentration has been calculated from the standard curve.

2.5.2. Glutathione Peroxidase (GSHPx)

GSHPx activity was estimated by the method of Sazuka *et al.*, [36]. Briefly, 100 μL homogenate was mixed with 200 μL each of EDTA, sodium azide, GSH, H_2O_2 and 400 μL buffer. The reaction mixture was incubated at 37 °C for 10 min followed by the addition of 10% TCA. After centrifugation, the supernatant was collected and mixed with 3 mL disodium hydrogen phosphate and 1000 μL DTNB. The absorbance of the sample/s was recorded against the blank at 412 nm using UV-Visible Spectrophotometer. The activity has been expressed as μmol GSH/mg protein.

2.5.3. Superoxide dismutase (SOD)

The SOD activity was measured by the method of Fried [37]. Briefly, 900 µL buffer was mixed with 100 µL each of tissue homogenate (T), nitroblue tetrazolium (NBT), phenazine methosulphate and NADH. The control (C) consisted of all the reagents except the homogenate, whereas the blank (B) consisted of buffer and the homogenate without any reagents. The absorbance of T, C and B was measured at 560 nm using a UV-Visible Spectrophotometer and the enzyme activity has been expressed in units (1 U = 50% inhibition of NBT reduction).

2.5.4. Lipid Peroxidation (LOO)

LOO was measured by the method of Beuege and Aust [38]. Briefly, the tissue homogenate was mixed with TCA-TBA-HCl solution, butylated hydroxytoluene (BHT, 3.5 mmol, 0.1 mL) and diethylenetriaminopentaacetic acid (DETAPAC, 70 µmol, 0.1 mL). The mixture was heated for 15 min in a boiling water bath. After centrifugation the absorbance was recorded at 535 nm using a UV-Visible Spectrophotometer. The lipid peroxidation has been expressed as MDA in nmol per mg protein.

2.5.5. Estimation of Protein

Protein contents were measured by the method of Lowry *et al*., (1951) using bovine serum albumin (BSA) as a standard.

2.6. Analysis of Data

The statistical significance between various groups was determined using student's *t*-test. Solo 4 statistical package (BMDP Statistical Software, Inc., Los Angeles, CA, USA) was used for data analysis. All the data are expressed as mean ± SEM (standard error of the mean).

3. Results

3.1. Glutathione (GSH)

GSH content declined immediately after wound creation up to 3 h and then elevated at 6 h post-irradiation in CMC + SIR group. A second decrement in GSH level was observed at 48 h post-irradiation. However, treatment of mice with curcumin before sham-irradiation resulted in a significant ($p < 0.05$) elevation in the GSH contents for all post-irradiation times. The irradiation of animals to various doses of fractionated γ-radiation resulted in a drastic but dose dependent decline in the GSH contents when compared with CMC + SIR group and a nadir was reached at 3 and 6 h post-irradiation at all exposure doses in both the CMC + IR and CUM+IR groups (Figure 1). Curcumin treatment prior to irradiation caused a significant elevation ($p < 0.05$, up to 24 h post-irradiation for 40 Gy) in GSH concentration when compared with the concurrent CMC + IR group. However, normal levels could not be restored even by 144 h post-irradiation in both CMC + IR and CUM + IR groups (Figure 1).

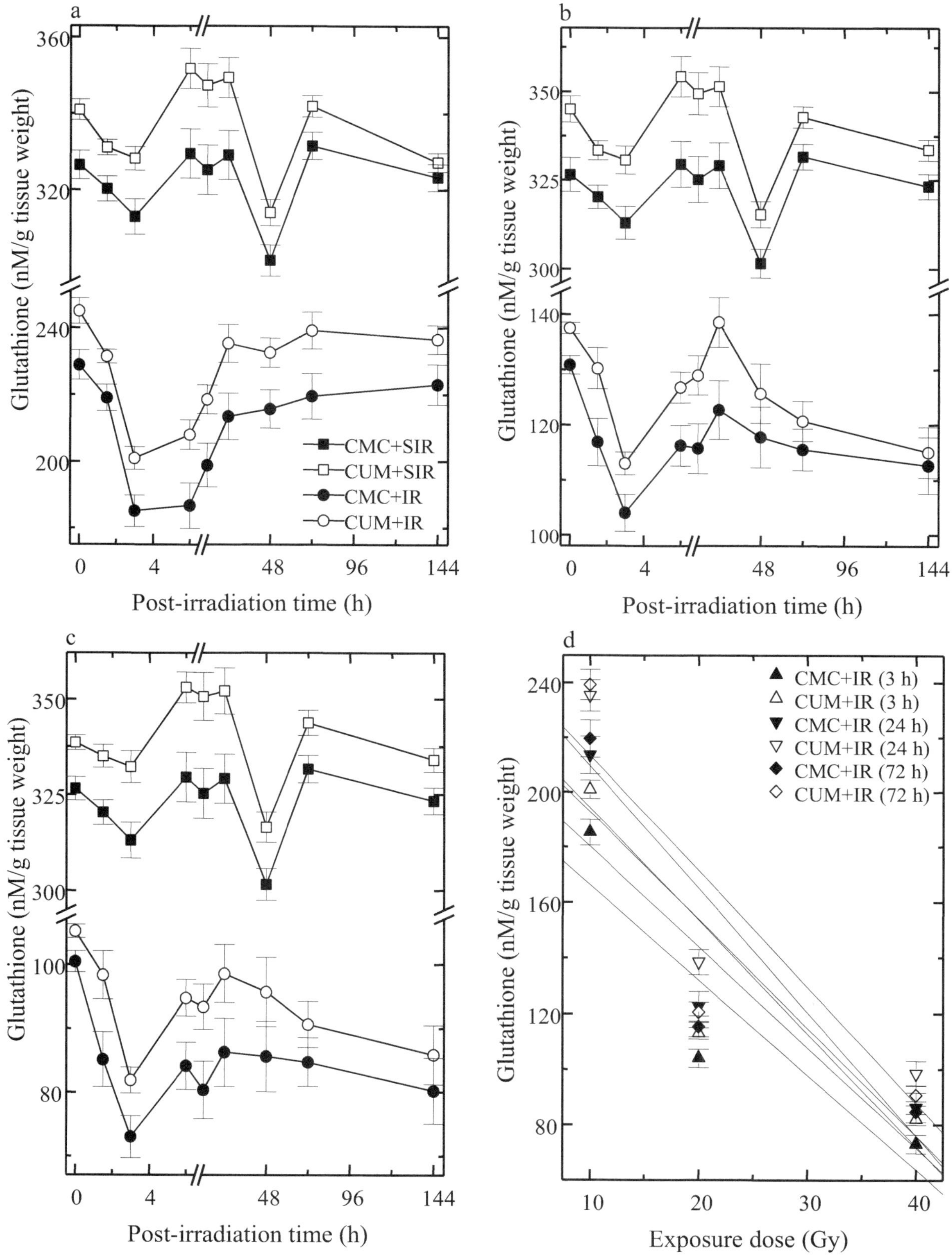

Figure 1. Effect of curcumin on glutathione concentration in the skin of mice exposed to fractionated doses of γ-radiation. (**a**) 10 Gy (**b**) 20 Gy (**c**) 40 Gy and (**d**) dose response relationship.

3.2. Glutathione Peroxidase (GSHPx)

The activity of GSHPx fluctuated with time in CMC + SIR group and a highest elevation was observed at 1.5 h post-irradiation. A second rise in GSHPx activity was observed at 24 h, which remained unaltered up to 72 h post-irradiation. Curcumin administration before sham-irradiation resulted in a significant elevation ($p < 0.05$ up to 72 h post-irradiation for five fractions of curcumin) in the GSHPx activity, when compared with CMC + SIR groups. The irradiation of animals to different doses of fractionated γ-radiation resulted in a dose dependent alleviation in the GSHPx activity in both the CMC + IR and CUM + IR groups when compared with the respective sham-irradiation groups (Figure 2). The pattern of fluctuation in GSHPx activity after exposure to different doses of fractionated γ-radiation was similar to that of sham-irradiation groups. The administration of curcumin before exposure to various doses of γ-radiation caused a drastic rise in the GSHPx activity and this increase was highest at 1.5 h ($p < 0.02$) followed by 24 h ($p < 0.03$) and 144 h post-irradiation in CUM + IR groups (Figure 2). However, spontaneous levels could not be restored even at 144 h post-irradiation.

3.3. Superoxide Dismutase (SOD)

The analysis of SOD activity showed a peak level at 1.5 that declined thereafter and attained a nadir at 48 h post-irradiation in CMC + SIR group. Treatment of mice with curcumin before sham-irradiation elevated the SOD activity significantly when compared with the CMC + SIR group. The exposure of mice to different doses of fractionated radiation resulted in a significant and dose dependent reduction in the SOD activity when compared with the CMC+SIR group, whereas curcumin treatment before exposure to various doses of fractionated radiation caused a significant augmentation ($p < 0.05$, up to 72 h post-irradiation for 10 Gy) in the SOD activity in CUM+IR group when compared with concurrent CMC + IR group (Figure 3). This elevation was approximately two-fold greater at 1.5 h post-irradiation for all exposure doses. The second rise in SOD activity was discernible at 24 h ($p < 0.05$) post-irradiation for 10, 20 and 40 Gy in CUM + IR group. The pattern of SOD activity in CUM + IR group was similar to that of CMC + IR group (Figure 3).

3.4. Lipid Peroxidation (LOO)

Infliction of excision wound caused an elevation in LOO in CMC + SIR group. LOO fluctuated with time in both CMC + SIR and CUM + SIR groups, where a highest elevation was observed at 3 h post-irradiation and a gradual decline thereafter. Curcumin treatment resulted in a significant ($p < 0.05$) decline in the spontaneous levels of LOO. Induction of LOO increased with an increase in irradiation dose (maximum for 40 Gy) as well as with assay time in both the CMC + IR and CUM + IR groups and a peak LOO was reached at 3 h post-irradiation. Thereafter, LOO declined steadily and reached a nadir at 144 h post-exposure (Figure 4). Curcumin pretreatment afforded a significant ($p < 0.05$, up to 24 h post-irradiation for 40 Gy) protection against the radiation-induced lipid peroxidation. However, the normal LOO levels could not be restored even by 144 h post-irradiation (Figure 4).

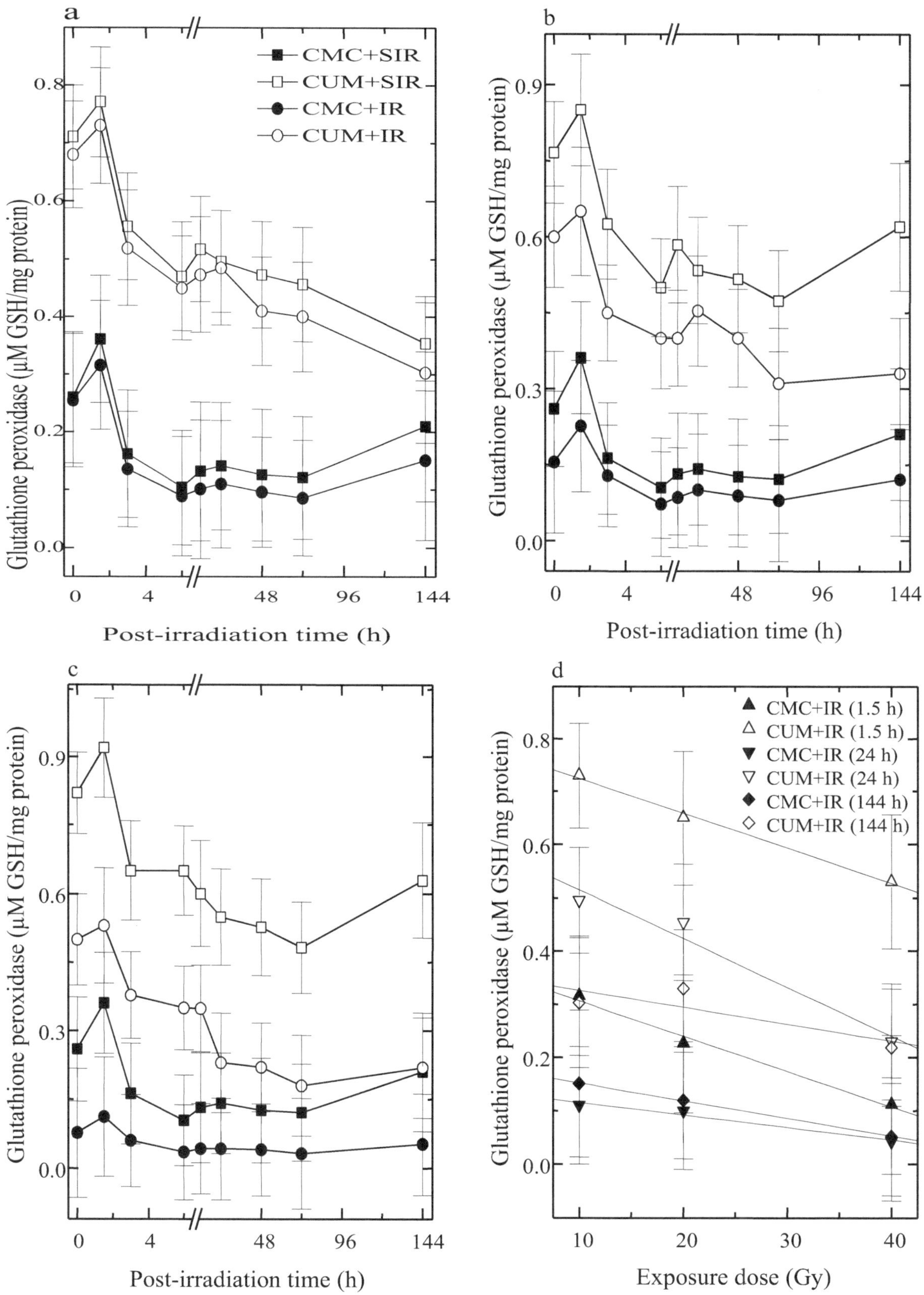

Figure 2. Effect of curcumin on glutathione peroxidase activity in the skin of mice exposed to different doses of fractionated γ-radiation. (**a**) 10 Gy (**b**) 20 Gy (**c**) 40 Gy and (**d**) dose response relationship.

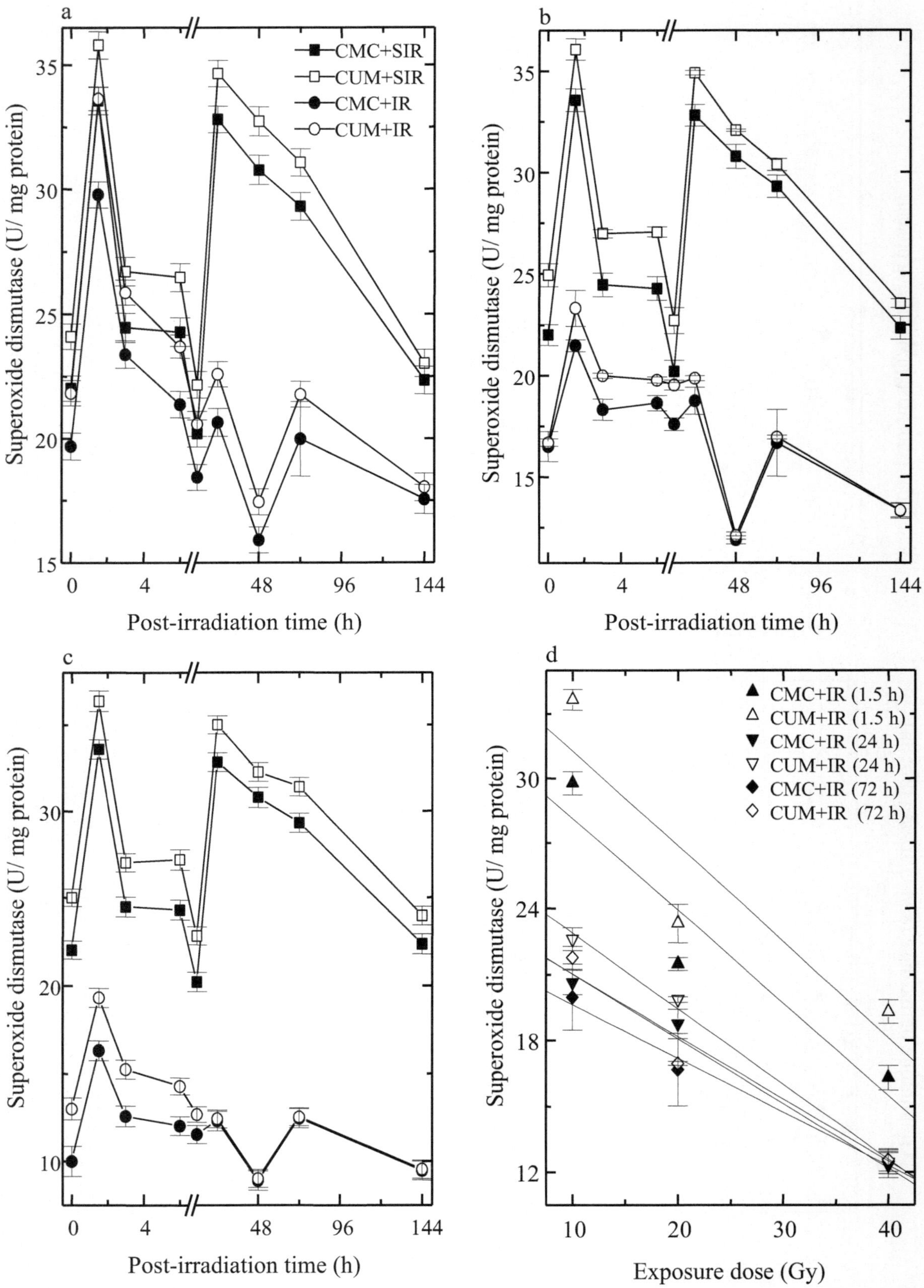

Figure 3. Effect of curcumin on superoxide dismutase activity in the skin of mice exposed to fractionated doses of fractionated γ-radiation. (**a**) 10 Gy (**b**) 20 Gy (**c**) 40 Gy and (**d**) dose response relationship.

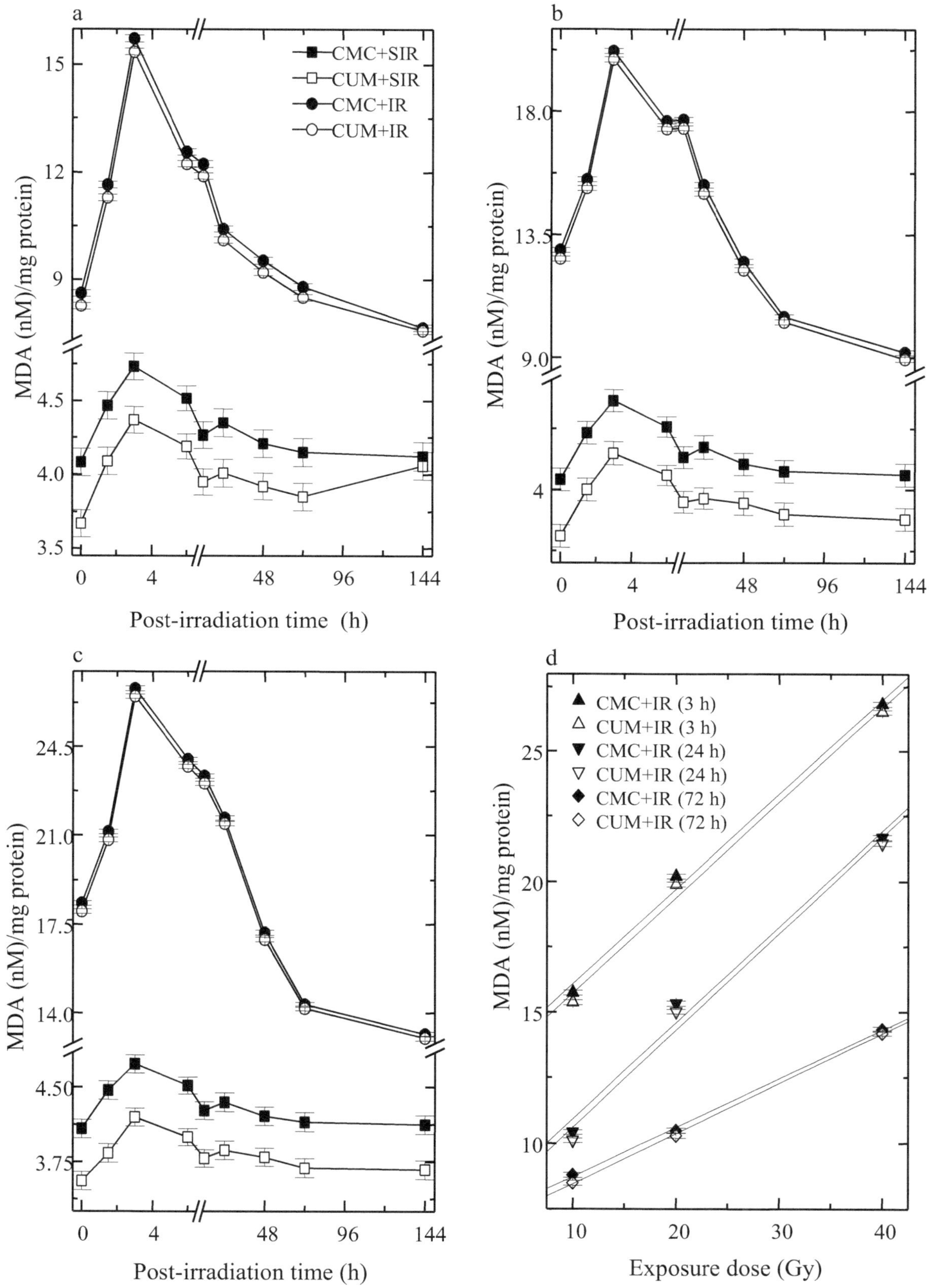

Figure 4. Effect of curcumin on lipid peroxidation level in the skin of mice exposed to fractionated doses of γ-radiation. (**a**) 10 Gy (**b**) 20 Gy (**c**) 40 Gy and (**d**) dose response relationship.

4. Discussion

In spite of the immense therapeutic gains produced by the fractionated irradiation regimens, radiation burden on the skin increases significantly. To a large extent, radiation injury to living cells is mediated by the generation of oxygen derived free radicals and hydrogen peroxide. Consequently, protection of skin by exogenous supply of antioxidants that scavenge ROS and restore normal redox state may allow increasing the radiation dose for better therapeutic gains. Curcumin—an active polyphenolic compound of turmeric, and a well-known culinary agent and curry spice, extensively used as a food additive to impart yellow color—was investigated for its efficacy to modulate radiation-induced alleviation of the antioxidant status in the skin of mice exposed to various doses of fractionated γ-radiation.

A direct quantitative comparison of the results of the present study to those reported by other investigators may not be possible, because of the use of different experimental protocols and conditions of assays (pH, temperature, reagent concentration) and different unit definitions. Nevertheless, results of the present investigation are qualitatively in good agreement with other studies, where similar effects have been reported [18,39]. Ionizing radiation induces ROS and lipid peroxidation that subsequently depletes antioxidant status in the skin [3,18]. Fractionated irradiation of mice skin caused a drastic decline in the GSH concentration and GSHPx and SOD, activities. A similar reduction in GSH concentration and GSHPx and superoxide dismutase activities has been reported earlier in mice skin exposed to fractionated γ-radiation [18]. A decline in the erythrocyte GSHPx and SOD activity has been observed in female rats during radiotherapy [40]. Whole body irradiation has been reported to reduce GSH concentration and the activities of GSHPx and SOD in the mouse liver earlier [41]. Ionizing radiation induces lipid peroxidation and a similar effect has been observed in the present study where, exposure of mice to various doses of fractionated gamma radiation resulted in an increase in lipid peroxidation and decreased the antioxidant status of the skin. Irradiation has been reported to increase the lipid peroxidation in mouse liver, stomach, small intestine and kidney and human peripheral blood lymphocytes earlier [41–45]. Curcumin pretreatment afforded protection against radiation-induced elevation in lipid peroxidation and arrested the radiation-induced decline in GSH concentration and GSHPx, and SOD activity. A similar observation has been reported earlier in mice skin treated with ascorbic acid before fractionated irradiation [18]. Curcumin has been reported to protect mouse liver against the radiation-induced decline in GSH concentration and GSHPx, and SOD activity and lipid peroxidation [45]. Similarly, ginger, bael, naringin and mangiferin have been reported to elevate the GSH concentration and GSHPx, and SOD activity and reduce radiation-induced lipid peroxidation [42–44].

The redox state of the cell is primarily a consequence of the precise balance between the levels of ROS and endogenous thiol buffers present in the cell, such as glutathione and thioredoxin, which protect cells from oxidative damage. Dramatic elevation of ROS, exceeding compensatory changes in the level of the endogenous thiol buffers, may result in the sustained activation of signaling pathways and expression of genes that induce apoptosis in affected cells [46]. Nuclear factor-(erythroid derived 2)-related factor-2 (Nrf2) resides in cytoplasm and translocates into nucleus to initiate antioxidant pathway [47]. Curcumin has been reported to upregulate Nrf2 gene in irradiated rat brain [48]. The upregulation of Nrf2 pathway may be involved in the rise in the GSH concentration, GSHPx and SOD activity after curcumin treatment in this study. Glutathione acts synergistically with other endogenous antioxidants and acts as a co-factor with the enzyme glutathione peroxidase to scavenge free radicals, and detoxify xenobiotics [49,50]. The depletion in GSH contents after exposure to γ-radiation may be due to the reaction of GSH with free radicals resulting in the formation of thiyl radicals that react to produce GSSG as reported earlier [51]. Depletion of glutathione *in vitro* and *in vivo* is known to cause inhibition of glutathione peroxidase activity and has been shown to increase lipid peroxidation [52]. A similar correlation between the depletion of GSH and elevation of LOO exists in the present investigation, which is consistent with the results of previous studies [18,53–55].

It is commonly accepted that SOD protects against the free radical damage by scavenging superoxide radical, converting, superoxide radical into H_2O_2 and prevents the formation of $^{\bullet}OH$ radical through superoxide driven Fenton reaction [56]. The H_2O_2 thus generated can be removed by catalase or GSHPx. However, radiation-induced decline in both SOD and GSHPx activity along with GSH promotes the formation of $^{\bullet}OH$ radicals, and initiation and propagation of LOO [57]. The increase in MDA levels and the concomitant decrease in antioxidant enzymes and GSH levels demonstrate the role of oxidative mechanisms in radiation-induced tissue damage. Glutathione peroxidase also protects the cell protein and membrane against oxidation [58]. The initial elevation of LOO levels seems to be due to the ROS-producing effect of radiation and the resultant formation of lipid peroxides from unsaturated fatty acids. The lower enzyme activities observed after irradiation were most likely due to the enzyme inactivating activity of ROS induced by radiation.

The mitigation of cytotoxic effect of ROS by curcumin may be due to the direct scavenging of free radicals and subsequent inhibition of oxygenation reaction as curcumin has been reported to be a good antioxidant, free radical scavenger and a radioprotective agent [27,59,60]. A similar free radical scavenging action of radiation-induced free radicals by curcumin seems to be operational in the present study. Curcumin may have lowered lipid peroxidation by maintaining the activities of antioxidant enzymes and glutathione at higher levels as these enzymes play an important role in the regulation of lipid peroxidation. This may have contributed to a rapid scavenging of radicals and consequently less damage to the skin. Curcumin has been reported to alleviate radiation-induced lipid peroxidation in the irradiated skin of mice [30]. It has been demonstrated that dietary supplementation of curcumin (2%, w/v) to male ddY mice for 30 days significantly increased activities of antioxidants and phase II-metabolizing enzymes in liver and kidney when compared to corresponding normal diet fed control mice [61]. Our earlier study has demonstrated that ascorbic acid treatment prior to irradiation significantly improved skin antioxidant status in mice after exposure to fractionated irradiation [18].

Our results suggest that oral administration of curcumin before irradiation significantly elevated the activity of glutathione concentration, glutathione peroxidase and superoxide dismutase activity and lowered the lipid peroxidation in mice skin exposed to various doses of fractionated γ-radiation. This activity of curcumin may be due to free radical scavenging and upregulation of Nrf2 expression. Our findings indicate that curcumin pretreatment may be one of the paradigms to reduce the effect of radiation on the skin of patients receiving radiotherapy for the treatment of cancer.

Acknowledgments

We are thankful to Mamadipudi Srinivas Vidyasagar, and J.G.R. Solomon, Department of Radiotherapy and Oncology, Kasturba Medical College Hospital, Manipal, India for providing the necessary irradiation facilities and for dosimetric calculations, respectively. The financial assistance in the form of Senior Research Fellowship to Golgod Krishnamurthy Rajanikant by the Indian Council of

Medical Research (ICMR), Government of India, New Delhi, India to carry out the above study is gratefully acknowledged.

Author Contributions

Ganesh Chandra Jagetia has designed the study and prepared the manuscript, whereas Golgod Krishnamurthy Rajanikant conducted the experiments.

Conflicts of Interest

The authors declare no conflict of interest.

References

1. Zhou, Y.; Ni, H.; Balint, K.; Sanzari, J.K.; Dentchev, T.; Diffenderfer, E.S.; Wilson, J.M.; Cengel, K.A.; Weissman, D. Ionizing Radiation Selectively Reduces Skin Regulatory T Cells and Alters Immune Function. *PLoS One* **2014**, *9*, e100800.
2. Monson, R.R.; Cleaver, J.E.; Abrams, H.L.; Bingham, E.; Buffler, P.A.; Cardis, E.; Cox, R.; Davis, S.; Dewey, W.C.; Gilbert, E.S.; *et al. Health Risks from Exposure to Low Levels of Ionizing Radiation: BEIR VII—Phase 2*; National Academies Press: Washigton, DC, USA, 2006.
3. Quintiliani, M. The oxygen effect in radiation interaction on DNA and enzymes. *Int. J. Radiat. Biol.* **1986**, *50*, 573–594.
4. Shindo, Y.; Witt, E.; Han, D.; Epstein, W.; Packer, L. Enzymic and non-enzymic antioxidants in epidermis and dermis of human skin. *J. Investig. Dermatol.* **1994**, *102*, 122–124.
5. Yu, B.P. Cellular defenses against damage from reactive oxygen species. *Physiol. Rev.* **1994**, *74*, 139–162.
6. Fuchs, J. Potentials and limitations of the natural antioxidants RRR-α tocopherol, L-ascorbic acid, and β-carotene in cutaneous photoprotection. *Free Radic. Biol. Med.* **1998**, *25*, 848–873.
7. Ichihashi, M.; Ahmed, N.U.; Budiyanto, A.; Wu, A.; Bito, T.; Ueda, M.; Osawa, T. Preventive effect of antioxidant on ultraviolet-induced skin cancer in mice. *J. Dermatol. Sci.* **2000**, *23*, 45–50.
8. Darr, D.; Fridovich, I. Free radicals in cutaneous biology. *J. Investig. Dermatol.* **1994**, *102*, 671–675.
9. Brenner, D.J.; Doll, R.; Goodhead, D.T.; Hall, E.J.; Land, C.E.; Little, J.B.; Lubin, J.H.; Preston, D.L.; Preston, R.J.; Puskin, J.S.; *et al.* Cancer risks attributable to low doses of ionizing radiation: Assessing what we really know. *Proc. Natl. Acad. Sci. USA* **2003**, *100*, 13761–13766.
10. Gagliano, N.; Bedoni, M.; Mantovani, G.; Chiriva-Internati, M.; Castelli, D.; Torri, C.; Donetti, E. Effect of a topical treatment in organotypic culture of human breast skin after exposure to gamma-rays. *Eur. J. Histochem.* **2007**, *51*, 283–290.
11. Chan, R.J.; Webster, J.; Chung, B.; Marquart, L.; Ahmed, M.; Garantziotis, S. Prevention and treatment of acute radiation-induced skin reactions: A systematic review and meta-analysis of randomized controlled trials. *BMC Cancer* **2014**, *14*, 53.
12. Hu, Z.P.; Kim, Y.M.; Sowa, M.B.; Robinson, R.J.; Gao, X.; Metz, T.O.; Morgan, W.F.; Zhang, Q. Metabolomic response of human skin tissue to low dose ionizing radiation. *Mol. Biosyst.* **2012**, *8*, 1979–1986.

13. Fuchs, J.; Hufljet, M.; Rothfuss, L.; Wilson, D.S.; Carcamo, G.; Packer, L. Impairment of enzymatic and non-enzymatic antioxidants in skin by UVB irradiation. *J. Investig. Dermatol.* **1989**, *93*, 769–773.
14. Meffert, H.; Diezel, W.; Sönnichsen, N. Stable lipid peroxidation products in human skin: Detection, ultraviolet induced increase, and pathogenic importance. *Experientia* **1976**, *32*, 1397–1398.
15. Buttke, T.M.; Sandstrom, P.A. Oxidative stress as a mediator of apoptosis. *Immunol. Today* **1994**, *15*, 7–10.
16. Sato, Y.; Kamazawa, N.; Suzuki, M.; Wang, C.M.; Ohte, S.; Shinoda, M. Studies on chemical protectors against radiation XXXIII. Protective mechanisms of various compounds against skin injury induced by radiation. *Yakugaku Zasshi* **1991**, *111*, 51–58.
17. Katiyar, S.K.; Afaq, F.; Perez, A.; Mukhtar, H. Green Tea polyphenol (−)- epigallocatechin-3-galate treatment of human skin inhibits ultraviolet radiation-induced oxidative stress. *Carcinogenesis* **2001**, *22*, 287–294.
18. Jagetia, G.C.; Rajanikant, G.K.; Rao, S.K.; Baliga, S.M. Alteration in the glutathione, glutathione peroxidase, superoxide dismutase and lipid peroxidation by ascorbic acid in the skin of mice exposed to fractionated gamma radiation. *Clin. Chim. Acta* **2003**, *332*, 111–121.
19. Jagetia, G.C.; Rajanikant, G.K. Acceleration of wound repair by curcumin in the excision wound of mice exposed to different doses of fractionated γ radiation. *Int. Wound J.* **2012**, *9*, 76–92.
20. Leung, A. *Encyclopedia of Common Natural Ingredients Used in Food, Drugs, and Cosmetics*; John Wiley: New York, NY, USA, 1980; pp. 313–314.
21. Jagetia, G.C.; Aggarwal, B.B. "Spicing Up" of the Immune System by Curcumin. *J. Clin. Immunol.* **2007**, *27*, 19–35.
22. Chang, H.; But, P.P. *Pharmacology and Applications of Chinese Materia Medica*, 2nd ed.; World Scientific Publishing Company: Singapore, 1987.
23. Ammon, H.P.; Wahl, M.A. Pharmacology of Curcuma longa. *Planta Med.* **1991**, *57*, 1–7.
24. Lin, J.K.; Pan, M.H.; Lin-Shiau, S.Y. Recent studies on the biofunctions and biotransformations of curcumin. *Biofactors* **2000**, *13*, 153–158.
25. Lao, C.D.; Ruffin, M.T.; Normolle, D.; Heath, D.D.; Murray, S.I.; Bailey, J.M.; Boggs, M.E.; Crowell, J.; Rock, C.L.; Brenner, D.E. Dose escalation of a curcuminoid formulation. *BMC Complem. Altern. Med.* **2006**, *6*, 10.
26. Susan, M.; Rao, M.N. Induction of glutathione-*S*-transferase activity by curcumin in mice. *Arzneim Forsch.* **1992**, *42*, 962–964.
27. Ak, T.; Gulcin, I. Antioxidant and radical scavenging properties of curcumin. *Chem. Biol. Interact* **2008**, *174*, 27–37.
28. Ruby, A.J.; Kuttan, G.; Babu, K.D.; Rajasekharan, K.N.; Kuttan, R. Anti-tumour and antioxidant activity of natural curcuminoids. *Cancer Lett.* **1995**, *94*, 79–83.
29. Sreejayan, N.; Rao, M.N.A. Curcuminoids as potent inhibitors of lipid peroxidation. *J. Pharm. Pharmacol.* **1994**, *46*, 1013–1016.

30. Jelveh, S.; Kaspler, P.; Bhogal, N.; Mahmood, J.; Lindsay, P.E.; Okunieff, P.; Doctrow, S.R.; Bristow, R.G.; Hill, R.P. Investigations of antioxidant-mediated protection and mitigation of radiation-induced DNA damage and lipid peroxidation in murine skin. *Int. J. Radiat. Biol.* **2013**, *89*, 618–627.
31. Jagetia, G.C.; Rajanikant, G.K. Role of curcumin, a naturally occurring phenolic compound of turmeric in accelerating the repair of excision wound in mice whole-body exposed to various doses of γ-radiation. *J. Surg. Res.* **2004**, *120*, 127–138.
32. Jagetia, G.C.; Rajanikant, G.K. Effect of curcumin on radiation-impaired healing of excisional wounds in mice. *J. Wound Care* **2004**, *13*, 107–109.
33. Jagetia, G.C.; Rajanikant, G.K. Curcumin treatment enhances the repair and regeneration of wounds in mice exposed to hemibody γ-irradiation. *Plast Reconstr. Surg.* **2005**, *115*, 515–528.
34. López-Jornet, P.; Camacho-Alonso, F.; Jiménez-Torres, M.J.; Orduña-Domingo, A.; Gómez-García, F. Topical curcumin for the healing of carbon dioxide laser skin wounds in mice. *Photomed. Laser Surg.* **2011**, *29*, 809–814.
35. Moron, M.S.; Depierre, J.W.; Mannervik, B. Levels of glutathione, glutathione reductase and glutathione-*s*-transferase activities in rat lung and liver. *Biochim. Biophys. Acta* **1979**, *582*, 67–78.
36. Sazuka, Y.; Tanizawa, H.; Takino, Y. Effect of adriamycin on the activities of superoxide dismutase, glutathione peroxidase and catalase in tissues of mice. *Jpn. J. Cancer Res.* **1989**, *80*, 89–94.
37. Fried, R. Enzymatic and non-enzymatic assay of superoxide dismutase. *Biochimie* **1975**, *57*, 657–60.
38. Beuege, J.A.; Aust, S.D. Microsomal lipid peroxidation. *Method Enzymol.* **1978**, *30*, 302–310.
39. Siems, W.; Gartner, C.; Kranz, D.; Schneider, W.; Grune, T.; Schimke, J.; Gau, S.; Wege, U.; Gerber, G. Long term effects of monthly low dose whole body irradiation on the glutathione status and thiobarbituric acid-reactive substance in different organs of male Wister rats. *Radiobiol. Radiother.* **1990**, *31*, 257–263.
40. Kaya, H.; Delibas, N.; Serteser, M.; Ulukaya, E.; Ozkaya, O. The effect of melatonin on lipid peroxidation during radiotherapy in female rats. *Strahlenther. Onkol.* **1999**, *175*, 285–258.
41. Jagetia, G.C.; Reddy, T.K. Modulation of radiation-induced alteration in the antioxidant status of mice by naringin. *Life Sci.* **2005**, *77*, 780–794.
42. Jagetia, G.C.; Baliga, M.S.; Venkatesh, P.; Ulloor, J.N. Influence of ginger rhizome (*Zingiber officinale* Rosc) on survival, glutathione and lipid peroxidation in mice after whole-body exposure to γ-radiation. *Radiat. Res.* **2003**, *160*, 584–592.
43. Jagetia, G.C.; Venkatesh, P.; Baliga, M.S. Evaluation of the radioprotective effect of bael leaf (*Aegle marmelos*) extract in mice. *Int. J. Radiat. Biol.* **2004**, *80*, 281–290.
44. Jagetia, G.C.; Venkatesha, V.A. Effect of mangiferin on radiation-induced micronucleus formation in cultured human peripheral blood lymphocytes. *Environ. Mol. Mutagen.* **2005**, *46*, 12–21.
45. Tawfik, S.S.; Abouelella, A.M.; Shahein, Y.E. Curcumin protection activities against γ-rays-induced molecular and biochemical lesions. *BMC Res. Notes* **2013**, *6*, 375.

46. Davis, W., Jr.; Ronai, Z.; Tew, K.D. Cellular thiols and reactive oxygen species in drug-induced apoptosis. *J. Pharmacol. Exp. Therapeut.* **2001**, *296*, 1–6.
47. Canales-Aguirre, A.A.; Gomez-Pinedo, U.A.; Luquin, S.; Ramırez-Herrera, M.A.; Mendoza-Magana, M.L.; Feria-Velasco, A. Curcumin protects against the oxidative damage induced by the pesticide parathion in the hippocampus of the rat brain. *Nutr. Neurosci.* **2012**, *15*, 62–69.
48. Xie, Y.; Zhao, Q.Y.; Li, H.Y.; Zhou, X.; Liu, Y.; Zhang H. Curcumin ameliorates cognitive deficits heavy ion irradiation-induced learning and memory deficits through enhancing of Nrf2 antioxidant signaling pathways. *Pharmacol. Biochem. Behav.* **2014**, *126*, 181–186.
49. Meister, A.; Anderson, M.E. Glutathione. *Annu. Rev. Biochem.* **1983**, *52*, 711–760.
50. Aquilano, K.; Baldelli, S.; Ciriolo, M.R. Glutathione: New roles in redox signaling for an old antioxidant. *Front. Pharmacol.* **2014**, *5*, 196.
51. Navarro, J.; Obrador, E.; Pellicer, J.A.; Aseni, M.; Vina, J.; Estrela, M. Blood glutathione as an index of radiation-induced oxidative stress in mice and humans. *Free Radic. Biol. Med.* **1997**, *22*, 1203–1207.
52. Younes, M.; Seigers, C.P. Mechanistic aspects of enhanced lipid peroxidation following glutathione depletion *in vivo*. *Chem. Biol. Interact.* **1981**, *34*, 257–266.
53. Miyachi, Y.; Imamura, S.; Niwa, Y. Decreased skin superoxide dismutase activity by a single exposure of ultraviolet radiation is reduced by liposomal superoxide dismutase pretreatment. *J. Investig. Dermatol.* **1987**, *89*, 111–112.
54. Record, I.R.; Dreosti, I.E.; Konstantinopoulos, M.; Buckley, R.A. The influence of topical and systemic vitamin E on ultraviolet light-induced skin damage in hairless mice. *Nutr. Cancer* **1991**, *16*, 219–225.
55. Iizawa, O.; Kato, T.; Tagami, H.; Akamatsu, H.; Niwa, Y. Long term follow-up study of changes in lipid peroxide levels and the activity of superoxide dismutase, catalase, and glutathione peroxidase in mouse skin after acute and chronic UV irradiation. *Arch. Dermatol. Res.* **1994**, *286*, 47–52.
56. Dickinson, D.A.; Forman, H.J. Cellular glutathione and thiols metabolism. *Biochem. Pharmacol.* **2002**, *64*, 1019–1026.
57. Altavilla, D.; Saitta, A.; Guarini, S.; Galeano, M.; Squadrito, G.; Cucinotta, D. Oxidative stress causes nuclear factor-κB activation in acute hypovolemic hemorrhagic shock. *Free Radic. Biol. Med.* **2001**, *30*, 1055–1066.
58. Brigelius-Fhole, R. Tissue-specific functions of individual glutathione peroxidases. *Free Radic. Biol. Med.* **1999**, *27*, 951–965.
59. Kunchandy, E.; Rao, M.N.A. Oxygen radical scavenging activity of curcumin. *Int. J. Pharm.* **1990**, *58*, 237–240.
60. Inano, H.; Onoda, M. Radioprotective action of curcumin extracted from *Curcuma longa* Linn: Inhibitory effect on formation of urinary 8-hydroxy-2′-deoxyguanosine, tumorigenesis, but not mortality, induced by γ-ray irradiation. *Int. J. Radiat. Oncol. Biol. Phys.* **2002**, *53*, 735–743.

61. Iqbal, M.; Sharma, S.D.; Okazaki, Y.; Fujisawa, M.; Okada, S. Dietary supplementation of curcumin enhances antioxidant and phase II metabolizing enzymes in ddY male mice: Possible role in protection against chemical carcinogenesis and toxicity. *Pharmacol. Toxicol.* **2003**, *92*, 33–38.

Permissions

All chapters in this book were first published in Antioxidants, by MDPI; hereby published with permission under the Creative Commons Attribution License or equivalent. Every chapter published in this book has been scrutinized by our experts. Their significance has been extensively debated. The topics covered herein carry significant findings which will fuel the growth of the discipline. They may even be implemented as practical applications or may be referred to as a beginning point for another development.

The contributors of this book come from diverse backgrounds, making this book a truly international effort. This book will bring forth new frontiers with its revolutionizing research information and detailed analysis of the nascent developments around the world.

We would like to thank all the contributing authors for lending their expertise to make the book truly unique. They have played a crucial role in the development of this book. Without their invaluable contributions this book wouldn't have been possible. They have made vital efforts to compile up to date information on the varied aspects of this subject to make this book a valuable addition to the collection of many professionals and students.

This book was conceptualized with the vision of imparting up-to-date information and advanced data in this field. To ensure the same, a matchless editorial board was set up. Every individual on the board went through rigorous rounds of assessment to prove their worth. After which they invested a large part of their time researching and compiling the most relevant data for our readers.

The editorial board has been involved in producing this book since its inception. They have spent rigorous hours researching and exploring the diverse topics which have resulted in the successful publishing of this book. They have passed on their knowledge of decades through this book. To expedite this challenging task, the publisher supported the team at every step. A small team of assistant editors was also appointed to further simplify the editing procedure and attain best results for the readers.

Apart from the editorial board, the designing team has also invested a significant amount of their time in understanding the subject and creating the most relevant covers. They scrutinized every image to scout for the most suitable representation of the subject and create an appropriate cover for the book.

The publishing team has been an ardent support to the editorial, designing and production team. Their endless efforts to recruit the best for this project, has resulted in the accomplishment of this book. They are a veteran in the field of academics and their pool of knowledge is as vast as their experience in printing. Their expertise and guidance has proved useful at every step. Their uncompromising quality standards have made this book an exceptional effort. Their encouragement from time to time has been an inspiration for everyone.

The publisher and the editorial board hope that this book will prove to be a valuable piece of knowledge for researchers, students, practitioners and scholars across the globe.

List of Contributors

Jean-Pierre Louboutin
Department of Pathology, Anatomy and Cell Biology, Thomas Jefferson University, Philadelphia, PA 19107, USA

Lokesh Agrawal
Department of Pathology, Anatomy and Cell Biology, Thomas Jefferson University, Philadelphia, PA 19107, USA

Beverly A. S. Reyes
Department of Neurosurgery, Farber Institute for Neurosciences, Thomas Jefferson University, Philadelphia, PA 19107, USA

Elisabeth J. Van Bockstaele
Department of Neurosurgery, Farber Institute for Neurosciences, Thomas Jefferson University, Philadelphia, PA 19107, USA

David S. Strayer
Department of Pathology, Anatomy and Cell Biology, Thomas Jefferson University, Philadelphia, PA 19107, USA

Rachel Shirley
Institute of Cardiovascular & Medical Sciences, College of Medical, Veterinary & Life Sciences, University of Glasgow, BHF GCRC, 126 University Place, Glasgow G12 8TA, UK

Emily N. J. Ord
Institute of Cardiovascular & Medical Sciences, College of Medical, Veterinary & Life Sciences, University of Glasgow, BHF GCRC, 126 University Place, Glasgow G12 8TA, UK

Lorraine M. Work
Institute of Cardiovascular & Medical Sciences, College of Medical, Veterinary & Life Sciences, University of Glasgow, BHF GCRC, 126 University Place, Glasgow G12 8TA, UK

Raghu C. Hariharapura
Department of Pharmaceutical Biotechnology, Manipal College of Pharmaceutical Sciences, Manipal University, Manipal 576 201, India

Ramamurthy Srinivasan
School of Pharmacy, International Medical University, Kuala Lumpur 57000, Malaysia

Godavarthi Ashok
Radiant Research Services Pvt. Ltd., Bangalore 560 050, India

Santoshkumar H. Dongre
Department of Chemical Technology, Dr. Babasaheb Ambedkar Marathwada University, Aurangabad 431001, India

Hitesh V. Jagani
Department of Pharmaceutical Biotechnology, Manipal College of Pharmaceutical Sciences, Manipal University, Manipal 576 201, India

Pottekkad Vijayan
Department of Pharmaceutical Biotechnology, Jagadguru Sri Shivarathreeshwara (JSS) College of Pharmacy, Ooty 643 001, India

Dharmendra Singh
Centre for Advanced Studies, Department of Zoology, University of Rajasthan, Jaipur 302 055, India
Department of Zoology, Dyal Singh College, University of Delhi, Lodhi Road, New Delhi 110 003, India

Priya Vrat Arya
Department of Zoology, Dyal Singh College, University of Delhi, Lodhi Road, New Delhi 110 003, India

Ved Prakash Aggarwal
Department of Zoology, Dyal Singh College, University of Delhi, Lodhi Road, New Delhi 110 003, India

Radhey Shyam Gupta
Centre for Advanced Studies, Department of Zoology, University of Rajasthan, Jaipur 302 055, India

Barbara Carletti
Unit of Neuromuscular and Neurodegenerative diseases, Children's Hospital and Research Institute "Bambino Gesù", 00165 Rome, Italy

Fiorella Piemonte
Unit of Neuromuscular and Neurodegenerative diseases, Children's Hospital and Research Institute "Bambino Gesù", 00165 Rome, Italy

Quan V. Vuong
Pancreatic Cancer Research, Nutrition Food & Health Research Group, School of environmental and Life Sciences, University of Newcastle, NSW 2258, Australia

Chloe D. Goldsmith
Pancreatic Cancer Research, Nutrition Food & Health Research Group, School of environmental and Life Sciences, University of Newcastle, NSW 2258, Australia

Trung Thanh Dang
Pancreatic Cancer Research, Nutrition Food & Health Research Group, School of environmental and Life Sciences, University of Newcastle, NSW 2258, Australia
Faculty of Food Technology, Nha Trang University, No. 2 Nguyen Dinh Chieu, Nha Trang, Khanh Hoa 8458, Vietnam

Van Tang Nguyen
Pancreatic Cancer Research, Nutrition Food & Health Research Group, School of environmental and Life Sciences, University of Newcastle, NSW 2258, Australia
Faculty of Food Technology, Nha Trang University, No. 2 Nguyen Dinh Chieu, Nha Trang, Khanh Hoa 8458, Vietnam

Deep Jyoti Bhuyan
Pancreatic Cancer Research, Nutrition Food & Health Research Group, School of environmental and Life Sciences, University of Newcastle, NSW 2258, Australia

Elham Sadeqzadeh
Pancreatic Cancer Research, Nutrition Food & Health Research Group, School of environmental and Life Sciences, University of Newcastle, NSW 2258, Australia

Christopher J. Scarlett
Pancreatic Cancer Research, Nutrition Food & Health Research Group, School of environmental and Life Sciences, University of Newcastle, NSW 2258, Australia

Michael C. Bowyer
Pancreatic Cancer Research, Nutrition Food & Health Research Group, School of environmental and Life Sciences, University of Newcastle, NSW 2258, Australia

Jennifer E. Slemmer
Bioscience Technology, Holland College, 140 Weymouth Street, Charlottetown, PE, C1A 4Z1, Canada

John T. Weber
School of Pharmacy, Memorial University of Newfoundland, 300 Prince Philip Drive, St. John's, NL, A1B 3V6, Canada

Sandra C. Gouveia-Figueira
Centro de Química da Madeira, CCCEE, Universidade da Madeira, Campus Universitário da Penteada, piso 0, Funchal 9000-390, Portugal.
Department of Chemistry, Umeå University, Umeå SE-901 87, Sweden
Department of Pharmacology and Clinical Neuroscience, Umeå University, Umeå SE-901 87, Sweden

Carla A. Gouveia
Centro de Química da Madeira, CCCEE, Universidade da Madeira, Campus Universitário da Penteada, piso 0, Funchal 9000-390, Portugal

Maria J. Carvalho
Centro de Química da Madeira, CCCEE, Universidade da Madeira, Campus Universitário da Penteada, piso 0, Funchal 9000-390, Portugal

Ana I. Rodrigues
Unidade de Geologia Marinha, Laboratório Nacional de Energia e Geologia, I.P., Estrada da Portela, Zambujal—Alfragide Apartado 7586, Amadoram 2720-866, Portugal

Malin L. Nording
Department of Chemistry, Umeå University, Umeå SE-901 87, Sweden

Paula C. Castilho
Department of Chemistry, Umeå University, Umeå SE-901 87, Sweden

Jean-Pierre Louboutin
Department of Pathology, Anatomy and Cell Biology, Thomas Jefferson University, 1020 Locust street, Philadelphia, PA 19107, USA

David Strayer
Department of Pathology, Anatomy and Cell Biology, Thomas Jefferson University, 1020 Locust street, Philadelphia, PA 19107, USA

Ashutosh Sharma
Department of Chemistry, University of Rajasthan, Jaipur 302 055, India

Mahabeer Prasad Dobhal
Department of Chemistry, University of Rajasthan, Jaipur 302 055, India

Erika K. Ross
Department of Biological Sciences and Eleanor Roosevelt Institute, University of Denver, 2199 S. University Blvd., Denver, CO 80208, USA

Aimee N. Winter
Department of Biological Sciences and Eleanor Roosevelt Institute, University of Denver, 2199 S. University Blvd., Denver, CO 80208, USA

Heather M. Wilkins
Department of Biological Sciences and Eleanor Roosevelt Institute, University of Denver, 2199 S. University Blvd., Denver, CO 80208, USA

Whitney A. Sumner
Department of Biological Sciences and Eleanor Roosevelt Institute, University of Denver, 2199 S. University Blvd., Denver, CO 80208, USA

Nathan Duval
Department of Biological Sciences and Eleanor Roosevelt Institute, University of Denver, 2199 S. University Blvd., Denver, CO 80208, USA

David Patterson
Department of Biological Sciences and Eleanor Roosevelt Institute, University of Denver, 2199 S. University Blvd., Denver, CO 80208, USA

Daniel A. Linseman
Department of Biological Sciences and Eleanor Roosevelt Institute, University of Denver, 2199 S. University Blvd., Denver, CO 80208, USA
Research Service, Veterans Affairs Medical Center, 1055 Clermont St., Denver, CO 80220, USA
Division of Clinical Pharmacology and Toxicology, Department of Medicine and Neuroscience Program, University of Colorado Denver, 12700 E 19th Ave., Aurora, CO 80045, USA

Bruno Moukette Moukette
Laboratory of Biochemistry, Department of Biochemistry and Physiological Sciences; Faculty of Medicine and Biomedical Sciences, University of Yaoundé I, P.O. Box 1364 Yaounde, Cameroon

Constant Anatole Pieme
Laboratory of Biochemistry, Department of Biochemistry and Physiological Sciences; Faculty of Medicine and Biomedical Sciences, University of Yaoundé I, P.O. Box 1364 Yaounde, Cameroon

Prosper Cabral Nya Biapa
Laboratory of Medecinal plant Biochemistry, Food Science and Nutrition, Department of Biochemistry, Faculty of Science, University of Dschang, P.O. Box 67 Dschang, Cameroon

Jacques Romain Njimou
Department of Chemical Materials Environmental Engineering, Via Eudossiana 18, University of Rome "La Sapienza", 00185 Rome, Italy

Vicky Jocelyne Ama Moor
Laboratory of Biochemistry, Department of Biochemistry and Physiological Sciences; Faculty of Medicine and Biomedical Sciences, University of Yaoundé I, P.O. Box 1364 Yaounde, Cameroon

Marco Stoller
Department of Chemical Materials Environmental Engineering, Via Eudossiana 18, University of Rome "La Sapienza", 00185 Rome, Italy

Marco Bravi
Department of Chemical Materials Environmental Engineering, Via Eudossiana 18, University of Rome "La Sapienza", 00185 Rome, Italy

Jeanne Yonkeu Ngogang
Laboratory of Biochemistry, Department of Biochemistry and Physiological Sciences; Faculty of Medicine and Biomedical Sciences, University of Yaoundé I, P.O. Box 1364 Yaounde, Cameroon

Ganesh Chandra Jagetia
Department of Zoology, Mizoram University, Aizawl-796 004, India

Golgod Krishnamurthy Rajanikant
School of Biotechnology, National Institute of Technology, Calicut-673 601, India